Personality Assessment in the DSM-5

The DSM-5 promises to be a major reformulation of psychopathology, and no section had been proposed for a more drastic change than the personality disorder section. Unlike the DSM-IV, the DSM-5 personality disorders had been conceptualized as involving core deficits in interpersonal and self-functioning, and were to have utilized a hybrid assessment model involving both pathological trait dimensions and a limited set of personality disorder types. These changes were based on empirical and theoretical work conducted during the era of DSM-III/IV. Nevertheless, there was significant disagreement among personality assessors regarding the DSM-5 proposal, and ultimately, at the end of 2012, the American Psychiatric Association Board of Trustees voted to retain the current DSM-IV personality disorders but to consider further how a trait-based system might be implemented into the assessment and diagnosis of personality pathology. In this volume, several members of the DSM-5 Work Group offer rationales for their proposal and offer empirical evidence regarding suggested changes. Several personality assessment researchers critique the proposal and offer alternative conceptualizations

This book was originally published as a special issue of the *Journal of Personality Assessment*.

Steven K. Huprich, Ph.D,. is Professor of Psychology at Eastern Michigan University, USA. He is an Associate Editor for the *Journal of Personality Disorders* and studies the assessment and classification of personality disorders.

Christopher J. Hopwood, Ph.D., is an Assistant Professor of Clinical Psychology at Michigan State University, USA. He is an Associate Editor for the *Journal of Personality Disorders* whose research and clinical practice focus on the assessment and treatment of personality pathology.

Personality Assessment in the DSM-5

Edited by
Steven K. Huprich and Christopher J. Hopwood

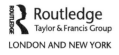
Routledge
Taylor & Francis Group

LONDON AND NEW YORK

First published 2013
by Routledge
2 Park Square, Milton Park, Abingdon, Oxon, OX14 4RN

Simultaneously published in the USA and Canada
by Routledge
711 Third Avenue, New York, NY 10017

Routledge is an imprint of the Taylor & Francis Group, an informa business

© 2013 Taylor & Francis

This book is a reproduction of the *Journal of Personality Assessment*, volume 93, issue 4. The Publisher requests to those authors who may be citing this book to state, also, the bibliographical details of the special issue on which the book was based.

British Library Cataloguing in Publication Data
A catalogue record for this book is available from the British Library

ISBN13: 978-0-415-63453-3

Typeset in Times New Roman
by Taylor & Francis Books

Publisher's Note
The publisher would like to make readers aware that the chapters in this book may be referred to as articles as they are identical to the articles published in the special issue. The publisher accepts responsibility for any inconsistencies that may have arisen in the course of preparing this volume for print.

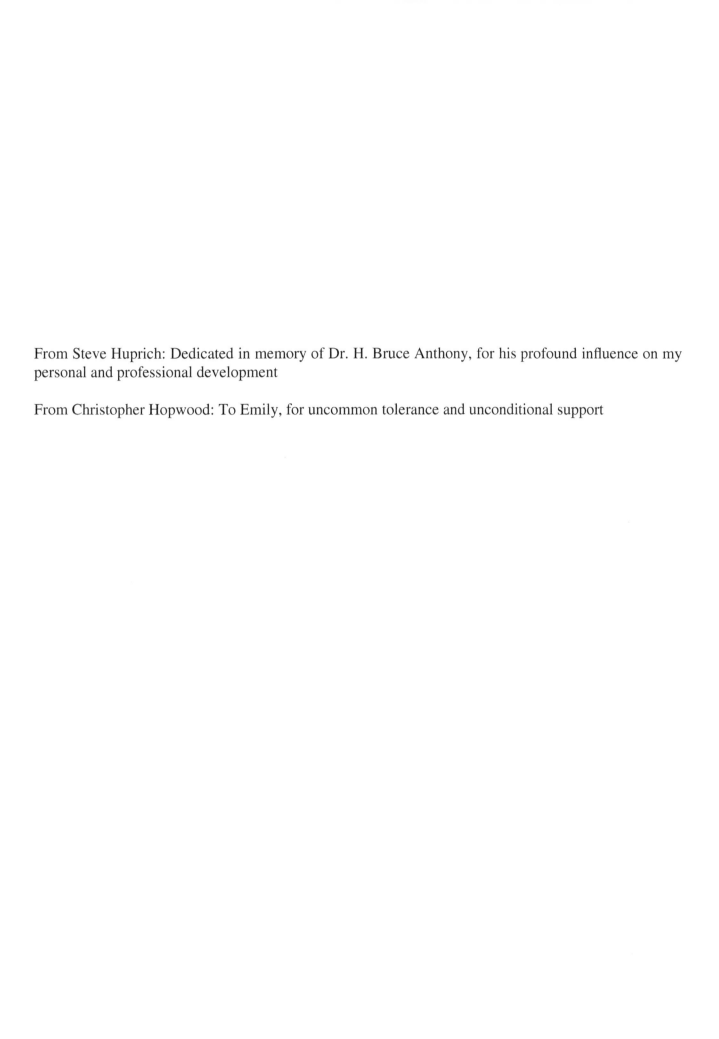

Contents

Citation Information

The chapters in this book were originally published in the *Journal of Personality Assessment*. When citing this material, please use the original issue information and page numbering for each article, as follows:

Chapter 2
An Overview of Issues Related to Categorical and Dimensional Models of Personality Disorder Assessment
Steven K. Huprich and Robert F. Bornstein
Journal of Personality Assessment, volume 89, issue 1 (August 2007) pp. 3–15

Chapter 3
Assessing Normal and Abnormal Personality Functioning: Strengths and Weaknesses of Self-Report, Observer, and Performance-Based Methods
Ronald J. Ganellen
Journal of Personality Assessment, volume 89, issue 1 (August 2007) pp. 30–40

Chapter 4
Personality in DSM–5: Helping Delineate Personality Disorder Content and Framing the Metastructure
Robert F. Krueger, Nicholas R. Eaton, Jaime Derringer, Kristian E. Markon, David Watson and Andrew E. Skodol
Journal of Personality Assessment, volume 93, issue 4 (July–August 2011) pp. 325–331

Chapter 5
Toward a Model for Assessing Level of Personality Functioning in DSM–5, Part I: A Review of Theory and Methods
Donna S. Bender, Leslie C. Morey and Andrew E. Skodol
Journal of Personality Assessment, volume 93, issue 4 (July–August 2011) pp. 332–346

Chapter 6
Toward a Model for Assessing Level of Personality Functioning in DSM–5, Part II: Empirical Articulation of a Core Dimension of Personality Pathology
Leslie C. Morey, Han Berghuis, Donna S. Bender, Roel Verheul, Robert F. Krueger and Andrew E. Skodol
Journal of Personality Assessment, volume 93, issue 4 (July–August 2011) pp. 347–353

Chapter 7
Assessing Personality in the DSM–5: The Utility of Bipolar Constructs
Douglas B. Samuel
Journal of Personality Assessment, volume 93, issue 4 (July–August 2011) pp. 390–397

Notes on Contributors

Donna S. Bender, Department of Psychiatry, University of Arizona College of Medicine, USA

Han Berghuis, Symfora Groep Psychiatric Center, Amersfoort, The Netherlands

Robert F. Bornstein, Derner Institute of Advanced Psychological Studies, Adelphi University, USA

Jaime Derringer, Psychology Department, University of Minnesota, USA

Nicholas R. Eaton, Psychology Department, University of Minnesota, USA

Ronald J. Ganellen, Department of Psychiatry and Behavioral Sciences, Northwestern University Medical School, USA

Lewis R. Goldberg, Oregon Research Institute, Eugene, Oregon, USA

Kathryn H. Gordon, Department of Psychology, North Dakota State University, USA

Christopher J. Hopwood, Department of Psychology, Michigan State University, USA

Steven K. Huprich, Department of Psychology, Eastern Michigan University, USA

Robert F. Krueger, Psychology Department, University of Minnesota, USA

Kristian E. Markon, Department of Psychology, University of Iowa, USA

Leslie C. Morey, Department of Psychology, Texas A & M University, USA

John E. Roberts, Department of Psychology, University at Buffalo, The State University of New York, USA

Michael D. Robinson, Department of Psychology, North Dakota State University, USA

Jane H. Rotterman, Department of Psychology, University at Buffalo, The State University of New York, USA

Douglas B. Samuel, Department of Psychiatry, Yale School of Medicine, USA and VA New England MIRECC, Connecticut, USA

Leonard J. Simms, Department of Psychology, University at Buffalo, The State University of New York, USA

Andrew E. Skodol, Department of Psychiatry, University of Arizona College of Medicine, USA

Roel Verheul, Faculty of Social and Behavioural Sciences–Clinical Psychology, University of Amsterdam, The Netherlands

David Watson, Department of Psychology, University of Notre Dame, USA

John Welte, Research Institute on Addictions, University at Buffalo, The State University of New York, USA

Aidan G. C. Wright, Department of Psychology, The Pennsylvania State University, USA

Introduction: Personality Assessment in the *DSM–5*

Steven K. Huprich
Department of Psychology
Eastern Michigan University

Christopher J. Hopwood
Department of Psychology
Michigan State University

Many personality assessors have expressed significant dissatisfaction with the *Diagnostic and Statistical Manual of Mental Disorders* (3rd ed. [*DSM–III*]; American Psychiatric Association, 1980; and 4th ed. [*DSM–IV*]; American Psychiatric Association, 1994) framework for conceptualizing personality disorders (e.g., Bornstein, 1998; Clark, 2007; Widiger & Trull, 2007). Common concerns have involved the categorical nature of the disorders, the use of arbitrary diagnostic cutoffs, diagnostic overlap, unclear distinctions between Axis I and II, the overly atheoretical nature of the criteria, the mix of traits and behaviours in those criteria, limited validity support for the overall model and some specific diagnoses, and limited associations with personality models commonly used in basic research and clinical practice. Despite the recommended changes, and the expectation that the *DSM-5* personality disorder section would look considerably different than what it has in the past, the American Psychiatric Association (APA) decided at the end of 2012 to reject the proposal of the PPDWG and to retain the current DSM-IV personality disorders, in spite of the fact that this system is replete with shortcomings. However, they opted to retain for further consideration the proposed trait system for how it might inform the assessment and diagnosis of personality pathology.

The *DSM–5* Personality and Personality Disorders Work Group (PPDWG) thus had a very difficult task on its hands. After some initial revisions, they eventually proposed a hybrid model of personality pathology for *DSM-5*, in which six of the extant categories would be retained as diagnostic types (Schizotypal, Antisocial, Borderline, Narcissistic, Avoidant, and Obsessive-Compulsive; Skodol et al., 2011a–c). Four of the current personality disorders (PDs) (Paranoid, Schizoid, Histrionic, and Dependent) were eliminated for lack of empirical support, and an empirically derived trait system was developed, which reflected a wide body of research that supported a hierarchical organization of universally identifiable traits (Allik, 2005; Markon, Krueger, & Watson, 2005; Widiger & Simonsen, 2005). Furthermore, the PPDWG introduced the need to assess an individual's level of functioning as part of their personality structure. Drawing upon the extensive object relations, interpersonal, and empirical literatures, level of functioning is assessed among the following dimensions: the extent to which the self is viewed as integrated and positively viewed, the individual's level of personal agency, the extent to which others can be perceived and related to empathically, and the capacity to experience intimacy with others. Thus, the personality disorder section in *DSM-5* is likely to look considerably different than what it has in the past.

Discussion about the *DSM-5* personality disorders has been ongoing for some time (e.g., Widiger & Clark, 2000), and a number of researchers and clinicians have commented on how the field can move forward. Because of the need to advance the field's knowledge of the personality disorders, particularly given the ongoing debate about the needed transition to a dimensionalized model of personality pathology, Steven Huprich and Robert Bornstein organized in 2007 a Special Issue of the *Journal of Personality Assessment*—"Dimensional versus Categorical Personality Disorder Diagnosis: Implications from and for Psychological Assessment." Not long after that, Christopher Hopwood and Steven Huprich organized two symposia on the future of personality disorder assessment that were presented at the 2010 Midwinter Meeting of the Society for Personality Assessment. Collectively, they combined papers from these symposia into another Special Issue of the *Journal of Personality Assessment* in 2011—"Personality Assessment in the *DSM-5*." This book, therefore, is a compilation of two papers from the former series and the entirety of papers from the latter series. It also includes two other papers relevant to the issue of assessing personality in a *DSM-5* era; one focusing upon the passive aggressive and negativistic personality disorder proposals and another on the social cognitive literature and how this field of experimental psychology should inform future research on the assessment of personality pathology.

Thus, with the support of Taylor & Francis Publishers, we are pleased to present this book on personality assessment in the *DSM-5* era. We have organized the book into three sections. First, we present a series of papers on how the personality assessment literature has led to the development of *DSM-5*, including an extended discussion of DSM-5 personality disorder assessment. The opening paper by Steven Huprich and Robert Bornstein presents a discussion of the categorical and dimensional framework for assessing personality disorders and considers the implications of what movement toward this framework means. Next, Ronald Ganellen reviews the strengths and limits of self-report, observer-based, and performance-based personality assessment for both normative and abnormal personality functioning. This is followed with three papers presented by members of the PPDWG. Robert Krueger and colleagues introduce the rationale for a trait structure in the *DSM-5* and what such a structure looks like. Donna Bender and Les Morey then each take the lead in two respective papers that discuss the theory, methods, and empirical support for assessing the level of functioning of the individual and why this type of assessment can be useful for advancing our assessment of personality pathology.

Second, we present three papers on how trait assessment can be advanced in *DSM-5* and beyond. Douglas Samuel begins with a critique of the trait model proposed for *DSM–5* for deviating significantly from the models commonly used in basic personality research, and highlights, in particular, concerns with using unipolar as opposed to bipolar personality traits. This is followed by Christopher Hopwood's argument for the utility of separating normative and pathological elements of personality traits explicitly in the *DSM–5* to increase the importance of personality assessment for psychiatric diagnosis in general and in line with recent empirical research regarding differences between normative and pathological personality features. Finally, Leonard Simms and colleagues provide some preliminary data from their Computerized Adaptive Assessment of Personality Disorder, a study funded by the National Institute of Mental Health which capitalizes upon the methodologies of computerized adaptive testing and item-response theory. Such a method allows the researcher to efficiently identify those items most likely to characterize the construct of interest, as well as the severity or extremity to which this trait exists in those who possess the construct.

In the final section of the book, we present a series of papers that introduces several issues related to how personality disorder assessment has been and should be conducted in the future. First, Steven Huprich begins by describing two issues relevant to personality assessment in the *DSM–5*: the limitations of several assessment methods that have informed existing models of personality pathology and the potential for psychoanalytic theory to usefully inform personality disorder nosology. Second, a unique and stimulating paper is offered by Michael Robinson and Kathryn Gordon on how social cognitive methodologies and the extant literature provide important insight into what and how personality pathology should be assessed. They critique the extensive use of self-report methodologies and demonstrate what experimentally-based assessment offers to the dynamic understanding of personality processes. Robert Bornstein then describes an alternative model of personality disorders, which retains many of the virtues of the *DSM–III/DSM–IV*, with important additions such as the depiction of overall personality pathology and personality-related strengths. Fourth, Aidan Wright reframes debates regarding categorical versus dimensional approaches to diagnosis in a manner that highlights the need to examine more carefully dynamic processes. In doing so he proposes that interpersonal theory offers a viable theoretical and measurement framework for understanding the dynamics of personality pathology. Finally, Christopher Hopwood and Aidan Wright present a comparison of the passive aggressive and negativistic personality disorders, and argue that the move toward the broader construct of negativism weakened the construct and contributed to its demise in the DSM system, despite the clinical importance of passive-aggressive behavior.

These are just some of the issues that will affect the *DSM-5* era of personality and personality disorder assessment. For instance, some questioned the clinical utility of the proposed *DSM-5* model of personality disorder assessment (Clarkin & Huprich, 2011; Shedler et al., 2010). And, with the APA Board of Trustees' retention of the *DSM-IV* system, many ideas and questions remain unanswered about the nature of personality assessment and its relationship to psychopathology. Thus, what the future holds for personality assessment in this era is simultaneously unknown, exciting, and potentially concerning. Moving forward, we offer this book as a sampling of the issues before the field and in the deepest spirit of advancing the science and practice of understanding human personality.

REFERENCES

Allik, J. (2005). Personality dimensions across cultures. *Journal of Personality Disorders, 19*, 212–232.

American Psychiatric Association. (1980). *Diagnostic and statistical manual of mental disorders* (3rd ed.). Washington, DC: Author.

American Psychiatric Association. (1994). *Diagnostic and statistical manual of mental disorders* (4th ed.). Washington, DC: Author.

*Bender, D. S., Morey, L. C., & Skodol, A. E. (2011). Toward a model for assessing level of personality functioning in *DSM–5*, Part I: A review of theory and methods. *Journal of Personality Assessment, 93*, 332–346.

Bornstein, R. F. (1998). Reconceptualizing personality disorder diagnosis in the *DSM–V*: The discriminant validity challenge. *Clinical Psychology: Science and Practice, 5*, 333–343.

*Bornstein, R. F. (2011). Toward a multidimensional model of personality disorder diagnosis: Implications for *DSM–5*. *Journal of Personality Assessment, 93*, 362–369.

Clark, L. A. (2007). Assessment and diagnosis of personality disorder: Perennial issues and an emerging reconceptualization. *Annual Review of Psychology, 58*, 227–257.

Clarkin, J. F., & Huprich, S. K. (2011). Do the DSM-5 proposals for personality disorders meet the criteria for clinical utility? *Journal of Personality Disorders, 25*, 192–205.

*Ganellen, R. J. (2007). Assessing normal and abnormal personality functioning: Strengths and weaknesses of self-report, observer, and performance-based methods. *Journal of Personality Assessment, 89*, 30–40.

*Hopwood, C. J. (2011). Personality traits in the *DSM–5*. *Journal of Personality Assessment, 93*, 398–405.

*Hopwood, C. J., & Wright, A. G. C. (2012). A comparison of passive-aggressive and negativistic personality disorders. *Journal of Personality Assessment, 94*, 296–303.

*Huprich, S. K. (2011). Contributions from personality- and psychodynamically oriented assessment to the development of the *DSM–5* personality disorders. *Journal of Personality Assessment, 93*, 354–361.

*Huprich, S. K., & Bornstein, R. F. (2007). Categorical and dimensional assessment of personality disorders: A consideration of the issues. *Journal of Personality Assessment, 89*, 3–15.

*Krueger, R. F., Eaton, N. R., Derringer, J., Markon, K. E., Watson, D., & Skodol, A. E. (2011). Personality in *DSM–5*: Helping delineate personality disorder content and framing the metastructure. *Journal of Personality Assessment, 93*, 325–331.

Markon, K. E., Krueger, R. F., & Watson, D. (2005). Delineating the structure of normal and abnormal personality: An integrative hierarchical approach. *Journal of Personality and Social Psychology, 88*, 139–157.

*Morey, L. C., Berghuis, H., Bender, D. S., Verheul, R., Krueger, R. F., & Skodol, A. E. (2011). Toward a model for assessing level of personality functioning in *DSM–5*, Part II: Empirical articulation of a core dimension of personality pathology. *Journal of Personality Assessment, 93*, 347–353.

*Robinson, M. D., & Gordon, K. H. (2011). Personality dynamics: Insight from the personality social cognitive literature. *Journal of Personality Assessment, 93*, 161–176.

*Samuel, D. B. (2011). Assessing personality in the *DSM–5*: The utility of bipolar constructs. *Journal of Personality Assessment, 93*, 390–397.

Shedler, J., Beck, A., Fonagy, P., Gabbard, G. O., Gunderson, J., Kernberg, O., Michaels, R., & Westen, D. (2010). Personality disorders in DSM-5. *American Journal of Psychiatry, 167*, 1026–1028.

*Simms, L. J., Goldberg, L. R., Roberts, J. E., Watson, D., Welte, J., & Rotterman, J. H. (2011). Computerized adaptive assessment of personality disorder: Introducing the CAT–PD project. *Journal of Personality Assessment, 93*, 380–389.

Skodol, A. E., Bender, D. S., Morey, L. C., Clark, L. A., Oldham, J. M., Alarcon, R. D., Krueger, R. F., Verheul, R., Bell, C. C., & Siever, L. J. (2011a). Personality disorder types proposed for DSM-5. *Journal of Personality Disorders, 25*, 136–169.

Skodol, A. E., Clark, L. A., Bender, D. S., Krueger, R. F., Livesley, W. J., Morey, L. C., et al. (2011b). Proposed changes in personality and personality disorder assessment and diagnosis for DSM-5, Part I: Description and rationale. *Personality Disorders: Theory, Research, and Treatment, 2*, 4–22.

Skodol, A. E., Bender, D. S., Oldham, J. M., Clark, L. A., Morey, L. C., Verheul, R., et al. (2011c). Proposed changes in personality and personality disorder assessment and diagnosis for *DSM-5*. Part II: Clinical application. *Personality Disorders: Theory, Research, and Treatment, 2*, 23–40.

Widiger, T. A., & Clark, L. A. (2000). Toward *DSM-V* and the classification of psychopathology. *Psychological Bulletin, 126*, 946–963.

Widiger, T. A., & Simonsen, E. (2005). Introduction to the special section: The American Psychiatric Association's research agenda for the DSM-V. *Journal of Personality Disorders, 19*, 103–109.

Widiger, T. A., & Trull, T. J. (2007). Plate tectonics in the classification of personality disorder: Shifting to a dimensional model. *American Psychologist, 62*, 71–83.

*Wright, A. G. C. (2011). Qualitative and quantitative distinctions in personalitydis order. *Journal of Personality Assessment, 93*, 370–379.

*Included in the book

An Overview of Issues Related to Categorical and Dimensional Models of Personality Disorder Assessment

Steven K. Huprich

Department of Psychology
Eastern Michigan University

Robert F. Bornstein

Derner Institute of Advanced Psychological Studies
Adelphi University

Despite long-standing efforts to improve the current diagnostic system for Axis II, problems remain with the categorical conceptualization of personality disorders (PDs). Due in part to these problems, interest has developed in dimensional models of PD classification. In this article, we discuss four issues relevant to categorical vs. dimensional assessment of PDs: (a) problems with self-reports in PD patients, (b) methodological issues in behavioral and clinician assessment of PDs, (c) challenges that arise when dimensional models are applied to patient and nonpatient samples, and (d) clinical implications of categorical and dimensional PD models. We suggest that researchers and clinicians address these concerns to avoid implementing a new PD assessment model that—although different from the current system—would otherwise remain fraught with difficulties.

Most clinicians agree that assessing and diagnosing personality disorders (PDs) can be difficult. Through several editions of the *Diagnostic and Statistical Manual of Mental Disorders* (*DSM*), authors have attempted to improve the descriptive criteria used to assign PD diagnoses and have introduced more behaviorally referenced, atheoretical definitions of PD symptoms and clearer cutoffs for identifying PD patients. Within this general framework, both the *Diagnostic and Statistical Manual of Mental Disorders* (4th ed.,text revision [*DSM–IV–TR*]; American Psychiatric Association, 2000) and the *International Classification of Diseases* (10th edition; World Health Organization, 1994) conceptualize PD diagnoses as distinct categories that may be identified when a patient meets a predefined threshold for symptom pervasiveness and impairment. Similar to the common practice of ignoring most subthreshold Axis I symptoms, little attention is given to the clinical implications of subthreshold PD symptom levels.

Despite long-standing efforts to improve these diagnostic manuals and diagnoses, problems remain with categorical conceptualization of PDs (Widiger & Samuel, 2005; Widiger & Sanderson, 1995; Wiggins & Pincus, 1994). Due in part to these problems, interest has developed in dimensional mod-

els of PD classification wherein individuals are evaluated on various scales of personality and evaluated for potential psychopathology given their relative suppressions or elevations on different scale scores (e.g., Huprich, 2003; Saulsman & Page, 2004; Strack, Lorr, & Campbell, 1990). Such an approach has the potential to provide a more comprehensive description of patient functioning, improve the clinician's understanding of the person being assessed, and represent more accurately the natural organization of personality and personality pathology (Livesley, 2006; Widiger & Simonsen, 2005: Widiger, Trull, Clarkin, Sanderson, & Costa, 2002). In the sections to follow, we discuss four issues relevant to both categorical and dimensional assessment of PDs: problems with self-reports, methodological issues in behavioral and clinician assessment of PDs, challenges that arise when categorical and dimensional assessment models are applied to patient and nonpatient samples, and clinical implications of categorical and dimensional models. We highlight opportunities and pitfalls that may occur during the transition to a dimensional PD model and suggest that researchers and clinicians address these concerns as they consider how to improve diagnosis and assessment of PDs to avoid implementing a new model that—although different from the current system—would otherwise remain fraught with difficulties.

PROBLEMS WITH EXTANT MEASURES OF PD CATEGORIES AND DIMENSIONS

Certain challenges in the transition to dimensional models affect both categorical and dimensional PD assessments. Four issues stand out.

Overreliance on Self-Report Methodology

Most PD assessments rely almost exclusively on patient self-reports, typically obtained using paper-and-pencil questionnaires and/or diagnostic interviews. Even when these instruments have adequate psychometric properties, self-reports by individuals with PDs introduce significant limitations. These problems have been well documented and are reviewed by Ganellen (2007/this issue). They fall into four broad, interrelated categories:

1. Concerns about individuals with a PD being able to describe their personality traits accurately.
2. Deliberate attempts on the part of some individuals to distort their self-presentation in a positive or negative way.
3. Lack of correspondence between self-reports and reports of significant others.
4. Lack of insight into problematic aspects of one's characteristic patterns of behavior or interpersonal relating.

Although these issues typically have been articulated and analyzed separately, they often co-occur. For instance, poor self–other correspondence might be in part the result of poor insight and a desire to present oneself in an overly positive or negative way. Such concerns are relevant to both categorical and dimensional PD assessment tools as well as to measures of normal-range personality. For example, one common, categorical measure of PDs, the Structured Clinical Interview for *DSM* (4th ed. [*DSM–IV*]; American Psychological Association, 1994] Axis II Disorders (SCID–II; First et al., 1995), asks individuals about the presence of various *DSM–IV* PD symptoms. Given their lack of insight, many PD patients may simply disavow qualities they do not see in themselves. Consequently, a diagnostic cutoff score could easily not be reached because of poor insight.

Problems with Psychometrics

Problems with the internal consistency, retest, and interrater reliability of measures used to assess current *DSM* PD categories are well documented; we direct the interested reader to some of the many references on this literature (e.g., Bornstein, 2003; Clifton, Turkheimer, & Olt-

manns, 2003, 2005; Durbin & Klein, 2006 ; First et al., 1995; Hirschfeld et al., 1983; Huprich & Ganellen, 2006; Klein, 2003; Klonsky, Oltmanns, & Turkheimer, 2002; McAllister, Baker, Mannes, Stewart, & Sutherland, 2002; Nestadt et al., 2006; Zimmerman, 1994).

In general, dimensional measures of PDs tend to be psychometrically superior to categorical measures. This is particularly noticeable when looking at the degree of convergence found across dimensional measures and their hierarchical organization (Markon, Krueger, & Watson, 2005; Widiger & Simonsen, 2005), which supports the biogenetic underpinnings of personality. The reliability of such measures is also impressive. For example, Stepp, Trull, Burr, Wofenstein, and Vieth (2005) evaluated Five-factor model of personality (FFM) domains and facets in a mixed sample of 200 psychiatric outpatients and undergraduate students using the Structured Interview for the FFM (Trull & Widiger, 1997). Stepp et al. reported good internal consistency with domain reliabilities of .85 (Neuroticism), .83 (Extraversion), .77 (Openness and Agreeableness), and .81 (Conscientiousness). Averaged across facets, internal consistencies were less strong: .67 (Neuroticism), .65 (Extraversion), and .52 (Openness, Agreeableness, and Conscientiousness). An excellent discussion of the strengths of the FFM in assessing PDs is provided by Widiger and Lowe (2007/this issue).

Dimensional measures also have their limitations in normal (Harlan & Clark, 1999) and clinical populations (Oltmanns, Gleason, Konsky, & Turnkheimer, 2005). For example, Miller, Pilkonis, and Clifton (2005) assessed the agreement between self-reports and other reports in 69 psychiatric patients. Correlations between informants were .37 (Neuroticism), .39 (Extraversion), .71 (Openness), .23 (Agreeableness), and .57 (Conscientiousness); the median facet level correlation was .43. Hierarchical regression analyses evaluated the incremental gain of other-report domain scores when used in conjunction with self-report domain scores to predict symptoms for each PD, with five PD dimensions showing significant incremental gain: paranoid, antisocial, borderline, histrionic, and obsessive–compulsive. However, no PD had over 50% of its variance predicted by the combination of self and other domain scores. Moreover, on measures of romantic, work, and social impairment, domain and facet scores as reported by others were more highly correlated with impairment than were self-report domain and facet scores.[1]

---

[1]Outside PD assessment, it is well documented that there are problems in self–other agreement when assessing an individual's psychopathology. Thus, it should not be surprising that such problems occur when assessing PDs. For instance, in a large-scale meta-analytic review, Meyer et al. (2001) reported that convergence among raters (e.g., parents, peers, teachers) in studies with children and adolescents yielded *r*s of .14 to .34. When diagnostic agreement was reported, kappa values ranged between .13 and .39. In studies of adults, *r*s ranged between .04 and .44, and kappa values ranged between .12 and .34. A more recent meta-analysis by Achenbach, Kruskowski, Dumenci, and Ivanova (2005) found that the average self-informant

Determining Pathological Personality Traits: Number and Severity

DSM–IV diagnostic thresholds notwithstanding, most clinicians identify (at least informally) pathological traits that may not be present in sufficient combination to meet criteria for a given PD but still require clinical attention. Moreover, even those patients who do meet the threshold for a *DSM–IV* PD are often evaluated along a continuum of severity; many clinicians conceptualize personality pathology dimensionally and incorporate dimensional language into their assessment. Such a procedure is inherent in the interpretation of Minnesota Multiphasic Personality Inventory–2 (MMPI–2; Graham, 2000) T scores, Millon Clinical Multiaxial Inventory–III (MCMI–III; Millon, 1994) PD scales, and Revised NEO Personality Inventory (NEO–PI–R; Costa & McCrae, 1992) facet scores (Widiger & Lowe, 2007/this issue) as well as in a clinician's in vivo integration of test data (Lerner & Lerner, 2007/this issue) or even nontest data (Silverstein, 2007/this issue). As discussion continues over the transition to a dimensional model for assessing and classifying PDs, the challenge remains to identify clinically significant PD pathology (see Trull, 2005, for suggestions regarding this issue).

Quantifying Pathognomic Trait Configurations

Although Costa and Widiger (2002) suggested that PDs are associated with a predictable pattern of FFM facets, Livesley (2006) and Widiger, Simonsen, Krueger, Livesley, and Verheul (2005) have pointed out that merely having a high or low level of one of more PD-related facets does not, in and of itself, imply pathology. This may be due to the fact that the FFM and its corresponding measures were designed to assess normal-range personality and not a wider range of personality pathology. When O'Connor (2005) evaluated empirically how FFM domains were associated with scores on each MCMI–III PD scale (Millon, 1994) he concluded

> Perhaps the most consistent and disconcerting finding was that the most deviant FFM elevations at the high ends of the PD continuums were generally only modestly deviant from the zero means.... Only rarely did FFM elevations project beyond one standard deviation from the means. (p. 292)

Furthermore, when facets were evaluated across PDs, there was a considerable range of deviation scores. O'Connor (2005) reported that the mean z score deviation of the facets

was .91 but that the range was large (.53), and there were numerous instances in which z values for the facets were elevated where no a priori prediction had been made.[2]

Although trait dimensions could be used to provide more comprehensive descriptions, there are multiple ways this might play out, such as the addition of new PDs beyond those already described, or elimination of PDs altogether with only a description of maladaptive components of traits. It is difficult for us to imagine that the current PDs would completely disappear from clinical use and hard to envision talking about personality pathology without employing some category label that describes the problem succinctly. It is also possible that categories proposed for inclusion in the *DSM* (e.g., passive–aggressive, self-defeating, depressive) or categories proposed within different theoretical frameworks (e.g., the narcissistic-masochistic character; Cooper, 1989), may be detected via empirically derived measures of personality and its disorders. In the end, every profession creates its own jargon; and once the practical implications of facet-by-facet descriptions of PD patients become clear, it seems likely that a new shorthand set of descriptors would emerge to group PD patients in efficient and clinically meaningful ways.

PSYCHOLOGICAL FACTORS AFFECTING SELF-REPORTED PERSONALITY PATHOLOGY

Limitations in the assessment of PD symptoms and PD-related traits stem in part from lack of attention to findings from other areas of psychology. Social, cognitive, and personality researchers have provided insights into human behavior and mental life that have important implications for how PDs are (or should be) assessed. In the following sections, we elucidate these research findings in four broad domains.

Triadic Reciprocal Determinism

Several decades ago, Mischel (1968) pointed out that personality traits (including maladaptive personality traits) may only be conceptualized meaningfully and assessed accurately with reference to the situations wherein trait-relevant

---

correlation among parallel instruments were .43 and .44, respectively, for internalizing and externalizing disorders. When different instruments were used, the mean cross-informant rating was .30.

[2]The LOESS procedure used by O'Connor (2005) is complex, utilizing

a series of local regression analyses that permits the form of a curve to vary across the variable continua ... ideal for revealing potentially complex, unanticipated patterns of association between variables. The procedure produces a smoothed, non-linear curve fit to the data that is analogous to the moving averages that are computed in time series analyses ... [and yields an] unbiased depiction of the patterns in the data. (p. 291) behaviors are exhibited. More recently, Bandura (1986, 1999) has described a theory of human behavior—triadic reciprocal determinism—which extends this line of reasoning. Bandura suggested that broad-based, decontextualized descriptions of personality traits are misguided insofar as they omit the impact of the situation and behaviors evoked by this situation. Bandura (1999) wrote

> Efficacious personality disposition is a dynamic, multi-faceted belief system that varies across different activity domains and under different situational demands rather than being a decontextualized conglomerate. The patterned individuality of efficacy beliefs represents the unique dispositional makeup . . . for any given person. (p. 161)

Although many of Bandura's original ideas about the limitations of broad-based personality descriptors have been empirically refuted (Kenrick & Funder, 1988), it is important to note that this framework does not deny the existence of stable behavioral dispositions but contends that predictable behavior patterns may be observed meaningfully and quantified accurately when context is taken into account. Thus, Bandura (1999) suggested that "personality measures that capture the contextualized and multifaceted nature of personal causation within an agentic model have greater explanatory and predictive power and provide more effective guides for personal change than do global trait measures" (p. 160).

The Cognitive-Affective Processing System

The central elements of Mischel and Shoda's (1995, 1999) cognitive-affective personality system (CAPS) are that (a) individuals differ with respect to cognitive and affective "mediating units" (e.g., encodings, expectancies, beliefs, affects, and goals); and (b) the interaction of these units differ across situations, even within an individual. Such differences produce an "if-then personality signature"—a unique pattern of trait-related behavior across different situations and settings (Kammarath, Mendoza-Denton, & Mischel, 2005; Mischel & Morf, 2003). Thus, the CAPS not only has noteworthy theoretical and practical implications in its own right but also suggests avenues for operationalizing and testing Bandura's (1968, 1999) conceptual framework.

For example, Shoda, Mischel, and Wright (1994) studied children's verbally aggressive behavior under different conditions: they compared two children across five interpersonal situations with a peer or adult and measured their level of verbal aggression in all five situations on two different occasions. Shoda et al. found a high degree of consistency within each child for each situation across time, yielding profile stability coefficients of .96 and .89. As Shoda et al. noted, this result simultaneously illustrates dispositional stability and situational specificity, a key feature of the CAPS model. Although it is rightfully noted that this approach focuses on idiographic

assessment—not nomothetic assessment that is found with many extant PD measures—research has suggested that the behavior of individuals with particular personality traits can be predicted using this framework. "Behavioral signatures" have been identified in highly dependent individuals by Bornstein, Riggs, Hill, and Calabrese (1996), and in narcissistic individuals by Morf and Rhodewalt (2001); in both sets of experiments, prototypic dependent and narcissistic behaviors (passivity/interpersonal yielding and anger in response to negative feedback) were exhibited only when situational context was such that PD-related responding was likely to further more basic underlying goals (strengthening of interpersonal ties in the case of dependency and self-promotion in the case of narcissism).

In discussing the future of the science of personality assessment, Mischel and Shoda (1999) questioned whether this "dispositional-trait and processing-dynamic" (p. 213 can be integrated into a unifying framework given longstanding assumptions about personality assessment. Mischel and Shoda (1999) wrote

> One of the most pernicious of these [previous assumptions about personality assessment] is the preemptive definition of personality psychology as a science of personality "traits," conceptualized as causal, genotypic entities that correspond to phenotypic behavioral dispositions. That automatically makes narrowly defined "traits" *the* target of investigation—as well as the bases for explanations. . . . [T]hese phenomena can be analyzed at [various] alternative and presumably complementary levels . . . allowing an ultimately more comprehensive and cumulative science conception of personality and its diverse manifestations and antecedents. (p. 213; italics added).

Unfortunately, few measures of Axis II disorders incorporate this degree of behavioral and contextual specificity. The SCID–II (First et al., 1995) asks context-free questions about stable dispositions such as "Do you have very high standards about what is right and what is wrong?" (obsessive–compulsive), Do you often get the feeling that things that have no special meaning to most people are really meant to give you a message?" (schizotypal), "Do you like to be the center of attention?" (histrionic), and "Have you all of a sudden changed your sense of who you are and where you are headed?" (borderline). These items solicit a verbal response and prompt the interviewer to seek examples or score the item simply by acknowledging the item's endorsement. Similar formats are used on the Personality Disorder Examination (Loranger, 1988), Diagnostic Interview for *DSM* Personality Disorders (Zanarini, Frankenburg, Chauncey, & Gunderson, 1987), and Personality Disorder Interview–IV (Widiger, Mangine, Corbitt, Ellis, & Thomas, 1995). To be sure, some diagnostic interviews or questionnaires attempt to solicit examples of situations when trait-relevant behavior is exhibited (e.g., SCID–II), but this level of specificity is not found with every item about every trait (nor does it guarantee the individual will accurately report his or her behavior).

Because patients with a PD tend to be limited in their ability to self-report accurately, open-ended questions such as these may fail to capture the ways in which PD-relevant traits are expressed. For instance, a male patient with obsessive–compulsive PD may believe he does not have very high standards about what is right and wrong even though when describing his work habits, he reports working 12 hr a day at an hourly wage job, often being in the office 3 hr per day by himself because he wants his work to be done as well as possible. Thus, in this domain, the therapist or interviewer may determine this individual has high standards for what is right or wrong despite the patient's lack of awareness. In this scenario, as in all if-then scenarios, determination of the personality trait is made by an external observer after considering behavioral exemplars of the trait(s) in question.

How could a PD measure capture situational specificity without losing the generalized behavioral predispositions that characterize different PDs? One possibility is to retain the broad-based symptom questions that currently characterize most PD measures but follow up on positive responses (i.e., acknowledged symptoms) with more focused questions regarding situational context, antecedents, and behavioral "triggers." Such an approach has the advantage of capturing an array of PD-related behaviors with each screening question and then supplementing this information with situational detail.

Assessing the motivational and affective underpinnings of PD-related behaviors presents a different sort of challenge. Implicit (performance-based) measures of personality (described following) may aid in detecting affective and motivational elements that are not—and in some cases cannot be—directly acknowledged (McClelland, Kocstner, & Weinberger, 1989). Alternatively, it may be that such motives are deduced from the observations of a trained clinician in the context of a trusting relationship and with sensitivity that could elicit information not otherwise reported in a first-time meeting or self-report instrument (Lerner & Lerner, 2007/this issue; Shedler & Westen, 2007/this issue).

Constructive Processes in Self-Understanding and Information Processing

It is widely accepted among personality psychologists that how individuals view themselves and make sense of their experience is a product of an active, constructive, psychological process. This idea is inherent in both psychodynamic (Cramer, 2000; Weinberger, 1998) and cognitive theories of PDs (Beck, Freeman, Davis, & Associates , 2004; Huprich, 2004). There also is an abundant literature on the manner in which the sense of self is established and maintained (Baumeister, 1998; Robins & John, 1997; Sedikides

& Strube, 1997). In one recent count, Robins, Norem, and Cheek (1999) identified 37 different self-concept theories. Similarly, attribution researchers have demonstrated repeatedly that in processing information about the self and others, individuals skew or selectively filter information to construct their experience in a way that minimizes negative affect and threats to the self. Mechanisms such as self-handicapping, hedonic bias, self-serving bias, and the actor–observer effect (Robins et al., 1999) all affect the accuracy of what is experienced and reported. Conversely, individuals may filter information in ways to present themselves as distressed so that they obtain the help they need (e.g., elevated F and suppressed K scales on the MMPI–2). Studies have documented how these constructive processes are related to specific PDs.

For example, McAllister et al. (2002) asked 425 undergraduates to learn a selection of material from a textbook and then tested them and provided false feedback about their performance. Individuals scoring high on the MCMI–III Narcissistic and Histrionic scales displayed the self-serving bias more than did other students when accounting for their performance on the test, whereas those with elevations on the Dependent and Avoidant scales showed little evidence of self-serving attributions.

Similarly, when Dolan (1995) examined blame attributions for criminal acts in a sample of 52 men in a treatment program as part of probation, she found that externalized blame was associated with elevations on the Revised Personality Diagnostic Questionnaire Schizoid, Avoidant, Obsessive–Compulsive, Passive–Aggressive, and Borderline scales (Hyler et al., 1988). Attributions to the individual's mental state were associated with elevations in avoidant PD, whereas attributions related to guilt were associated with schizotypal, avoidant, and dependent PDs.

Along somewhat different lines, twin studies provide indirect support for the importance of the constructive process in assessing PD-relevant traits. A widely cited study (Loehlin & Nicholls, 1976) found a moderate degree of genetic influence on the expression of a broad range of personality traits, with monozygotic (MZ) twins sharing approximately 50% of the variance across measures. Specifically, across 24,000 twin pairs, MZ twins had a correlation of .51 on Neuroticism and .46 on Extraversion, whereas corresponding dizygotic twins had respective correlations of .18 and .20. A more recent study by Riemann, Angleitner, and Strelau (1997) measured the Big Five traits in almost 1,000 twin pairs. Reimann et al. found that across the five factors, approximately 50% of the variance was shared by MZ twins; for those twins that shared the same environment, an additional 5% of variance was accounted for in Extraversion, Agreeableness, and Openness to Experience. This left approximately 50% of the variance to be accounted for by nonshared environment, which would include self-perceptions of the aforementioned traits (as well as measurement error).

Tellegen et al. (1988) assessed 14 personality traits with the Multidimensional Personality Questionnaire (Tellegen, 1982) in over 400 twin pairs. Like the prior studies, Tellegen et al. reported that approximately 50% of variance in personality cannot be attributed to genetic factors, with a substantial portion of this variance accounted for by what they termed "unshared familial variance." Tellegen et al. alluded to the fact that idiosyncratic, constructive processes help account for this variance. Tellegen et al. (1988) stated "Particularly helpful would be research on individual rearing environments that would identify *psychologically meaningful components* [italics added] of the unshared environment" (p. 1037). Even in genetically similar individuals raised in the same environment, a substantial amount of variability in self-reports is affected by their unique psychological understanding of themselves and their experiences.

Thus, when examining the literature on the psychological constructive processes as related to self-reports of personality, it appears that a substantial amount of variation in these measures may be accounted for by such processes. Furthermore, it has not yet been determined to what extent many of these processes affect self-reported PD symptoms and features nor how well such processes can be detected even when they are more directly identified. Although genetic influences on self-reported personality traits are quite significant, even in genetically similar individuals, a substantial amount of variability in self-reports may be attributable to their unique psychological understanding of themselves, others, and their experiences. Consequently, additional strategies are needed to improve the assessment of personality traits and PDs.

Unconscious and Affective Influences on Personality Reports

It is widely accepted that unconscious (or implicit) processes affect motivation, memory, learning, perception, thought, affect, and behavior (see Baumeister, 1998; Bornstein, 2002). As Kihlstrom (1999) noted, "contemporary cognitive psychology has begun to offer a clear theoretical framework for studying the relations between conscious and nonconscious mental life" (p. 437). Kihlstrom (1999) went on to suggest that as implicit processes in perception, learning, and memory become increasingly established, researchers should examine more closely "unconscious emotional and motivational life [and] . . . the role of unconscious processes in personality and social interaction" (p. 438).

In a pioneering review almost two decades ago, McClelland et al. (1989) differentiated explicit from implicit motivation. *Implicit* motive measures assess an individual's automatic, unconscious patterns of behavior, whereas *explicit* measures assess an individual's self-attributed motives (which do not always correspond to the person's expressed behavior). McClelland et al. added that implicit measures provide a more direct measure of one's motivational and emotional experiences than do explicit measures because

they are less strongly affected by conscious bias and are a product of early preverbal affective experiences. Stated differently, information derived from implicit measures provides information about patterns of thinking, reacting, and behaving that individuals may not recognize as being characteristic of them (Bornstein, 2002; Meyer, 2000; Weiner, 2005; see also Bornstein, 1999, for meta-analytic data regarding the construct validity of widely used implicit dependency tests).

Given the modest intercorrelations of scores on self-report and free-response measures of a given trait or need state, one might reasonably ask whether these two types of measures are in fact assessing the same underlying construct. Meta-analytic reviews of the validity of self-report and free-response measures of dependency (Bornstein, 1999) and need for achievement (Spangler, 1992) have suggested that they are, with divergences in the behaviors predicted by the two types of measures primarily a function of contextual influence. As Weinberger and McClelland (1990) noted, implicit motive scores typically predict spontaneous behavioral trends exhibited in a wide variety of situations and settings, whereas self-attributed motive scores predict focused, goal-directed responses exhibited primarily in situations in which the implications of a given motive or need state are highly salient to the actor (see also Bornstein, 2002, for a discussion of this issue).

One example of a study in which the explicit–implicit distinction yielded important information about the expression of PD-relevant personality features was conducted by Bornstein (1998a). Using an implicit measure, the Rorschach Oral Dependency Scale (ROD; Masling, Rabie, & Blondheim, 1967) and an explicit measure, the Interpersonal Dependency Inventory (IDI; Hirschfeld et al., 1977), Bornstein (1998a) identified four groups of individuals: high dependency (HD; high scores on both the IDI and the ROD), unacknowledged dependency (UAD; high ROD and low IDI), dependent self-presentation (DSP; high IDI and low ROD), and low dependency (low scores on both the IDI and ROD). Bornstein (1998a) then assigned individuals in each of these categories to one of two experimental groups. In one group, individuals were told that they were in a study of problem solving , whereas the other was told that they were in a study of dependency and help seeking. As predicted, study instructions interacted with dependency status to predict trait-relevant behavior. Specifically, the UAD group engaged in help seeking at rates similar to the HD group when they believed they were involved in a problem-solving task; however, the UAD group did not show high rates of help seeking when they believed they were in a study of dependency. In contrast, the DSP group engaged in moderate amounts of help seeking when they believed they were in a problem-solving task; however, when told they were in a study of dependency, the DSP group engaged in help-seeking behavior at a rate similar to that of the HD group.

Mood state can also affect the measurement of PD-relevant traits. Hirschfeld et al. (1983) evaluated a group of psychiatric outpatients who were being treated for major depression and assessed their underlying personality with five different self-report inventories. One year later, Hirschfeld et al. (1983) reassessed patients for major depression and readministered the personality inventories. They found that patients who had recovered from depression differed at retest from those who had not recovered. Specifically, emotional lability, hypersensitivity, passivity, resiliency, extraversion, and interpersonal dependency all changed in an adaptive direction in those who had recovered from depression.

The effect of mood state on measures of personality is notable even when more modest changes in mood occur. Bornstein, Bowers, and Bonner (1996) induced a positive, negative, or neutral mood in participants using the Velten (1968) and Baker and Gutterfreund (1993) mood induction procedures. Bornstein, Bowers, et al. (1996) hypothesized that implicit dependency scores should increase when a negative mood was induced, whereas self-reported dependency would remain unchanged. These hypotheses were based on findings that had demonstrated that depressed mood increases individuals' underlying dependent feelings (e.g., Hirschfeld, Klerman, Andreason, Clayton, & Keller, 1986; Zuroff & Mongrain, 1987). In both studies, ROD scores increased significantly in a negative mood, whereas IDI scores remained unchanged.

Other studies have demonstrated the stability of personality despite variations in depression. Santor, Bagby, and Joffe (1997) evaluated the extent to which scores on the NEO–PI (Costa & McCrae, 1985, 1989) changed as a function of treatment for depression in a sample of 71 outpatients receiving pharmacotherapy over the course of 5 weeks. They found that Neuroticism, Extraversion, and depression scores all changed toward a more "healthy" level over the course of treatment. The greatest change was found in depression scores, whereas less change was found for Neuroticism and Extraversion. More specifically, the correlations between from baseline to the end of treatment were .76 for Neuroticism and .80 for Extraversion, whereas correlations between depression measures across both time periods were .41 and .43, respectively. Santor et al. (1997) interpreted these findings as demonstrating the relative stability of personality traits despite significant absolute changes in the scores.

Along somewhat different lines, Chamberlain, Huprich, and Erdodi (2006) attempted to differentiate state and trait components of the Depressive Personality Disorder Inventory (DPDI; Huprich, Margrett, Barthelemy, & Fine, 1996) by factor analyzing scores from 362 nonclinical, clinical, and primary care participants who completed the DPDI and the Beck Depression Inventory–II (BDI–II; Beck, Steer, & Brown, 1996). Chamberlain et al. (2006) found five factors, three of which loaded most heavily on items associated with depressive PD (self-criticism, pessimism, worrying/brooding), whereas two were most associated with the

BDI–II (fatigue/self-contempt). Moreover, items that stated a negative quality in the affirmative ("I frequently think something is about to go wrong") were those most associated with the DPDI and not the BDI–II. Chamberlain et al. suggested that depressive PD may be associated with a tendency to agree with negative statements describing one's experiences and qualities; that is, there could be a response bias for negative qualities that accounts for the manner with which congruent self-statements are accepted.

Collectively, these studies have illustrated four important issues regarding the role of unconscious processes and the impact of mood on personality and PD assessment. First, there are elements of personality that are not fully accessible to conscious awareness yet still influence personality test scores. Second, mood has a significant and meaningful impact on self-reported personality traits. Third, although some personality traits generally remain stable, personality test scores associated with these traits do change over time. Fourth, the wording of questions used to assess aspects of personality associated with and related to mood may play an important role in determining what is reported.

Although dimensional measures and categorical-based measures of PDs (e.g., SCID–II) are designed to capture broadband, pervasive aspects of personality and its disorders, there appears to be an asymptotic level of variance that can be explained with current dimensional and categorical measures. Thus, any effort to improve the manner by which PDs are assessed should incorporate issues such as those we describe for the science of PD assessment to advance.

IMPROVING PD DIAGNOSIS: BEHAVIORAL AND CLINICIAN ASSESSMENT

Given the limitations described previously, what can be done to improve the assessment of PDs? In the following, we offer six strategies, some of which may be more relevant to dimensional models, some to categorical models, and some to both. All, however, offer ways of enhancing psychologists' understanding of PDs and improving PD diagnosis.

Use Behaviorally Referenced Symptom Criteria to Improve Diagnostic Accuracy

Although recent editions of the *DSM* include detailed descriptions of PD symptoms, in many cases, these symptom descriptions have not been derived from investigations of actual PD behavior but from interview data collected from patients and knowledgeable informants. Thus, many PD symptom criteria are not consistent with research on the behavioral correlates of theoretically related personality styles. For example, Bornstein (1997) noted that of the eight *DSM–IV* symptoms of dependent PD, four are supported by behaviorally referenced empirical data, two have never been tested directly, and two have been contradicted repeatedly. Exacerbating this problem, the vast majority of contemporary PD symptom validation studies (82% of those published in five major PD journals between 1991 and 2000) have not employed any sort of behavioral outcome criteria but assess the validity of PD symptoms solely with respect to questionnaire and/or interview data (Bornstein, 2003).

Bornstein (2003) outlined a framework for conducting behaviorally referenced PD symptom validation studies in future *DSM* field trials. This framework involves assessing the predictive validity of PD symptoms using two parallel strategies. First, in vivo sampling of PD-related behaviors via continuous monitoring and/or spot sampling procedures can be used to determine the frequency and situational specificity of various theoretically related responses. Second, laboratory studies can be used to ascertain what interpersonal and intrapersonal events trigger PD-related behaviors (e.g., rejection by a valued other, changes in mood state).

Operationalize PD Symptoms in Context-Specific Terms

In vivo and laboratory studies can help identify the contextual factors that exacerbate (or ameliorate) PD symptoms; these findings can then be used to modify PD symptom criteria in future versions of the *DSM*. Bornstein (1998b) proposed that—in addition to assigning separate PD intensity and pervasiveness ratings when rendering diagnoses—it would be useful to list those situations wherein a given PD symptom (or set of symptoms) was especially problematic for a particular patient, and those situations wherein a given PD symptom actually enhanced adaptation and functioning. It is possible, for example, that a patient's obsessive symptoms might cause difficulties in friendships and romantic relationships but be adaptive at work. Another patient's histrionic symptoms might lead to problems at the office but work well in certain social settings. Thus, effective operationalization of PD symptoms in context-specific terms involves (a) uncovering broad-based situational influences on a given PD symptom through nomothetic research studies and then (b) applying these findings to form hypotheses regarding context-driven PD dynamics in individual patients.

Assess Motivation and Affect Underlying PD-Related Behaviors

An important domain of future research involves assessing the motivation and affect underlying PD-related behaviors, but as Pervin (1999) noted, systematic examination of PD-related motivation and affect is scanty. This type of research may allow clinicians and researchers to determine the psychological processes that drive PD-related behaviors and de-

termine, for example, whether suspiciousness, guardedness, and social introversion are really the result of paranoid personality processes that serve to disavow aggressive and hateful feelings or if such traits and behaviors are the result some other cause not indicative of paranoia (e.g., an unrecognized anxiety disorder, concerns regarding self-protection in an environment in which real harm is possible).

Assess Defenses as Well as Behaviors and Thought Patterns

PDs are associated with a predictable constellation of defenses and coping strategies that serve to modulate affect, motives, and impulses. A significant literature has been developed on this topic (see Bornstein, 2005; Cramer, 1991, 2000; Lingiardi et al., 1999; Millon, 1990; Vaillant, 1985, 1992, 1994; Weinberger, 1998) with particular attention directed toward the etiological role defenses play in the development of certain PDs. For example, evidence suggests that overreliance on projection may be central to the development of paranoid PD, whereas excessive use of splitting is central to borderline pathology (Lerner, 2005; Vaillant, 1994). Moreover, recent empirical studies have demonstrated the utility of evaluating defenses when assessing PDs.

For example, Soldz, Budman, Demby, and Merry (1995) evaluated 257 psychiatric outpatients for defense style, PD symptoms, and FFM domain scores. Soldz et al. found that immature defenses were associated with Neuroticism and withdrawal defenses with Extraversion; mature defenses were associated only with Openness. Defense style also predicted substantial amounts of variance in Neuroticism (39%) and Extraversion (43%); smaller proportions of unique variance were accounted for in Agreeableness (14%), Conscientiousness (12%), and Openness (11%). Seven of the *DSM* (3rd ed., revised; American Psychiatric Association, 1987) PD symptom sets were predicted by defense level above and beyond FFM factor scores, with increases in R^2 ranging from .05 (Dependent) to .16 (Histrionic). For all indices of PD pathology combined, defense style scores predicted an additional 20% of the variance in PD scores beyond the five factors. A separate axis for coding of patients' defense style—the Defensive Functioning Scale (DFS)—has been proposed in the *DSM-IV-Text Revision* (American Psychiatric Association, 2000, pp. 807–813). Information coded on this axis includes a listing of each patient's characteristic defenses as well as an overall rating of that patient's predominant defense level (i.e., a rating of defense maturity/effectiveness). This information could enhance the predictive value of PD diagnoses by (a) allowing researchers to determine whether theoretically related defenses actually are linked with particular PD symptoms in a variety of patient populations and (b) enabling clinicians to ascertain which defenses are most commonly used by a particular PD patient. Furthermore, if the DFS functions like other measures of defense, it could be useful in understanding comorbidity

(J. C. Perry, 1988) and predicting treatment response (Blais, Conboy, Wilcox, & Norman, 1996, J. C. Perry, 1988, 2001; J. D. C. Perry & Perry, 2004; Vaillant, 1992, 1994). Preliminary evidence on the utility of the DFS has been reported in two studies (Blais et al., 1996; J. C. Perry et al., 1998).

Use Psychological Assessment Information That May Not Be Detected in Self-Report

In many instances, patients' reports of personality traits and expressed behaviors are consistent with data derived from alternative sources (e.g., free-response test data, archival data, reports of knowledgeable informants). However, in some instances, patients' self-reports are inconsistent with data derived from other sources. Although the traditional approach to personality assessment emphasizes seeking convergences among different data sources, in recent years, assessment researchers have shown that discontinuities between information derived from self-reports and that derived from other, less direct data sources can reveal important information regarding personality dynamics and PD pathology (see Bornstein, 2002; Ganellen, 1996; Huprich & Ganellen, 2006; Meyer, 1996, 1997; Viglione, 1999; Weiner, 1999, 2005). Much research in this area has focused on integrating Rorschach data to examine test score continuities and discontinuities (e.g., Meyer, 1996, 1997, 2000); other studies have explored convergences and divergences between behaviorally referenced test data and trait-specific self-report scales (see, e.g., McClelland et al.'s [1989] findings regarding implicit and self-attributed achievement motives and Bornstein's [2002] findings regarding implicit and self-attributed dependency needs).

In part as a response to the self–other discrepancies documented by Meyer et al. (2001) and others, interest in this issue has increased and research has shown that comparing other reports to self-reports allows for improved prediction of PDs. Clifton et al. (2004, 2005) have found that reports of interpersonal problems and ratings from others regarding a target individual's personality traits add to the ability to predict personality pathology. For example, Clifton et al. (2004) found that individuals who describe themselves as angry and hostile are described by peers as paranoid (see also Oltmanns et al., 2005, for similar results).

Use Clinicians' Prototypes of Personality Pathology to Refine PD Diagnostic Criteria

More than two decades ago, Cantor, Smith, and French (1980) found that to a surprising degree, clinical diagnoses were based not on systematic assessment of symptom profiles but on the extent to which a given patient matched the clinician's prototype for a particular disorder. When Westen (1997) surveyed over 400 clinicians regarding what types

of information they use to assess patients for a PD, he found that—independent of theoretical orientation—many clinicians rely largely on patients' narratives and in-session and out-of-session behaviors to assign a diagnosis. Furthermore, Shedler and Westen (2004a) found that clinicians have well-developed prototypes for the PDs and that clinicians' prototypes "placed greater emphasis on patients' mental life or inner experience" (p. 1350) than on a symptom criteria set.

Prototype matching may hold particular promise in the dimensional assessment of PDs. Westen and Shedler (1999a, 1999b) have empirically demonstrated that clinicians' cognitive prototypes of *DSM–IV* PDs correspond well with actual patients who receive treatment for a PD. Furthermore, prototype matching identified patients with personality problems commonly seen in practice that are not currently used as part of the standard PD diagnoses found in *DSM–IV* such as depressive PD (Shedler & Westen, 2004a, 2004b). Although it could be that findings from this line of research reflect the constructive processes that clinicians use in addition to actual patient behavior, it is hard to dismiss the ecological validity of these findings given that they were based on the responses of experienced clinicians across all major theoretical approaches. Furthermore, this method places greater priority on the trained clinician's ability to rate and assess personality pathology above and beyond patient self-reports[3] (Shedler & Westen, 2007/this issue).

TRANSITIONING FROM CATEGORICAL TO DIMENSIONAL PD ASSESSMENT

One practical advantage of moving from categorical to dimensional PD assessment is that dimensional data do not preclude making categorical decisions. Just as it is possible to quantify one's blood pressure or cholesterol level and also to know whether these values exceed an established cutoff for clinically significant elevation, it is possible to determine a patient's level of dependency or narcissism and to know whether these levels are significantly elevated. The reverse is not true: Just as merely knowing whether one's blood pressure is "high" does not provide any information regarding how high it may be, merely knowing that a patient meets the *DSM* criteria for avoidant PD tells the clinician nothing

---

[3]This conclusion does not imply that clinician or observer ratings of patients should take priority over self-reports. Training and experience notwithstanding, mental health professionals have attributional biases that affect their perception of patients. When Markham and Trower (2003) investigated psychiatric nurses' causal attributions about patient behavior, they found that patients diagnosed with borderline PD were rated as having more personal control over behavior than were patients diagnosed with major depression or schizophrenia. Numerous studies have documented the impact of patient gender on clinicians' interpretation of PD-relevant behavior and on their willingness to assign PD diagnoses (e.g., Widiger & Clark, 2000).

about the intensity of that patient's avoidance. In this respect, use of a dimensional PD assessment strategy represents an incremental gain in information with no loss of predictive capacity.

Even if clinicians and clinical researchers agree that a dimensional PD assessment model is warranted, disagreement is likely to persist regarding implementation of such a model. Recent work in this area has suggested several possibilities.

The PD Continuum Model

PD assessment using this approach would involve quantifying the intensity of symptoms in each PD domain and/or the number and type of PD symptoms experienced by the patient regardless of which PD category these symptoms are now classified (see, e.g., Bornstein, 1998b). Within this general framework, it might also be useful to (a) assign ratings on other PD-related dimensions to increase the precision of clinical description and prediction (e.g., impairment, pervasiveness, stability, longevity) and (b) enumerate those situations wherein PD symptoms are most problematic for a given patient (to capture contextual influences on PD dynamics).

The Underlying Factors Approach

Best represented by research involving the FFM, the underlying factors approach to dimensional PD assessment would involve delineating empirically validated profiles of underlying traits associated with each PD category and using these patterns to (a) help determine which PD syndromes a given patient is likely to exhibit and (b) understand the personality traits that underlie that patient's PD-related behavior. Although much research in this area has involved the FFM, other trait models (e.g., Cloninger's seven-factor model [Cloninger & Svrakic, 1994], Millon's biopsychosocial approach [Strack & Millon, 2007/this issue]) also offer promise in this area. Integrating across dimensional models, it has been suggested that four factors may account for most of the variance in PD diagnosis: emotional dysregulation, constraint/conscientiousness, antagonism/dissocial, and inhibition/introversion (Livesley, Jang, & Vernon, 1998; Widiger & Simonsen, 2005). Alternatively, dimensional models may actually be hierarchically organized and readily integrated[4] (Markon et al., 2005; see Figure 1).

---

[4]As a result of this integration, there appears to be the rebirth of an important idea from the earliest understanding of PDs. Westen, Gabbard, and Blagov (2006) noted that using personality as a basis for conceptualizing psychopathology represents a return to ideas initially set forth by Freud and other psychoanalytic theorists in understanding the basic interplay between personality structure and (dys)function. Weston et al., (2006) added that an understanding of psychological processes (e.g., object relations, defenses) are quite informative in understanding personality beyond surface traits.

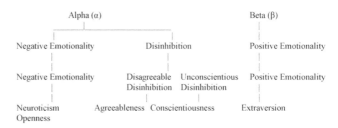

FIGURE 1.   Results from Markon, Kreuger, and Watson's (2005) meta-analysis demonstrating a hierarchical structure to personality dimensions.

The Multiple Levels Strategy

This strategy is based on the premise that multimodal assessment yields richer information than a diagnostic interview alone, so that in addition to using traditional interview and/or questionnaire PD measures, PD assessment should be supplemented with data derived from independent sources (e.g., free-response test data, information from knowledgeable informants). Implicit in this strategy is the assumption that patient self-reports yield useful—but limited—information regarding underlying dynamics and expressed behaviors and that exploration of divergences among different data sources can be as informative as exploration of convergences and consistencies:sometimes more so (Bornstein, 2002; Weiner, 2005). This suggests that PD assessment and diagnosis would regularly involve multiple measures to assess the patient and confirm whether personality pathology exists and if so, how that pathology is best characterized.

CONCLUSION

A dimensional model of assessing personality pathology has much to offer the science and practice of PD assessment. However, there are several challenges to the implementation of a dimensional model. For both categorical and dimensional approaches to PD assessment, exclusive use of self-report methods do not permit the assessment of the entire range of psychological processes affecting personality trait expression and trait–behavior links. We suggest that a combination of behavioral and clinician assessment of various domains of functioning may facilitate PD diagnosis. Thus, to improve the conceptualization and assessment of PDs, there is a need to expand the manner by which PDs are assessed and diagnosed. Such an approach should maximize psychological science's ability to diagnose and assess personality pathology in accurate and meaningful ways.

REFERENCES

Achenbach, T. M., Krukowski, R. A., Dumenci, L., & Ivanova, M. Y. (2005). Assessment of adult psychopathology: Meta-analyses and implications of cross-informant correlations. *Psychological Bulletin, 131,* 361–382.

American Psychiatric Association. (1952). *Diagnostic and statistical manual of mental disorders*. Washington, DC: Author.

American Psychiatric Association. (1987). *Diagnostic and statistical manual of mental disorders* (3rd ed., rev.). Washington, DC: Author.

American Psychiatric Association. (1994). *Diagnostic and statistical manual of mental disorders* (4th ed.). Washington, DC: Author.

American Psychiatric Association. (2000). *Diagnostic and statistical manual of mental disorders* (4th ed., text revision). Washington, DC: Author.

Baker, R. C., & Gutterfreund, D. G. (1993). The effects of written autobiographical recollection induction procedures on mood. *Journal of Clinical Psychology, 49*, 563–568.

Bandura, A. (1986). *Social foundations of thought and action: A social cognitive theory*. Englewood Cliffs, NJ: Prentice Hall.

Bandura, A. (1999). Social cognitive theory of personality. In L. A. Pervin & O. P. John (Eds.), *Handbook of personality* (2nd ed., pp. 154–196.). New York: Guilford.

Baumeister, R. F. (1998). The self. In D. T. Gilbert, S. T. Fiske, & G. Lindzey (Eds.), *The handbook of social psychology* (Vol. 2, 4th ed., pp. 680–740). Boston, MA: McGraw-Hill.

Beck, A. T., Freeman, A., Davis, D. D., & Associates. (2004). *Cognitive therapy of personality disorders* (2nd ed). New York: Guilford.

Beck, A. T., Steer, R. A., & Brown, G. K. (1996). *Beck Depression Inventory II Manual*. San Antonio, TX: Psychological Corporation.

Blais, M. A., Conboy, C. A., Wilcox, N., & Norman, D. K. (1996). An empirical study of the *DSM–IV* Defensive Functioning Scale in personality disordered patients. *Comprehensive Psychiatry, 37*, 435–440.

Bornstein, R. F. (1997). Dependent personality disorder in the *DSM–IV* and beyond. *Clinical Psychology: Science and Practice, 4*, 175–187.

Bornstein, R. F. (1998a). Implicit and self-attributed dependency strivings: Differential relationships to laboratory and field measures of help-seeking. *Journal of Personality and Social Psychology, 75*, 779–787.

Bornstein, R. F. (1998b). Reconceptualizing personality disorder diagnosis in the *DSM–V*: The discriminant validity challenge. *Clinical Psychology: Science and Practice, 5*, 333–343.

Bornstein, R. F. (1999). Criterion validity of objective and projective dependency tests: A meta-analytic assessment of behavioral prediction. *Psychological Assessment, 11*, 48–57.

Bornstein, R. F. (2002). A process dissociation approach to objective-projective test score interrelationships. *Journal of Personality Assessment, 78*, 47–68.

Bornstein, R. F. (2003). Behaviorally referenced experimentation and symptom validation: A paradigm for 21st century personality disorder research. *Journal of Personality Disorders, 17*, 1–18.

Bornstein, R. F. (2005). *The dependent patient: A practitioner's guide*. Washington, DC: American Psychological Association.

Bornstein, R. F., Bowers, K. S., & Bonner, S. (1996). Relationships of objective and projective dependency scores to sex role orientation in college student participants. *Journal of Personality Assessment, 66*, 555–568.

Bornstein, R. F., Riggs, J. M., Hill, E. L., & Calabrese, C. (1996). Activity, passivity, self-denigration, and self-promotion: Toward an interactionist model of interpersonal dependency. *Journal of Personality, 64*, 637–673.

Cantor, N., Smith, E. E., & French, R. D. (1980). Psychiatric diagnosis as prototype categorization. *Journal of Abnormal Psychology, 89*, 181–193.

Chamberlain, J., Huprich, S. K., & Erdodi, L. (2006, March). *The factor structure of the Depressive Personality Disorder Inventory*. Poster session presented at the annual midwinter meeting of the Society for Personality Assessment, San Diego, CA.

Clifton, A., Turkheimer, E., & Oltmanns, T. F. (2004). Contrasting perspectives on personality problems: Descriptions from self and others. *Personality and Individual Differences, 36*, 1499–1514.

Clifton, A., Turkheimer, E., & Oltmanns, T. F. (2005). Self- and peer perspectives on pathological personality traits and interpersonal problems. *Psychological Assessment, 117*, 123–131.

Cooper, A. M. (1989). Narcissism and masochism: The narcissistic-masochistic character. *Psychiatric Clinics of North America, 12*, 541–552.

Costa, P. T., Jr., & McCrae, R. R. (1985). *The NEO-PI Personality Inventory manual*. Odessa, FL: Psychological Assessment Resources.

Costa, P. T., Jr., & McCrae, R. R. (1989). *The NEO–PI/NEO–FFI manual supplement*. Odessa, FL: Psychological Assessment Resources.

Costa, P. T., Jr., & McCrae, R. R. (1992). *Revised NEO-Personality Inventory(NEO–PI–R) and the NEO Five-Factor Inventory (NEO–FFI professional manual*. Odessa, FL: Psychological Assessment Resources.

Costa, P. T., Jr., & Widiger, T. A. (2002). *Personality disorders and the Five-factor model of personality* (2nd ed.). Washington, DC: American Psychological Association.

Cloninger, C. R., & Svrakic, D. M. (1994). Differentiating normal and deviant personality by the seven-factor personality model. In S. Strack & M. Carr (Eds.), *Differentiating normal and abnormal personality* (pp. 40–64). New York: Springer.

Cramer, P. (1991). *The development of defense mechanisms: Theory, research, and assessment*. New York: Springer-Verlag.

Cramer, P. (2000). Defense mechanisms in psychology today: Further processes for adaptation. *American Psychologist, 55*, 637–646.

Dolan, B. (1995). The attribution of blame for criminal acts: Relationship with personality disorders and mood. *Criminal Behaviour and Mental Health, 5*, 41–51.

Durbin, C. E., & Klein, D. N. (2006). Ten-year stability of personality disorders among outpatients with mood disorders. *Journal of Abnormal Psychology, 115*, 75–44.

First, M. B., Spitzer, R. L., Gibbon, M., Williams, J. B. W., Davies, W. M., Borus, J., et al. (1995). The Structured Clinical Interview for *DSM–III–R* Personality Disorders (SCID–II): Part II. Multi-site test-retest reliability. *Journal of Personality Disorders, 9*, 92–104.

Ganellen, R. J. (1996). *Integrating the Rorschach and the MMPI-2 in personality assessment*. Mahwah, NJ: Lawrence Erlbaum Associates.

Ganellen, R. J. (2007/this issue). Assessing normal and abnormal personality functioning: Strengths and weaknesses of self-report, observer, and performance-based methods. *Journal of Personality Assessment, 89*, 30–40.

Graham, J. R. (2000). *MMPI–2: Assessing personality and psychopathology* (3rd ed.) New York: Oxford University Press.

Grilo, C., & McGlashan, T. (1999). Stability and course of personality disorders. *Current Opinion in Psychiatry, 12*, 157–162.

Harlan, E., & Clark, L. A. (1999). Short-forms of the Schedule for Nonadaptive and Adaptive Personality (SNAP) for self and collateral ratings: Development, reliability, and validity. *Assessment, 6*, 131–146.

Hathaway, S. R., & McKinley, J. C. (1943). *The Minnesota Multiphasic Personality Inventory*. Minneapolis: University of Minnesota Press.

Hirschfeld, R. M. A., Klerman, G. L., Andreason, N. C., Clayton, P. J., & Keller, M. B. (1986). Psychosocial predictors of chronicity in depressed patients. *British Journal of Psychiatry, 148*, 648–654.

Hirschfeld, R. M. A., Klerman, G. L., Clayton, P. J., Keller, M. B., McDonald-Scott, P., & Larkin, B. H. (1983). Assessing personality: Effects of the depressive state on trait measurement. *American Journal of Psychiatry, 140*, 695–699.

Hirschfeld, R. M. A., Klerman, G. L., Gough, H. G., Barrett, J., Korchin, S. J., & Chodoff, P. (1977). A measure of interpersonal dependency. *Journal of Personality Assessment, 41*, 610–618.

Huprich, S. K. (2003). Evaluating NEO–PI–R profiles of veterans with personality disorders. *Journal of Personality Disorders, 17*, 33–44.

Huprich, S. K. (2004). The evolution of cognitive therapy for personality disorders: Convergence in theories and therapies [Review of the book *Cognitive therapy for personality disorders* (2nd ed.). *PsycCRITIQUES*.

Huprich, S. K., & Ganellen, R. J. (2006). The advantages of using the Rorschach to assess personality disorders. In S. K. Huprich (Ed.), *Rorschach assessment of the personality disorders* (pp. 27–53). Mahwah, NJ: Lawrence Erlbaum Associates.

Huprich, S. K., Margrett, J., Barthelemy, K., & Fine, M. A. (1996). The Depressive Personality Disorder Inventory: An initial examination of its psychometric properties. *Journal of Clinical Psychology, 52*, 153–159.

Hyler, S. E., Rieder, R. O., Williams, J. B. W., Spitzer, R. L., Hendler, J., & Lyons, M. (1988). The Personality Diagnostic Questionnaire: Development and preliminary results. *Journal of Personality Disorders, 2,* 229–237.

Kammarath, L. K., Mendoza-Denton, R., & Mischel, W. (2005). Incorporating *If . . . then . . .* personality signatures in person perception: Beyond the person-situation dichotomy. *Journal of Personality and Social Psychology, 88,* 605–618.

Kenrick, D. T., & Funder, D. C. (1988). Profiting from controversy: Lessons from the person-situation debate. *American Psychologist, 43,* 23–34.

Klein, D. N. (2003). Patients' versus informants' reports of personality disorders in predicting 7¹/₂-year outcome in outpatients with depressive disorder. *Psychological Assessment, 15,* 216–222.

Klonsky, E. D., Oltmanns, T. F., & Turkheimer, E. (2002). Informant-reports of personality disorder: Relation to self-reports and future research directions. *Clinical Psychology: Science and Practice, 9,* 300–311.

Lerner, P. M. (2005). Defense and its assessment: The Lerner Defense Scale. In R. F. Bornstein & J. M. Masling (Eds.), *Scoring the Rorschach: Seven validated systems* (pp. 237–269). Mahwah, NJ: Lawrence Erlbaum Associates.

Lerner, P. M., & Lerner, H. D. (2007/this issue). A psychoanalytic clinician looks at diagnostic labels and diagnostic classification systems. *Journal of Personality Assessment, 89,* 70–81.

Lingiardi, V., Lonati, C., Delucchi, F., Fossati, A., Vanzulli, L., & Maffei, C. (1999). Defense mechanisms and personality disorders. *Journal of Nervous and Mental Disease, 187,* 224–228.

Livesley, W. (2006). Behavioral and molecular genetic contributions to a dimensional classification of personality disorders. *Journal of Personality disorders, 19,* 131–155.

Livesley, W. J., Jang, K. L., & Vernon, P. A. (1998). Phenotypic and genetic structure of traits delineating personality disorder. *Archives of General Psychiatry, 55,* 941–948.

Loehlin, J. C., & Nicholls, J. (1976). *Heredity, environment, and personality.* Austin: University of Texas.

Loranger, A. W. (1988). *Personality Disorder Examination (PDE) manual.* Yonkers, NY: DV Communications.

Markham, D., & Trower, P. (2003). The effects of the psychiatric label "borderline personality disorder" on nursing staff's perceptions and causal attributions for challenging behaviors. *British Journal of Clinical Psychology, 42,* 243–256.

Markon, K. E., Krueger, R. F., & Waston, D. (2005). Delineating the structure of normal and abnormal personality: An integrated hierarchical approach. *Journal of Personality and Social Psychology, 88,* 139–157.

Masling, J. M., Rabie, L., & Blondheim, S. H. (1967). Obesity, level of aspiration, and Rorschach and TAT measures of oral dependence. *Journal of Consulting Psychology, 31,* 233–239.

McAllister, H. A., Baker, J. D., Mannes, C., Stewart, H., & Sutherland, A. (2002). The optimal margin of illusion hypothesis: Evidence from the self-serving bias and personality disorders. *Journal of Social and Clinical Psychology, 21,* 414–426.

McClelland, D. C., Koestner, R., & Weinberger, J. (1989). How do self-attributed and implicit motives differ? *Psychological Review, 96,* 690–702.

Meyer, G. J. (1996). The Rorschach and MMPI: Toward a more scientific understanding of cross-method assessment. *Journal of Personality Assessment, 67,* 558–578.

Meyer, G. J. (1997). On the integration of personality assessment methods: The Rorschach and MMPI. *Journal of Personality Assessment, 68,* 297–330.

Meyer, G. J. (2000). Incremental validity of the Rorschach Prognostic Rating Scale over the MMPI Ego Strength Scale and IQ. *Journal of Personality Assessment, 74,* 356–370.

Meyer, G. J., Finn, S. E., Eyde, L. D., Kay, G. G., Moreland, K. L., Dies, R. R. et al. (2001). Psychological testing and psychological assessment. A review of evidence and issues. *American Psychologist, 56,* 128–165.

Miller, J. D., Pilkonis, P. A., & Clifton, A. (2005). Self- and other-reports of traits from the Five factor model: Relations to personality disorder. *Journal of Personality Disorders, 19,* 400–419.

Millon, T. (1990). *Toward a new personology: An evolutionary model.* New York: Wiley.

Millon, T. (1994). *Manual for the MCMI–III.* Minneapolis, MN: National Computer Systems.

Mischel, W. (1968). *Personality assessment.* New York: Wiley.

Mischel, W., & Morf, C. C. (2003). The self as a psycho-social dynamic processing system: A meta-perspective on a century of the self in psychology. In M. R. Leary & J. P. Tangney (Eds.), *Handbook of self and identity* (pp. 15–43). New York: Guilford.

Mischel, W., & Shoda, Y. (1995). A cognitive-affective system theory of personality: Reconceptualizing situations, dispositions, dynamics, and invariance in personality structure. *Psychological Review, 102,* 246–268.

Mischel, W., & Shoda, Y. (1999). Integrating dispositions and processing dynamics within a unified theory of personality: The cognitive-affective personality system. In L. A. Pervin & O. P. John (Eds.), *Handbook of personality* (2nd ed., pp. 197–218). New York: Guilford.

Morf, C. C., & Rhodewalt, F. (2001). Unraveling the paradoxes of narcissism: A dynamic self-regulatory processing model. *Psychological Inquiry, 12,* 177–196.

Nestadt, G., Hsu, F. C., Samuels, J., Bienvenu, O. J., Reti, I., Costa, P. T., Jr., et al. (2006). Latent structure of the *Diagnostic and Statistical Manual of Mental Disorders,* fourth edition, personality disorder criteria. *Comprehensive Psychiatry, 47,* 54–62.

O'Connor, B. (2005). Graphical analysis of personality disorders in Five-factor model space. *European Journal of Personality, 19,* 287–305.

Oltmanns, T. F., Gleason, M. E. J., Konsky, E. D., & Turnkheimer, E. (2005). Meta-perception for pathological personality traits: Do we know when others think that we are difficult? *Consciousness and Cognition: An International Journal, 14,* 739–751.

Perry, J. C. (1988). A prospective study of life stress, defenses, psychotic symptoms, and borderline and antisocial personality disorders and bipolar II type affect. *Journal of Personality Disorders, 2,* 49–51.

Perry, J. C. (2001). A pilot study of defenses in adults with personality disorders entering psychotherapy. *Journal of Nervous and Mental Disease, 189,* 651–660.

Perry, J. C., Hoglend, P., Shear, K., Vaillant, G. E., Horowitz, M., Kardos, M. D., et al. (1998). Field trial of a diagnostic axis for defense mechanisms for *DSM–IV. Journal of Personality Disorders, 12,* 56–68.

Perry, J. D. C., & Perry, J. C. (2004). Conflicts, defenses, and the stability of narcissistic personality features. *Psychiatry: Interpersonal and Biological Processes, 67,* 310–330.

Pervin, L. (1999). *Handbook of personality: Theory and research* (2nd ed.). New York: Guilford.

Riemann, R., Angleitner, A., & Strelau, J. (1997). Genetic and environmental influences on personality: A study of twins reared together using the self- and peer report NEO–FFI scales. *Journal of Personality, 65,* 449–476.

Robins, R. W., & John, O. P. (1997). The quest for self-insight: Theory and research on accuracy and bias in self-perception. In R. Hogan, J. Johnson, & S. Briggs (Eds.), *Handbook of personality psychology* (pp. 649–679). New York: Academic.

Robins, R. W., Norem, J. K., & Cheek, J. M. (1999). Naturalizing the self. In L. A. Pervin & O. P. John (Eds.), *Handbook of personality: Theory and research* (2nd ed., pp. 443–477). New York: Guilford.

Santor, D. A., Bagby, R. M., & Joffe, R. T. (1997). Evaluating stability and change in personality and depression. *Journal of Personality and Social Psychology, 73,* 1354–1362.

Saulsman, L. M., & Page, A. C. (2004). The five-factor model and personality disorder empirical literature: A meta-analytic review. *Clinical Psychology Review, 23,* 1055–1085.

Sedikides, C., & Strube, M. J. (1997). Self-evaluations: To thine own self be good, to thine own self be sure, to thine own self be true, and to thine own self be better. In M. P. Zanna (Ed.), *Advances in experimental social psychology* (Vol. 29, pp. 209–269). New York: Academic.

Shedler, J., & Westen, D. (2004a). Refining personality disorder diagnosis: Integrating science and practice. *American Journal of Psychiatry, 161,* 1350–1365.

Shedler, J., & Westen, D. (2004b). Dimensions of personality pathology: An alternative to the Five-factor model. *American Journal of Psychiatry, 161*, 1743–1754.

Shedler, J., & Westen, D. (2007/this issue). The Shedler–Westen Assessment Procedure (SWAP): Making personality diagnosis clinically meaningful. *Journal of Personality Assessment, 89*, 41–55.

Shoda, Y., Mischel, W., & Wright, J. C. (1994). Intra-individual stability in the organization and patterning of behavior: Incorporating psychological situations into the idiographic analysis of personality. *Journal of Personality and Social Psychology, 56*, 41–53.

Silverstein, M. (2007/this issue). Diagnosis of personality disorders: A case study. *Journal of Personality Assessment, 89*, 82–94.

Soldz, S., Budman, S., Demby, A., & Merry, J. (1995). The relation of defensive style to personality and the big five personality factors. *Journal of Personality Disorders, 9*, 356–370.

Spangler, W. D. (1992). Validity of questionnaire and TAT measures of need for achievement: Two meta-analyses. *Psychological Bulletin, 112*, 140–154.

Stepp, S. D., Trull, T. J., Burr, R. M., Wofenstein, M., & Vieth, A. Z. (2005). Incremental validity of the Structured Interview for the Five-factor model of personality (SIFFM). *European Journal of Personality, 19*, 343–357.

Strack, S., Lorr, M., & Campbell, L. (1990). An evaluation of Millon's circular model of personality disorders. *Journal of Personality Disorders, 4*, 353–361.

Strack, S., & Millon, T. (2007/this issue). Contributions to the dimensional assessment of personality disorders using Millon's model and the Millon Clinical Multiaxial Inventory (MCMI–III). *Journal of Personality Assessment, 89*, 56–69.

Tellegen, A. (1982). *Brief manual for the Differential Personality Questionnaire*. Unpublished manuscript, University of Minnesota, Minneapolis.

Tellegen, A., Lykken, D. T., Bouchard, T. J., Jr., Wilcox, K. J., Segal, N., & Rich, S. (1988). Personality similarity in twins reared apart and together. *Journal of Personality and Social Psychology, 54*, 1031–1039.

Trull, T. J. (2005). Dimensional models of personality disorder: Coverage and cutoffs. *Journal of Personality Disorders, 19*, 262–282.

Trull, T. J., & Widiger, T. A. (1997). *The semi-structured interview for the Five-factor model*. Odessa, FL: Psychological Assessment Resources.

Vaillant, G. (1985). An empirically derived hierarchy of adaptive mechanisms and its usefulness as a potential diagnostic axis. *Acta Psychiatrica Scandinavia, 71*, 171–180.

Vaillant, G. (1992). The beginning of wisdom is never calling a patient borderline: Or The clinical management of immature defenses in the treatment of individuals with personality disorders. *Journal of Psychotherapy Practice & Research, 1*, 117–134.

Vaillant, G. (1994). Ego mechanisms of defense and personality psychopathology. *Journal of Abnormal Psychology, 103*, 44–50.

Velten, E. (1968). A laboratory task for induction of mood states. *Behavior Research and Therapy, 6*, 473–482.

Viglione, D. J. (1999). A review of recent research addressing the utility of the Rorschach. *Psychological Assessment, 11*, 251–265.

Weinberger, D. A. (1998). Defenses, personality structure, and development: Integrating psychodynamic theory into a typological approach to personality. *Journal of Personality, 66*, 1061–1080.

Weinberger, J., & McClelland, D. C. (1990). Cognitive versus traditional motivational models: Irreconcilable or complementary? In R. Sorrentino & E. T. Higgins (Eds.), *Handbook of motivation and cognition* (pp. 562–597). New York: Academic.

Weiner, I. B. (1999). What the Rorschach can do for you: Incremental validity in clinical applications. *Assessment, 6*, 327–339.

Weiner, I. B. (2003). *Principles of Rorschach Interpretation* (2nd ed.). Mahwah, NJ: Lawrence Erlbaum Associates.

Weiner, I. B. (2005). Integrative personality assessment with self-report and performance-based measures. In S. Strack (Ed.), *Handbook of personology and psychopathology* (pp. 317–331). New York: Wiley.

Westen, D. (1997). Divergences between clinical and research methods for assessing personality disorders: Implications for research and the evolution of Axis II. *American Journal of Psychiatry, 154*, 895–903.

Westen, D., Gabbard, G. O., & Blagov, P. (2006). Back to the future: Personality structure as a context for psychopathology. In R. F. Krueger & J. L. Tackett (Eds.), *Personality and psychopathology: Building bridges* (pp. 335–384). New York: Guilford.

Westen, D., & Shedler, J. (1999a). Revising and assessing Axis II, Part I: Developing a clinically and empirically valid assessment method. *American Journal of Psychiatry, 156*, 258–272.

Westen, D., & Shedler, J. (1999b). Revising and assessing Axis II, Part II: Toward an empirically based and clinically useful classification of personality disorders. *American Journal of Psychiatry, 156*, 273–285.

Widiger, T. A., & Clark, L. A. (2000). Toward *DSM–V* and the classification of psychopathology. *Psychological Bulletin, 126*, 946–963.

Widiger, T. A., & Lowe, J. A. (2007/this issue). Five-factor model assessment of personality disorder. *Journal of Personality Assessment, 89*, 16–29.

Widiger, T. A., Mangine, S., Corbitt, E. M., Ellis, C. G., & Thomas, G. V. (1995). *Personality disorder interview–IV*. Odessa, FL: Psychological Assessment Resources.

Widiger, T. A., & Samuel, D. B. (2005). Diagnostic categories or dimensions? A question for the *Diagnostic and Statistical Manual of Mental Disorders—Fifth Edition*. *Journal of Abnormal Psychology, 114*, 494–504.

Widiger, T. A., & Sanderson, C. J. (1995). Toward a dimensional model of personality disorders. In W. J. Livesley (Ed.), *The DSM–IV personality disorders* (pp. 433–458). New York: Guilford.

Widiger, T. A., & Simonsen, E. (2005). Introduction to the special section: The American Psychiatric Association's research agenda for the *DSM–V*. *Journal of Personality Disorders, 19*, 103–109.

Widiger, T. A., Simonsen, E., Krueger, R., Livesley, W. J., & Verheul, R. (2005). Personality disorder research agenda for the *DSM–V*. *Journal of Personality Disorders, 19*, 315–338.

Widiger, T. A., Trull, T. J., Clarkin, J. F., Sanderson, C., & Costa, P. T., Jr. (2002). A description of the *DSM–IV* personality disorders with the Five-factor model of personality. In P. T. Costa, Jr. & T. A. Widiger (Eds.), *Personality disorders and the Five factor model of personality* (pp. 89–102). Washington, DC: American Psychiatric Press.

Wiggins, J. S., & Pincus, A. L. (1994). Personality structure and the structure of personality disorders. In P. T. Costa, Jr. & T. A. Widiger (Eds.), *Personality disorders and the Five-factor model of personality* (pp. 73–93). Washington, DC: American Psychiatric Press.

World Health Organization. (1994). *International classification of diseases* (10th ed.) Author.

Zanarini, M. C., Frankenburg, F. R., Chauncey, D. L., & Gunderson, J. G. (1987). The Diagnostic Interview for Personality Disorders: Interrater and test-retest reliability. *Comprehensive Psychiatry, 28*, 467–480.

Zimmerman, M. (1994). Diagnosing personality disorders: A review of issues and research methods. *Archives of General Psychiatry, 51*, 225–245.

Zuroff, D. C., & Mongrain, M. (1987). Dependency and self-criticism: Vulnerability factors for depressive affective states. *Journal of Abnormal Psychology, 96*, 14–22.

Steven K. Huprich
Department of Psychology
Eastern Michigan University
537 Mark Jefferson Buildin
Ypsilianti, MI 48197
Email: shuprich@emich.edu

Received February 3, 2006
Revised Revised January 5, 2007

Assessing Normal and Abnormal Personality Functioning: Strengths and Weaknesses of Self-Report, Observer, and Performance-Based Methods

Ronald J. Ganellen

Department of Psychiatry and Behavioral Sciences
Northwestern University Medical School

Assessing personality characteristics; distinguishing the boundaries between normal and abnormal functioning; identifying impairment in the domains of work, interpersonal relationships, and emotional state due to maladaptive personality traits; and translating these findings into effective, appropriate treatment interventions is a complicated endeavor. Valid, reliable conclusions about an individual's personality functioning and adjustment cannot be reached unless one has accurate information about that person's patterns of behavior, cognitions, emotions, and interpersonal relationships. I discuss strengths and weaknesses of assessment approaches utilizing explicit assessment methods, such as self-report measures and clinical interviews; information obtained from knowledgeable observers; and performance-based, implicit assessment methods such as the Rorschach Comprehensive System (Exner, 2003). In contrast to explicit methods of assessment, implicit methods can provide salient information about a personality construct whether or not individuals have accurately conceptualized that construct, have weighed how the construct describes them, are self-aware, and are willing to openly provide information relevant to that construct. I propose that the accuracy of conclusions about an individual's personality style, problems in adjustment, and treatment needs may be improved if conclusion are based on a multimethod assessment approach that incorporates information gathered using explicit assessment methods, information provided by significant others, and data from performance-based or implicit measures of personality.

Dear Dr. Psychologist,

I am referring Mr. N to you for an evaluation. Mr. N was referred for psychotherapy by his internist who thought the physical symptoms he reported were hard to pin down and were likely secondary to anxiety and stress caused by friction with his wife. After meeting with him twice I am puzzled how to conceptualize his situation and dynamics and am unsure how to be most helpful to him.

Mr. N initially impressed me as a very bright, articulate man. I was taken aback when he rather quickly became visibly flushed and angry while describing a recent, upsetting interaction with his wife and then quite suddenly became tearful. There were similar abrupt shifts in his emotional state both times we met.

When I asked whether he had talked with his wife about their problems, Mr. N replied that he felt talking to her is

pointless as, in his view, she blames him for everything that goes wrong, attacks him for making her unhappy, and holds grudges. He then proceeded to give a very detailed account of ways in which he feels she has let him down as a partner. His tone of voice while providing this account was rather dramatic and his voice dripped with sarcasm and bitterness. Although certain his wife knows how he feels, Mr. N thinks talking to his wife will only make things worse. The only way he can imagine things will get better is for him and his wife to separate when their youngest child, a freshman in high school, moves out of the house to go to college.

Although I anticipated treating Mr. N for anxiety based on the information provided by his physician, I am concerned about his level of depression and personality functioning. Frankly, I'm puzzled how to conceptualize Mr. N's presentation. I've considered the possibility of histrionic features given his emotional intensity, narcissistic dynamics given the sensitivity to criticism he described, as well as passive–aggressive characteristics given his reluctance to address problems and indirect manner of expressing anger. I'd appreciate a consultation.

This brief clinical vignette provides an example of the complexities clinicians face in understanding the interplay among their patients' presenting problems, relationship difficulties, personality characteristics, and emotional reactions. It can be particularly challenging to get a handle on whether the problems an individual experiences are due to significant maladaptive personality traits associated with a personality disorder (PD) based on observation and the information obtained during a clinical interview and psychotherapy sessions. This can occur for a variety of reasons including the possibility that mood states may influence or distort what individuals report about themselves and how they appear. For instance, someone who is depressed may appear dependent, passive, withdrawn, self-conscious, and vulnerable (Barnett & Gotlib, 1988), whereas someone who is angry may appear forceful, agitated, demanding, mistrustful, and unwilling to listen to what others have to say. This may be one reason why the psychologist meeting with Mr. N was uncertain what to make of Mr. N's passivity and withdrawal; these behaviors could be attributed to longstanding personality characteristics or to his current mood. Furthermore, determining whether Mr. N's description of his wife as a critical, demeaning malcontent was accurate or was a function of a persisting sensitivity to feeling criticized and misunderstood may also be difficult.

A number of theoretical models and assessment methods are available to clinicians and researchers to identify maladaptive personality traits and diagnose PDs. Although there is wide recognition that maladaptive personality traits are clinically and theoretically important, there is considerable controversy within the field concerning how best to conceptualize and assess these characteristics (Widiger, Simonsen, Krueger, Livesley, & Verheul, 2005). Controversy exists, for instance, as to whether PDs should be viewed in categorical or dimensional terms; the boundaries between personality and other mental disorders such as depression and anxiety; and whether characteristics and symptoms of PDs fall on a continuum ranging from normal to abnormal variants of personality functioning as opposed to being separate and distinct phenomena (Livesley, 2003; Widiger & Simonsen, 2005).

In terms of assessment of PDs, differences of opinion exist as to which methods should be used to assess relevant characteristics. Some approaches advocate obtaining information from a patient, which may be supplemented by observations, and information provided by a person who is familiar with patient, such as a partner or family member. Others advocate administration of semistructured clinical interviews, such as the Personality Disorder Examination (Loranger, 1988) or the Structured Clinical Interview for *DSM* (3rd ed., rev.; American Psychological Association, 1987) (First, Spitzer, Gibbon, & Williams, 1995); self-report inventories, such as the Minnesota Multiphasic Personality Disorder–2

(MMPI–2; Butcher, Dahlstrom, Graham, Tellegen, & Kaemmer, 1989) or Millon Clinical Multiaxial Inventory–III (Millon, 1994); and methods of integrating information obtained from multiple sources including clinical observation over time, patient self-report, and interviews with a close friend, romantic partner, or family member such as the Longitudinal Expert and All Data method (Spitzer, 1983). Furthermore, assuming that relevant personality characteristics can be assessed reliably, some writers have questioned how information concerning personality traits and PDs impacts on clinical decision making and contributes to developing effective treatment interventions that are tailored to an individual patient's needs (Verheul, 2005).

A number of researchers have concluded that the level of agreement among different approaches to diagnosing PDs is moderate to low (Zimmerman, 1994). For instance, studies that have examined convergent validity across self-report inventories and semistructured interviews have reported moderately strong associations, at best, or inconsistent agreement, at worst (Renneberg, Chambless, Dowdall, & Fauerbach, 1992). This conclusion is illustrated by a recent meta-analysis conducted by Widiger and Coker (2002). They examined agreement between self-report and semistructured interviews ratings of specific PDs and found the following median convergent validity coefficient values: .30 for paranoid PD; .37 for schizoid PD; .33 for antisocial PD; .51 for borderline PD; .29 for histrionic PD; .29 for narcissistic PD; .51 for avoidant PD; .39 for dependent PD; and .12 for obsessive–compulsive PD (Widiger & Coker, 2002).

Research has also shown that rates of agreement between patient and informant reports are typically low (Bernstein et al., 1997; Ferro & Klein, 1997; Klonsky, Oltmanns, & Turkheimer, 2002; Riso, Klein, Anderson, Ouimette, & Lizardi, 1994; Zimmerman, 1994; Zimmerman, Pfohl, Coryell, Stangl, & Corenthal, 1988). After reviewing the literature, Klonsky et al. (2002) characterized the agreement between self-ratings and informant ratings of features of PD as "modest at best" (p. 300), with values ranging from .18 to .80 and a median value of .36. Low levels of agreement have been found not only when different sources of information, such as patients and knowledgeable informants, are asked to rate the presence or absence of specific PDs but also, on a more general level, when asked simply whether or not a PD exists (Dreessen, Hildebrand, & Arntz, 1998; Riso et al., 1994; Zimmerman et al., 1988). Ready and Clark (2002) concluded that studies have "routinely found poor agreement for categorical PD diagnoses and moderate agreement for dimensional measures of PD criteria" (p. 40).

Different explanations have been offered to account for these disappointing findings. In addition to theoretical and methodological critiques concerning the validity and limitations of current approaches to classifying PDs, such as those made by proponents of a dimensional as opposed to categorical model of PDs (Costa & Widiger, 2002; Widiger & Simonsen, 2005), important questions have been raised about the strengths and weaknesses of different methodologies used to assess adaptive and maladaptive features of personality functioning. One aim of this article is to consider the advantages and disadvantages of assessment approaches that rely solely on explicit assessment methods including clinical interviews of patients and knowledgeable informants, semistructured interviews, and self-report methods. In the remainder of this article, I contrast explicit and implicit methods of psychological assessment and attempt to demonstrate that assessment approaches utilizing implicit or performance-based measures of personality and psychological functioning, such as the Rorschach Comprehensive System (CS; Exner, 2003), can make important contributions to assessment of personality functioning and treatment planning that complements the information that can be obtained from assessment relying on explicit methods. Although in a considerable part of this article, I discuss weakness and limitations in the use of explicit approaches, it is not my intent to claim that one method is superior to the other. One reason for outlining these potential limitations is that, in my opinion, the literature concerning assessment of personality functioning in recent years has focused to a great extent on the development, validation, and application of self-report instruments and interview methods developed specifically to diagnose PDs or measure different dimensions of personality, with little attention paid to the contribution implicit approaches may make. Although these efforts have resulted in significant progress in a number of respects, given the complexities of assessment of personality characteristics, it is my hope that discussion of the issues I present following will stimulate researchers and clinicians to consider the possibility that, at least in some cases, a more complete, refined understanding of adaptive and maladaptive personality functioning may be reached by integrating information obtained using both explicit and performance-based assessment approaches.

I acknowledge from the outset that unlike some methods developed specifically to diagnose *DSM* (4th ed., [*DSM–IV*]; American Psychiatric Association, 1994) PDs or to assess different dimensions of personality functioning, the information derived from the CS does not link directly to each criteria required by the *DSM–IV* to diagnose a PD nor to each factor defined by dimensional models of personality. Furthermore, a number of features of *DSM–IV* Axis II disorders and some facets of dimensional models of personality functioning may not be measured at all by the CS. For instance, no CS variables directly assesses whether an individual is unable to discard useless or worthless items that have no sentimental value, a characteristic of an obsessive–compulsive PD, and no CS variables directly identify the personality dimension of positive emotionality that is related to being outgoing, sociable, and active (Clark & Watson, 1999).

As I discuss following, however, CS variables can identify and describe many of the enduring patterns of inner experience, interpersonal dysfunction, and behaviors asso-

ciated with some but not all of the *DSM–IV* PD diagnostic criteria. These include characteristic ways of perceiving oneself and others; interpreting events in an accurate as opposed to a distorted manner; effectiveness in managing emotional responses and affective intensity; capacity to relate to other people in an appropriate, prosocial manner; and exerting control over one's impulses. Similarly, a number of CS variables are conceptually related to the features of the domains of personality defined in dimensional models. For instance, dimensional models identify a domain of aggressive or antagonistic interpersonal relatedness that may be captured by CS variables revealing mistrustful, suspicious attitudes and a tendency to react to others with resentment, hostility, and antagonism. Stated differently, I take the position that CS variables provide useful information about many of the theoretical constructs underlying both categorical and dimensional models of PDs.

I am not claiming that a diagnosis of a PD or an assessment of all domains of personality functioning can or should be made on the basis of the CS alone. However, I hope to demonstrate that in combination with information that may be obtained from interviews, self-report, other report, and clinician–therapist interactions, Rorschach data can make a meaningful contribution to the complex process of determining first, whether an individual exhibits enduring, maladaptive personality characteristics that hinder effective functioning or cause significant subjective distress, information necessary to reach a determination as to the presence or absence of a PD; and second, to using this formulation to improve clinical decision making. Even though there may not be a direct, one-to-one correspondence between *DSM–IV* criteria and Rorschach variables, I argue following that information provided by the CS (a) complements the information obtained from other sources when a diagnosis of a PD is being investigated; (b) can, in some instances, supply data other sources do not provide; and (c) can be useful in developing and tailoring treatment interventions for individual patients.

Some authors have questioned the empirical basis of the CS and its clinical utility (cf. Hunsely & Bailey, 2001). These concerns appear to be unwarranted, however, as the results of several meta-analyses (e.g., Hiller, Rosenthal, Bornstein, Berry, & Brunell-Neuleib, 1999; Meyer & Archer, 2001) have shown that the construct validity of the Rorschach is equivalent to that of the MMPI (Hathaway & McKinley, 1943) and Wechsler Adult Intelligence Scale (Wechsler, 1955). The debate concerning use of the Rorschach and its clinical utility underscores the importance of using CS variables that are both theoretically relevant to the domain of personality functioning being measured and that have adequate empirical support. As Meyer and Archer (2001) succinctly stated, the results of the meta-analysis they conducted showed that "Rorschach scales can provide valid information. Like all tests, the Rorschach is more valid for some purposes than others" (p. 499).

IMPLICIT VERSUS EXPLICIT PERSONALITY ASSESSMENT

Writers have distinguished among different approaches to psychological assessment. These include unstructured clinical interviews, structured clinical interviews; self-report instruments, observer rating scales, and performance-based personality tests (Meyer et al., 2001. Unstructured clinical interviews, for instance, elicit an individual's account of their functioning, concerns, and thematic life narratives, whereas structured clinical interviews and self-report instruments elicit information about the problems and symptoms an individual experiences overtly and the individual's conscious understanding of themselves. In contrast, performance-based measures of personality, such as the CS or Thematic Apperception Test (Murray, 1943), elicit information about personality characteristics, cognitive functioning, and interpersonal dynamics using relatively unstructured tasks that tap into an individual's templates of perception, cognition, and representations of self and others. Each of these methods of information gathering has their strengths and weaknesses. As I discuss in more detail following, methods that rely on information provided directly by an individual, such as data obtained during a clinical interview or self-report inventory, may accurately show what individuals know about themselves but may be limited by the individual's willingness to communicate openly and frankly and to describe themselves in unfavorable terms; their ability to make accurate judgments about themselves; and their insight into their emotional world, patterns of thinking, interpersonal style, or behavior. Information obtained by observers, such as family members or romantic partners, during an interview or from an observer-rating scale may be limited by what the observer knows about the person being rated as well as by the dynamics of the relationship between the observer and the person being rated.

Performance-based measures of personality, in contrast, may not provide specific details about an individual's history or specific symptoms but can provide meaningful, valid, and clinically relevant information about normal and abnormal personality characteristics, patterns of thinking, regulation of affect, and interpersonal functioning that may parallel or complement information obtained from other sources (Ganellen, 1996, 2006). This occurs because performance-based measures, such as the CS, use a different method of gathering information than interview, self-report, or observer ratings. McClelland, Koestner, and Weinberger (1989) distinguished between two broad approaches to personality assessment, those that use explicit measures, such as self-report instruments or clinical interviews, and those that use implicit measures, such as performance-based measures. McClelland et al. (1989) argued that explicit measures assess an individual's self-attributed motives and information accessible to conscious introspection, whereas implicit measures assess an individual's automatic, unconscious patterns of behav-

ior, perception, motivation, and cognition. Stated differently, without requiring an individual to verbalize or describe aspects of their psychological functioning, data derived using implicit assessment methods provide information about patterns of thinking, reacting, and behaving that individuals may not recognize as being characteristic of them or may not be able to consciously articulate.

Given these differences, McClelland et al. (1989) concluded that in contrast to explicit methods of personality assessment, implicit measures of personality functioning are less subject to being filtered or consciously controlled and are therefore less susceptible to self-presentational biases than explicit measures. As a result, performance-based measures may yield information relevant to personality characteristics that are not consciously accessible to a patient when responding to questions asked during an interview or when completing a self-report measure. For instance, a man may readily acknowledge that he is troubled by symptoms of depression during a clinical interview and obtain elevated scores on self-report measures of depression but may not be able to articulate the relationship between these emotional reactions and his need to obtain affirmation, admiration, and recognition, characteristics that may be identified on the CS by an elevated number of reflection responses (Exner, 2003). This finding should alert the clinician to the role that narcissistic dynamics play in this man's life as well as his involvement in the treatment process.

The literature on interpersonal dependence needs provides a number of well-documented examples of the distinction between implicit and explicit methods of personality assessment and illustrates how performance-based methods can provide meaningful information about real-world behaviors that may not be apparent using self-report methods. Furthermore, consistent with McClelland et al.'s (1989) position, this literature also provides evidence that implicit or performance-based assessment approaches may not be as susceptible to self-report bias as explicit approaches. I summarize in the following several such studies, which used the Rorschach Oral Dependency Scale (ROD; Masling, Rabie, & Blondheim, 1967) and the Interpersonal Dependency Inventory (IDI; Hirschfeld et al., 1977). The ROD is a well-validated, widely used, reliable implicit measure of interpersonal dependency (Bornstein, 1996), whereas the IDI is a well-validated, widely used, reliable explicit measure of dependence.

Bornstein (2002) reviewed studies on the relationship between the ROD and IDI and concluded first, that these two measures are modestly correlated (mean $r = .29$) and second, that consistent with predictions based on theoretical distinctions between explicit and implicit dependence needs, each measure is associated with different aspects of interpersonal dependency. For example, Bornstein (1998) evaluated the implicit–explicit distinction in a study examining help-seeking behavior during an experimental session. In this study, participants with different dependency needs were assigned to different experimental conditions. Based on scores on the ROD and IDI, Bornstein (1998) identified the following four groups: a low dependency (LD) group defined by low scores on both the IDI and ROD; a high dependency (HD) group, defined by high scores on both the IDI and ROD; an unacknowledged dependency (UAD) group, defined by high score on the ROD and low score on the IDI; and a dependent self-presentation (DSP) group, defined by high score on the IDI and low score on the ROD. Participants in each group were assigned to one of two experimental conditions. In one condition, participants were told that the purpose of the study was to observe problem-solving skills, whereas in the other condition, participants were told that the purpose of the study was to observe dependency and help-seeking behaviors. These instructions made help-seeking behavior explicit in the second as opposed to the first experimental condition.

Bornstein (1998) predicted that participants in the four groups would produce different levels of *help-seeking behavior,* defined as the number of times a participant asked for help or guidance, in the two experimental conditions. Consistent with predictions, Bornstein (1998) found an interaction between study instructions and dependency group status. Specifically, participants in the UAD group engaged in help-seeking at rates similar to the HD group when told that problem-solving was being studied but engaged in low rates of help-seeking behavior when told that help-seeking behavior was being studied. In fact, ratings of help-seeking behavior did not significantly differ between the UAD and LD group in the latter condition. In contrast, participants in the DSP group engaged in moderate amounts of help seeking when they believed they were in a problem-solving task but engaged in help-seeking behavior at a rate similar to the HD group when told that help-seeking behavior was being studied in the second condition. Thus, as predicted, individuals who consciously described themselves as having high or low dependency needs objectively acted differently when the salience of dependent behavior was experimentally manipulated.

Bornstein, Rossner, Hill, and Stepanian (1994) conducted three studies examining whether scores on the IDI and ROD were affected by experimental conditions in which dependence was described in either positive or negative terms. Findings from these studies consistently showed that scores on explicit but not implicit measures of dependency were affected by experimental manipulations. As predicted, when dependency was presented as being a positive characteristic, IDI ratings of dependency increased, and when dependency was presented as a negative characteristic, IDI ratings of dependency decreased. In contrast, ROD scores were not influenced by experimentally manipulated evaluative sets. Bornstein et al. (1994) concluded that although self-reported dependency scores are affected by conscious self-monitoring of reported dependency, implicit measures of dependency are not. This suggests that whereas self-report

measures of dependency can be deliberately skewed by self-presentational pressures, implicit measures of dependency, such as the ROD, are less susceptible to impression management strategies. One implication of these findings for assessment of adaptive and maladaptive personality traits is that reliable, accurate information about some personality characteristics, such as dependency, may be obtained using an implicit or performance-based approach even though an individual may be consciously reluctant to provide accurate information when those characteristics are assessed used a direct, explicit assessment method.

SELF-REPORT METHODS

According to the *DSM–IV* (text revision; American Psychological Association, 2001), a PD is diagnosed if an individual has "an enduring pattern of inner experience and behavior that deviates markedly from the expectations of the individual's culture" (p. 603). These problematic reactions can be manifested in terms of inappropriate or distorted ways of viewing oneself or others, difficulties in managing emotional responses, difficulties in establishing and maintaining mutually satisfying interpersonal relationships, or behavior demonstrating problems with impulse control (Criterion A). Not only must the clinician identify persisting patterns of cognition, affect, interpersonal functioning, and impulse control, but the patterns have to be determined to be inflexible and pervasive across a broad range of personal and social situations (Criterion B) and to lead to "clinically significant distress in impairment in social, occupational, or other important areas of functioning" (Criterion C).

Reading these criteria suggests some reasons individuals may have difficulty describing themselves accurately when responding to questions or probes concerning characteristics associated with PDs during a clinical interview, semistructured interview, or self-report inventory. One reason is that for many people, the concepts and terminology contained in the *DSM–IV* may be unfamiliar, abstract, or hard to conceptualize. If an individual is not familiar with or does not understand the general guidelines used to identify PDs or the specific criteria required to diagnose specific *DSM–IV* PDs, they may understandably have trouble providing accurate, reliable information. For example, unless a person grasps what impressionistic speech is, a feature of histrionic PD, it may be difficult for that person to rate whether his or her speech is overly vague, imprecise, and lacking in detail. Perhaps for this reason, many explicit assessment methods do not assess impressionistic speech with a direct probe (e.g., "Is your speech excessively impressionistic?") but instead make judgments about this construct based on samples of behaviors exhibited during a semistructured interview. For instance, the Personality Disorder Interview–IV (Widiger, Mangine, Corbitt, Ellis, & Thomas, 1995) rates this item based on observations of the person's speech during the interview or when responding to probes such as asking for a description of another person. Note that rating of this construct is not based on self-description, an explicit approach that requires familiarity with this dimension, but instead on a sample of behavior, a performance-based approach incorporated into a semistructured interview. As discussed previously, implicit measures similarly obtain samples of behavior that can be rated for certain personality characteristics independent of an individual's familiarity with that construct.

The impact of the abstract nature of diagnostic criteria and the degree to which individuals are familiar with these concepts may be mitigated if interview or test items are clearly written in everyday language and are anchored by easily understood examples. Assuming an individual has a sound conceptual understanding of the characteristics being probed, neither the *DSM–IV* criteria nor most dimensional models of personality functioning provide any clear guidelines to gauge whether the individual's patterns of thinking, feeling, and acting conform to or deviate from cultural norms and expectations. In other words, neither approach provides explicit, agreed-on points of demarcation between normal and abnormal personality functioning (Widiger et al., 2005). For instance, an individual may report viewing people with suspicious mistrust and a wary expectation others will try to take advantage of him. This description may be quite accurate. There clearly is considerable room for judgment, however, in determining whether these attitudes and expectations are deviant, as required for a diagnosis of a paranoid PD, as opposed to reflecting a cynical perspective of human nature and how the world operates. Similarly, the demarcation between a robust sense of self-confidence and an inflated view of one's importance, a feature of a narcissistic PD, is not well defined in the *DSM–IV.*

Note that these brief examples concerning suspicious mistrust and impressionistic speech do not involve the issue of insight, an issue that I discuss following. Instead, I presented these examples to illustrate the following general point: There is considerable room for interpretation when an individual is asked to make a judgment as to whether a pattern of thinking, behaving, or reacting is normal or abnormal and whether that pattern causes either significant distress or difficulties in functioning.

Assuming that individuals understand both the terms and concepts involved when responding during a clinical interview or when taking a self-report inventory as well as the guidelines to distinguish when a pattern of thinking, emotional reactions, and behavior is persistent and maladaptive, accurate self-reports depend on truthful and realistic responding. Patients' accounts of their functioning may be skewed consciously or unconsciously in ways that render self-report untrustworthy or unreliable. Individuals may consciously and deliberately misrepresent their history for a variety of reasons. For instance, Widiger et al. (1995) observed that some individuals with an antisocial PD (ASPD) intentionally attempt to mislead and deceive clinicians "simply for their own amusement and pleasure" (p. 21).

It is also possible that some individuals will deny some maladaptive personality characteristics or features of a PD not because it is not true but because they are aware that admitting to that characteristic would involve making an unflattering statement about themselves. For instance, how many people are likely to describe themselves as someone who expresses emotions in a shallow manner, one of the criteria used to diagnose a histrionic PD? Similarly, most people would likely be reluctant to say they have little empathy for others, a feature of ASPD, even if they knew this was true of them because this description is uncomplimentary. This is one reason that most self-report and semistructured interviews do not use single questions to specifically address these and other characteristics but in addition to asking questions that are phrased more tactfully, rely on observations made by an interviewer during an interview. As noted previously, obtaining and then rating a sample of behavior during a semistructured interview is a form of performance-based assessment as opposed to a purely explicit assessment approach. This underscores the general point that conclusions about personality functioning may be more complete and accurate if based on information integrating both explicit and implicit methods rather than relying exclusively on one or the other.

Individuals may give biased descriptions of their functioning that are not as blatant or deliberate as the examples provided previously. Some individuals may sincerely attempt to describe themselves accurately but give incomplete or inaccurate information because of unconscious defenses or impression management strategies that limit their awareness of how others are affected by their behavior. For instance, a male individual who frequently spends most of his waking hours engaged in work-related tasks may perceive himself as a conscientious, responsible, productive employee without recognizing that his behavior interferes with developing close bonds with others. Even if he feels he is not as involved with others as he would wants to be, this person is not likely to rate himself as being excessively devoted to work; to the contrary, he may consider his self-discipline as worthy of praise and be troubled that his behavior does not elicit the approval he anticipates. In this example, the individual does not recognize the impact obsessive–compulsive characteristics have; stated differently, he does not appreciate the toll his choices, priorities, and actions take on interpersonal relationships. A similar lack of insight may cause individuals who are suspicious or mistrustful to deny reading too much into benign remarks or events not because this description is inaccurate but because there is no doubt in their minds that words, behaviors, and events are anything but benign. Thus, persistent, maladaptive patterns of thinking, feeling, and behaving characteristic of a PD may contribute to psychological blind spots or a lack of self-awareness that leads an individual to deny having maladaptive personality traits that are obvious to others.

The previous discussion identifies reasons why, in some cases, relying on self-report methods alone may not produce accurate or complete information concerning maladaptive personality characteristics and may have limited utility in distinguishing between normal and abnormal variants of a dimension of personality functioning. In addition to deliberately providing inaccurate information, some individuals may be unaware they exhibit certain characteristics, may not realize the consequences of their customary ways of structuring their lives, or may not want to acknowledge traits or behaviors they consider unflattering or socially undesirable. Moreover, findings from self-report approaches may be skewed if individuals are unfamiliar with or do not understand the concepts and terms being investigated. Given the possibility that information obtained using explicit methods of personality functioning may be limited, incomplete, self-serving, or inaccurate, it seems reasonable to consider the possibility that information from other sources, such as information provided by others or results from performance-based methods, could make assessment of personality functioning and diagnosis of PDs more valid and reliable. As discussed previously, although degree of self-awareness and self-presentational concerns can bias responses on self-report inventories, this is less likely to be a concern for findings obtained using implicit measures of certain dimensions of personality functioning (Bornstein et al., 1994).

For example, one characteristic that can be difficult to assess is the tendency to react to situations with considerable emotional intensity, a characteristic associated with a histrionic personality style. Widiger et al. (1995) pointed out some challenges in assessing this trait including the possibility that some persons will describe their lives in an overly exaggerated manner when they are in the midst of an emotional crisis but not at other times and "because the threshold for what is exaggerated or excessive (expression of emotions) is unclear" (p. 129). Information provided by a performance-based assessment approach may be helpful when considering these issues. One CS variable relevant to this aspect of psychological functioning is the FC:CF + C ratio; significant associations between skewed scores on this ratio and ratings of histrionic personality features have been reported (Blais, Hilsenroth, Castlebury, Fowler, & Baity, 2001). A tendency for an individual to have strong, unrestrained emotional reactions may be identified if he or she produces a skewed score on this ratio, even if that individual does not see himself or herself as having this characteristic. This brief example is presented not to "prove" that implicit assessment methods are superior to explicit methods but instead to illustrate how integrating these methods may result in learning about aspects of adaptive and maladaptive personality functioning that could not be reached relying on one approach alone.

INFORMANT RATINGS

As noted previously, ratings of personality characteristics made by patients about themselves and ratings of them made by others who know them well often do not match well (Klonsky et al., 2002; Zimmerman, 1994). Similarly, Meyer et al. (2000) summarized a number of studies and meta-analytic reviews examining convergence between information provided by an individual about himself or herself and information provided by a wide range of informants, such as peers, family members, spouses, teachers, and clinicians. Meyer et al. (2000) found "relatively low to moderate associations between independent methods of assessing similar constructs" (p. 145) in both child and adult populations in diverse settings. Based on these findings, Meyer et al. concluded

> First, at best, any single assessment method provides a partial or incomplete representation of the characteristics it intends to measure. Second, in the world of applied clinical practice, it is not easy to obtain accurate or consensually agreed on information about patients. (p. 145)

Zimmerman, Pfohl, Stangl, and Corenthal (1986) illustrated how differences in information provided by individuals about themselves and others can have a marked impact in clinical practice. Zimmerman et al. (1986) reported that they initially made a diagnosis concerning the presence and type of PD based on information provided by the patient. However, Zimmerman et al. (1986) changed the initial diagnosis in 20% of their cases after they obtained additional information from an informant. The change in diagnosis usually occurred because the informant provided information concerning pathology not reported by the patient.

Even in nonclinical populations, the correlation between self-report ratings and ratings made by knowledgeable others is relatively modest, ranging from .30 to .55 (Ready & Clark, 2002). Modest levels of self-observer agreement have been found consistently regardless of the assessment method employed (i.e., questionnaire as opposed to structured interview), sample characteristics (clinical vs. nonclinical), and relationship between the person being rated and the informant (e.g., family member vs. teacher). Ready and Clark (2002) observed that self-informant ratings are generally highest for personality traits that involve easily observed behaviors and lowest for characteristics involving internal processes or subjective experiences that are not as readily accessible such as characteristic patterns of thinking and emotional reactions.

Although the relatively modest levels of agreement between self-ratings and informant ratings may be seen as a function of the biases and inaccuracies in self-report discussed previously, this does not explain the well-documented finding that there is frequently substantial disagreement among ratings of an individual provided by different informants. For instance, ratings of a child made by different adults (e.g., parents as opposed to teachers, mothers as opposed to fathers) more often disagree than agree (Achenbach, McConaughy, & Howell, 1987; Meyer et al., 2001; Zucker, Morris, Ingram, Morris, & Bakeman, 2002). These studies have repeatedly shown that different informants provide nonoverlapping and possibly contradictory information about the same individual. There have been a number of reasons offered to explain disagreements between different raters including the possibility that one informant simply may know the individual being rated better than the other. Along this vein, in the Child Behavior Checklist literature (CBCL; Achenbach, 1991), some authors have suggested that mothers' ratings of their children may be more valid than ratings made by fathers, as in general, mothers spend more time with their children than fathers (Fitzgerald, Zucker, Maguin, & Reider, 1994). This is an important consideration when assessing whether an individual should be diagnosed with a PD; one might naturally put more stock in ratings made by the person most familiar with that individual, particularly when discrepant reports are obtained from different informants.

Another explanation has been offered to explain the discrepancies frequently found between ratings of children made by their mothers and fathers: Fathers may be more tolerant of certain behaviors, such as roughhousing or play fighting, than mothers, whereas mothers may be more tolerant than fathers of other behaviors such as a daughter's moodiness. Stated in more general terms, disagreements in ratings made by different informants may occur not because observers disagree as to whether the person exhibits a pattern of behavior but because of differences in observers' tolerance for a personality characteristic and evaluation as to whether the characteristic is adaptive or maladaptive. This may be seen in reactions to behaviors typical of a histrionic PD; although some people may enjoy spending time with a person they see as being lively, spontaneous, and emotionally expressive, others may react with irritation if they view the person as being attention seeking and expressing emotions in an overly dramatic but shallow manner.

Other, more complex explanations for disagreements between raters exists. One might argue that it is natural for different people to have divergent views of the same individual because people do not have the same type of relationship with everyone in their lives. Rather, individuals develop unique relationships with others that are shaped by the give and take that occurs between people over time and that are colored by each person's needs, expectations, and behaviors. Thus, for instance, one would not expect a man to act the same with his boss as he does with his poker buddies. Because different relationships elicit different reactions and behaviors, it is natural that certain problematic patterns of thinking, reacting, and social behavior may be more readily observed by some people than others, not because one person knows the person better than the other but as a function of the dynamics of a specific dyadic relationship.

Research that has examined the low levels of agreement between parents' ratings of their own child has also suggested that disagreements between parents occur frequently when one parent exhibits signs of a psychological disorder (Achenbach et al., 1987). Depression, for instance, may influence how parents evaluate their children's behavior and how tolerant they are of their child's strengths and weaknesses. In addition, some researchers have observed that informants' ratings of personality characteristics are correlated with characteristics of any PD exhibited by that observer (Zimmerman, 1993). Widiger et al. (1995) commented that although "narcissistic persons may devalue the subject, a borderline informant may idealize the subject" (p. 32). More generally, these observations suggest that because information provided by knowledgeable informants may be colored by the observers' personal dynamics, not all informants are able to provide a balanced, objective account of another person's strengths and weaknesses. For example, a dependent woman may excuse or justify her partner's sexual infidelities and financial irresponsibility if she is motivated by a fear of abandonment, whereas a very different description may be provided by the man's sister who is fed up with the impact his selfish behavior has had on their family. This brief vignette illustrates the general point that the data given by any informant about another person is likely to represent a mixture of objective facts and subjective interpretation of those facts that has been shaped by the dynamics of the relationship between the observer and the person being rated.

IMPLICATIONS FOR ASSESSMENT OF ADAPTIVE AND MALADAPTIVE PERSONALITY FUNCTIONING

The issues I discussed previously have a number of important implications for the assessment of personality style and diagnosis of PDs and for treatment planning. Obviously, valid, reliable conclusions about an individual's personality characteristics, interpersonal functioning, and adjustment cannot be reached unless one has accurate information about that person's patterns of behavior, cognitions, emotions, and interpersonal relationships. Ready and Clark (2002) convincingly argued that accurate assessment is critical for "planning effective intervention, developing realistic expectations for change, and creating opportunities for increased self-awareness" (p. 46). Given the issues discussed previously, one should expect to find that although some individuals may provide accurate information about their personality traits, others may provide inaccurate, biased, or limited information because of familiarity with the constructs being asked about, self-awareness, or willingness to be candid. One should also anticipate finding discrepancies among information provided by an individual about himself or herself as opposed to information provided by a knowledgeable observer, such as a family member or close friend, as well as discrepancies among different observers.

It is reasonable to consider whether one source of information (self-report vs. observer ratings vs. implicit methods) consistently provides more accurate data than other sources of information (Zimmerman, 1994). It is not clear from the available literature whether to weight data provided by an individual about himself or herself more heavily than material provided by knowledgeable informants. Alternatively, one might argue that it is essential to obtain information from multiple sources given the complexities of diagnosing PDs. For example, the discrepancies found between different informants in the child assessment literature discussed previously have led some researchers to recommend that the most complete picture of an individual's problems and behavior will be obtained if information is gathered from multiple sources rather than relying on material provided using one method alone. Similar suggestions have been made by authors who have concluded that self-reports and other reports provide independent, valid information about personality functioning, social behaviors, self-image, patterns of thinking, and functional impairment that contributes incrementally to developing a full understanding of an individual's psychological characteristics (Klein, 2003; Meyer et al., 2001; Miller, Pilkonis, & Clifton, 2005; Ready, Watson, & Clark, 2002). These findings suggest that relying solely on explicit assessment methods may produce a useful but incomplete picture of an individual's personality functioning, strengths, and the maladaptive characteristics that contribute to emotional distress, impairment in managing adult demands, and developing healthy interpersonal relationships.

Rather than attempting to determine which assessment method is the most accurate, it may be more productive to conclude that data obtained using one method may be more informative than a different method in some situations and vice versa. Individuals may be a better source of information than observers if one is interested in their subjective, inner experience, for example, whereas observers may better recognize the impact of maladaptive behaviors and attitudes associated with personality pathology. Miller et al. (2005), for instance, reported that although narcissistic individuals perceived themselves as being interpersonally warm and engaged, others rated them as being socially aversive because of objectionable interpersonal behaviors that the narcissistic individuals apparently were not aware of. Similarly, Klein (2003) found that informant ratings of features of passive–aggressive PD were significantly related to measures of psychological and social functioning, whereas self-report ratings of the same passive–aggressive features were not associated with any of these outcome measures. Klein reasoned this occurred because observers were more aware of the impact of anger expressed via passive–aggressive maneuvers than were patients.

Although the literature reviewed previously highlights potential limitations of relying on self-report information alone, the reality of clinical practice is that clinicians typically do not have an opportunity to gather personality information from significant others (Miller et al., 2005). It therefore seems reasonable to incorporate an assessment method that contributes useful, valid information to assessment of personality functioning that does not share the limitations of self-report assessment methods and that can complement information obtained using explicit methods or provided by the person's significant others, if available. For the reasons discussed previously, performance-based assessment procedures, such as the CS, should be viewed as appropriate methods to include in assessments of personality functioning. In particular, data from the CS provides valid information about relevant domains of personality functioning that, in some cases, may not be revealed by self-report methods or that an individual may be motivated to conceal. The observation made by Ready and Clark (2002) that agreement between self–other ratings are strongest for easily observed behavior and weakest for internal processes—such as characteristic patterns of thinking, emotional reactions, self-concept, and schemata used to organize reactions to others—suggests another potential contribution of performance-based methods: Implicit assessment approaches may provide a means to access information about important internal processes that are less available using self-report or observer ratings.

The literature contrasting implicit and explicit assessment of dependence discussed previously suggests that performance-based measures of personality characteristics, such as the CS, can, in some situations, provide information about personality functioning that may not be obtained using explicit assessment methods. As the study conducted by Bornstein et al. (1994) showed, when explicit assessment methods are used, some individuals may be reluctant to acknowledge certain characteristics if they consider the characteristics to be negative, unflattering, or unfavorable. Bornstein et al.'s (1994) results demonstrate that valid information about some personality characteristics may be obtained using implicit methods in spite of these self-presentational concerns. The utility of the CS in such instances will depend, of course, on whether the dimension of psychological functioning in question is adequately represented by CS variables.

As noted previously, another distinction between implicit and explicit methods of personality assessment concerns the extent to which an individual has developed an adequate definition of a particular dimension of personality functioning and consciously recognizes where he or she falls on that dimension. Direct, explicit assessment of a specific characteristic requires that individuals understand a particular construct, such as the dimension of conscientiousness as opposed to disinhibition, and if they do, have evaluated themselves in terms of that dimension. In contrast, implicit measures can complement information obtained using explicit assessment methods by providing salient information about aspects of adaptive and maladaptive personality functioning whether or not an individual has accurately conceptualized a construct such as reacting to events with considerable emotional intensity (Blais et al., 2001, and weighed how that construct describes them. (For a discussion of relationships between CS variables and specific dimensions of personality functioning, see Huprich, 2006).

In addition to providing meaningful information concerning adaptive and maladaptive aspects of personality functioning, CS data can also provide valuable findings that can be useful for treatment planning, information that may complement or not be obvious from self-report methods (Blais et al., 2001). For instance, CS data may alert a therapist that a patient is likely to express emotions in a highly exaggerated manner, highlight a potential for impulsive behavior, or reveal conflicts about an individual's self-image that may be masked by a self-confident demeanor during a clinical interview. Huprich and Ganellen (2006) illustrated ways in which data from the CS may have clinical utility in treatment of patients with PDs, in general, and borderline PD (BPD) in particular. Huprich and Ganellen noted that although psychotherapy is frequently the primary modality of treatment for patients with BPD, some patients require a combination of psychotherapy and medication and that different classes of medication may be indicated depending on whether a patient exhibits significant affective dysregulation, impulsivity, and behavioral dyscontrol, or impaired cognitive-perceptual functioning such as paranoia or ideas of reference; treatment with antipsychotic medication is recommended for BPD patients when cognitive-perceptual symptoms predominate, whereas SSRIs are recommended for patients with affective dysregulation (c.f., Gabbard, 2000; Oldam, 2006; Oldham et al., 2002; Soloff, 2000). CS findings may be quite helpful in identifying these different domains of symptom patterns. Future research investigating this issue would be quite valuable. In addition, the CS may provide useful information concerning a patient's potential to engage in self-destructive or suicidal behavior (Fowler, Piers, Hilsenroth, Holdwick, & Padawer, 2001; Ganellen, 2004).

In summary, assessment of adaptive and maladaptive personality characteristics; distinguishing the boundaries between normal and abnormal functioning; identifying impairment in the domains of work, interpersonal relationships, and emotional state; and translating these findings into effective, appropriate treatment interventions is inherently complicated. These efforts may be biased, incomplete, or inaccurate if a clinician or researcher relies exclusively on explicit assessment methods such as self-report instruments or observer ratings. Hopefully, the preceding discussion illustrates that the accuracy of conclusions about an individual's personality functioning, problems in adjustment, and treatment needs may be improved if conclusions are based on a multimethod assessment approach that incorporates information gathered using explicit assessment methods—including data obtained from interviews, self-report questionnaires, and information provided by significant others—and data from performance-based, implicit measures of personality such as the CS.

REFERENCES

Achenbach, T. M. (1991). *Manual for the Child Behavior Checklist and 1991 profile*. Burlington: University of Vermont, Department of Psychiatry.

Achenbach, T. M., McConaughy, S. H., & Howell, C. T. (1987). Child/adolescent behavioral and emotional problems: Implications of cross-informant correlation for situational specificity. *Psychological Bulletin, 101,* 213–232.

American Psychiatric Association. (1987). *Diagnostic and statistical manual of mental disorders* (3rd ed., rev.). Washington, DC: Author.

American Psychiatric Association. (2001). *Diagnostic and statistical manual of mental disorders* (4th ed.). Washington, DC: Author.

American Psychiatric Association. (2001). *Diagnostic and statistical manual of mental disorders* (4th ed., text revision). Washington, DC: Author.

Barnett, P., & Gotlib, I. (1988). Psychosocial functioning and depression: Distinguishing antecedents, concomitants, and consequences. *Psychological Bulletin, 104,* 97–126.

Bernstein, D. P., Kasapis, C.H., Bergman, A., Weld, E., Mitropoulou, V., Horvath, T., et al.(1997). Assessing Axis II disorders by informant interview. *Journal of Personality Disorders, 11,* 158–167.

Blais, M. A., Hilsenroth, M. J., Castelbury, F., Fowler, J. C., & Baity, M. R. (2001). Predicting DSM-IV Cluster B Personality Disorder criteria from MMPI–2 and Rorschach data: A test on incremental validity. *Journal of Personality Assessment, 76,* 150–168.

Bornstein, R. F. (1996). Construct validity of the Rorschach Oral Dependency scale: 1967–1995. *Psychological Assessment, 8,* 200–205.

Bornstein, R. F. (1998). Implicit and self-attributed dependency strivings: Differential relationships to laboratory and field measures of help-seeking. *Journal of Personality and Social Psychology, 75,* 779–787.

Bornstein, R. F., Rossner, S. C., Hill, E. L., & Stepanian, M. L. (1994). Face validity and fakability of objective and projective measures of dependency. *Journal of Personality Assessment, 63,* 363–386.

Butcher, J. N., Dahlstrom, W. G., Graham, J. R., Tellegen, A., & Kaemmer, B. (1989). *MMPI–2: Minnesota Multiphasic Personality Inventory–2: Manual for administration and scoring.* Minneapolis: University of Minnesota Press.

Clark, L. A., & Watson, D. (1999). Temperament: A new paradigm for trait psychology. In L. Pervin & O. John (Eds.), *Handbook of personality. Theory and research* (2nd ed., pp. 399–423). New York: Guilford.

Costa, P. T., Jr., & Widiger, T. A. (2002). *Personality disorders and the five-factor model of personality* (2nd ed.). Washington, DC: American Psychological Association.

Dreesen, L., Hildebrand, M., & Arntz, A. (1998). Patient-informant concordance on the Structured Clinical Interview for *DSM–III–R* personality disorders (SCID–II). *Journal of Personality Disorders, 12,* 149–161.

Exner, J. E., Jr. (2003). *The Rorschach: A comprehensive system: Vol. 1: Basic foundations* (4th ed.). New York: Wiley.

Ferro, T., & Klein, D. N. (1997). Family history assessment of personality disorders: I. Concordance with direct interview and between pairs of informants. *Journal of Personality Disorders, 11,* 123–136.

First, M. B., Spitzer, R. L., Gibbon, M., & Williams, J. B. W. (1995). The Structured Clinical Interview for *DSM–III–R* Personality Disorders (SCID–II). *Journal of Personality Disorders, 9,* 83–91.

First, M. B., Spitzer, R. L., Gibbon, M., Williams, J. B. W., Davies, M., Borus, J., et al.(1995). The Structured Clinical Interview for *DSM–III–R* Personality Disorders (SCID–II). Part II: Multi-site test–retest reliability study. *Journal of Personality Disorders, 9,* 92–104.

Fitzgerald, H. E., Zucker, R. A., Maguin, E. T., & Reider, E. E. (1994). Time spent with child and parental agreement about preschool children's behavior. *Perceptual and Motor Skills, 79,* 336–338.

Fowler, J. C., Piers, C., Hilsenroth, M. J., Holdwick, D. J., & Padawer, J. R. (2001). The Rorschach Suicide Constellation: Assessing various degrees of lethality. *Journal of Personality Assessment, 76,* 333–351.

Gabbard, G. O. (2000). Combining medication with psychotherapy in the treatment of personality disorders. In J. G. Gunderson & G. O. Gabbard (Eds.), *Psychotherapy for Personality Disorders* (pp. 65–90). Washington, DC: American Psychiatric Press.

Ganellen, R. J. (1996). *Integrating the Rorschach and the MMPI–2 in Personality Assessment.* Mahwah, NJ: Lawrence Erlbaum Associates, Inc.

Ganellen, R. J. (2004). Rorschach contributions to assessment of suicide risk. In R. Yufit & D. Lester (Eds.), *Assessment, treatment, and prevention of suicide* (pp. 93–120). New York: Wiley.

Ganellen, R. J. (2006). Rorschach assessment of normal and abnormal personality. In S. Strack (Ed.), *Differentiating normal and abnormal personality* (pp. 473–500). Springer-Verlag.

Hathaway, S. R., & McKinley, J. C. (1943). *The Minnesota Multiphasic Personality Inventory.* Minneapolis: University of Minnesota Press.

Hiller, J. B., Rosenthal, R., Bornstein, R. F., Berry, D. T. R., & Brunell-Neuleib, S. (1999). A comparative meta-analysis of Rorschach and MMPI validity. *Psychological Assessment, 11,* 278–296.

Hirschfeld, R. M. A., Klerman, G. L., Gough, H. G., Barrett, J., Korchin, S. J., & Chodoff, P. (1977). A measure of interpersonal dependency. *Journal of Personality Assessment, 41,* 610–618.

Hunsley, J., & Bailey, J. M. (2001). Whither the Rorschach? An analysis of the evidence. *Psychological Assessment, 13,* 472–485.

Huprich, S. (2006). *Rorschach assessment of personality disorders.* Mahwah, NJ: Lawrence Erlbaum Associates.

Huprich, S., & Ganellen, R. J. (2006). Clinical utility of the Rorschach Inkblot Method in the assessment of personality disorders. In S. Huprich (Ed.), *Rorschach assessment of personality disorders* (pp. 27–53). Mahwah, NJ: Lawrence Erlbaum Associates.

Klein, D. N. (2003). Patients' versus informants' reports of personality disorders in predicting 7 1/2-year outcome in outpatients with depressive disorder. *Psychological Assessment, 15,* 216–222.

Klonsky, E. D., Oltmanns, T. F., & Turkheimer, E. (2002). Informant-reports of personality disorder: Relation to self-reports and future research directions. *Clinical Psychology: Science and Practice, 9,* 300–311.

Loranger, A. W. (1988). *Personaliity Disorder Examination (PDE) manual.* Yonkers, NY: DV Communications.

Masling, J. M., Rabie, L., & Blondheim, S. H. (1967). Obesity, level of aspiration, and Rorschach and TAT measures of oral dependency. *Journal of Consulting Psychology, 31,* 233–239.

McClelland, D. C., Koestner, R., & Weinberger, J. (1989). How do self-attributed and implicit motives differ? *Psychological Review, 96,* 690–702.

Meyer, G. J., & Archer, R. P. (2001). The hard science of Rorschach research: What do we know and where do we go? *Psychological Assessment, 13,* 486–502.

Meyer, G. J., Finn, S. E., Eyde, L. D., Kay, G. G., Moreland, K. L., Dies, R. R., et al. (2001). Psychological testing and psychological assessment: A review of evidence and issues. *American Psychologist, 56,* 128–165.

Miller, J. D., Pilkonis, P. A., & Clifton, A. (2005). Self- and other-reports of traits from the Five-factor model: Relations to personality disorder. *Journal of Personality Disorders, 19,* 400–419.

Millon, T. (1994). *Manual for the MCMI–III.* Minneapolis, MN: National Computer Systems.

Murray, H. A. (1943). *Thematic Apperception Test.* Cambridge, MA: Harvard University Press.

Oldham, J. M. (2006). Integrated treatment for borderline personality disorder. *Psychiatric Annals, 36,* 361–369.

Oldham, J. M., Gabbard, G. O; Goin, M. K, Gunderson, J., Soloff, P., Spiegel, D., et al. (2002). Practice guideline for the treatment of patients with borderline personality disorder. *American Psychiatric Association practice guidelines for the treatment of psychiatric disorders: Compendium 2002* (pp. 767-855). Washington, DC: American Psychiatric Association.

Ready, R. E., & Clark, L. A. (2002). Correspondence of psychiatric patient and informant ratings of personality traits, temperament, and interpersonal problems. *Psychological Assessment, 14,* 39–49.

Ready, R. E., Watson, D., & Clark, L. A. (2002). Psychiatric patient- and informant-reported personality predicting concurrent and future behavior. *Assessment, 9,* 361–372.

Riso, L. P., Klein, D. N., Anderson, R. L., Ouimette, P. C., & Lizardi, H. (1994). Concordance between patients and informants on the personality disorder examination. *American Journal of Psychiatry, 151,* 568–573.

Soloff, P. H. (2000). Psychopharmacology of borderline personality disorder. *The Psychiatric Clinics of North America, 23,* 169–192.

Spitzer, R. L. (1983). Psychiatric diagnosis: Are clinicians still necessary? *Comprehensive Psychiatry, 24,* 399–411.

Verheul, R. (2005). Clinical utility for dimensional models of personality pathology. *Journal of Personality Disorders, 19,* 283–302.

Wechsler, D. (1955). *Manual for the Wechsler Adult Intelligence Scale.* New York: Psychological Corporation.

Widiger, T. A., & Coker, L. A. (2001). Assessing personality disorders. In J. N. Butcher (Ed.), *Clinical personality assessment: Practical approaches* (2nd ed., pp. 407–434). New York: Oxford University Press.

Widiger, T. A., Mangine, S., Corbitt, E. M., Ellis, C. G., & Thomas, G. V. (1995). *Personality Disorder Interview–IV: A semistructured interview for the assessment of personality disorders.* Odessa, FL: Psychological Assessment Resources.

Widiger, T. A., & Simonsen, E. (2005). Alternative dimensional models of personality disorder: Finding a common ground. *Journal of Personality Disorders, 19,* 110–130.

Widiger, T. A., Simonsen, E., Krueger, R., Livesley, J., & Verheul, R. (2005). Personality disorder research agenda for the *DSM–V. Journal of Personality Disorders, 19,* 315–338.

Zimmerman, M. (1993, September). *Interstudy rater variance: A major problem in diagnosing personality disorders.* Paper presented at the 3rd International Congress on the Disorders of Personality, Cambridge, MA.

Zimmerman, M. (1994). Diagnosing personality disorders: A review of issues and research methods. *Archives of General Psychiatry, 51,* 225–245.

Zimmerman, M., Pfohl, B., Coryell, W., Stangl, D., & Corenthal, C. (1988). Diagnosing personality disorder in depressed patients: A comparison of patient and informant interviews. *Archives of General Psychiatry, 45,* 733–737.

Zimmerman, M., Pfohl, B., Stangl, D., & Corenthal, C. (1986). Assessment of DSM-III personality disorders: The importance of interviewing an informant. *Journal of Clinical Psychiatry, 47,* 261–263.

Zucker, M., Morris, M. K., Ingram, S. M., Morris, R. D., & Bakeman R. (2002). Concordance of self- and informant ratings of adults' current and childhood attention-deficit/hyperactivity disorder symptoms. *Psychological Assessment, 14,* 379–389.

Ronald J. Ganellen
405 N. Wabash Avenue, #2810
Chicago, IL 60611-3591
Email: r-ganellen@northwestern.edu

Received March 20, 2006
Revised July 19, 2006

Personality in *DSM–5:* Helping Delineate Personality Disorder Content and Framing the Metastructure

Robert F. Krueger,[1] Nicholas R. Eaton,[1] Jaime Derringer,[1] Kristian E. Markon,[2] David Watson,[3] and Andrew E. Skodol[4]

[1]*Psychology Department, University of Minnesota*
[2]*Department of Psychology, University of Iowa*
[3]*Department of Psychology, University of Notre Dame*
[4]*Department of Psychiatry, University of Arizona*

The transition from the *Diagnostic and Statistical Model of Mental Disorders* (4th ed., text revision [*DSM–IV–TR*]; American Psychiatric Association, 2000) to the fifth edition (*DSM–5*) represents an unprecedented opportunity to integrate dimensional personality trait models into the official nosology. Not surprisingly, a variety of issues have arisen in contemplating this challenging integration. In this article, we address how a dimensional personality trait model could be a helpful component of *DSM–5,* from the perspective of our roles as work group members and advisors involved in the creation of a trait model and corresponding assessment instrument. We focus in particular on two potential roles for a trait model in *DSM–5* that are under official consideration. First, a dimensional personality trait model might be helpful in delineating the content of personality disorders. Second, a trait model might assist in organizing the "metastructure" of *DSM–5* (i.e., the arrangement of chapters and other broader classificatory rubrics).

Personality is an indispensible construct in clinical settings. It is difficult to imagine effective assessment and intervention in the absence of personality as an organizing construct for both kinds of endeavors. Nevertheless, the extensive literature on clinical personality assessment—and the multidimensional personality models that are a major focus of this literature—exists largely in isolation from official psychiatric nosologies. The *Diagnostic and Statistical Model of Mental Disorders* (4th ed., text revision [*DSM–IV–TR*]; American Psychiatric Association, 2000) reflects this disjuncture, in that personality disorder (PD) is defined in terms of traits, but diagnosed in the form of 10 putatively separate and categorical PDs, each with its own criterion set. Quoting from the *DSM–IV–TR,* "*Personality traits* are enduring patterns of perceiving, relating to, and thinking about the environment and oneself that are exhibited in a wide range of social and personal contexts. Only when personality traits are inflexible and maladaptive and cause significant functional impairment or subjective distress do they constitute Personality Disorders" (American Psychiatric Association, 2000, p. 686).

The problems with the *DSM–IV–TR* system for specific PD conceptualization and diagnosis are well known and are reviewed extensively elsewhere (see, e.g., Krueger & Eaton, 2010, for a recent account). As multiple scholars have noted (e.g., Clark, 2007; Livesley, 2007; Trull & Durrett, 2005; Widiger, Simonsen, Krueger, Livesley, & Verheul, 2005), many of the problems with the *DSM–IV–TR* approach to PDs could be solved by conceptualizing key aspects of PDs using dimensional models of personality (see Huprich & Bornstein, 2007, for a discussion

of issues relevant to categorical and dimensional approaches to PDs).

This, however, is just the beginning. The relevance of personality to the classification of psychopathology extends well beyond conceptualization of PD. Multidimensional models of personality variation could play a central role in shifting the entire *DSM* toward a more empirically based (and etiologically based) nosology. This is because the organization of psychopathological tendencies has notable parallels with the organization of the personality dimensions that underlie those tendencies. Indeed, these connections constitute a major theme in current discussions regarding the form and structure of *DSM–5,* as well as discussions surrounding National Institute of Mental Health funding priorities (e.g., as part of the Research Domain Criteria [RDoC] initiative; Insel & Cuthbert, 2009).

The focus of this article is, therefore, twofold. First, we briefly review official *DSM–5* efforts to create a personality trait model and corresponding assessment instrument, and related discussions surrounding how empirically based models of personality variation might be helpful in conceptualizing key features of PDs. Second, we describe how personality models can be used to frame the overall "metastructure" of *DSM–5.* We are writing this article from our perspectives as Personality and Personality Disorders Work Group participants (R. F. Krueger, member, and A. E. Skodol, chair), graduate students of Work Group members (N. R. Eaton, J. Derringer), and Work Group advisors appointed because of their expertise in personality trait models (K.E. Markson, D. Watson). The article thereby reports on current official *DSM–5* activities in which we have participated.

PDs and Dimensional Models of Personality in the *DSM–5* Process

One shortcoming of the *DSM–IV–TR* approach to conceptualizing PD is the assertion that PD is well conceptualized as a set of 10 categories. In contrast to this assertion, there is little evidence that PDs constitute categories in nature; rather, the preponderance of the evidence demonstrates that PD variation is more continuous than discrete (e.g., Eaton, Krueger, South, Simms, & Clark, 2011; Haslam, in press). Many of the limitations of the *DSM–IV–TR* model (e.g., low reliability, artificial thresholds for diagnosis, high comorbidity; Clark, 2007; Trull & Durrett, 2005) likely stem from assuming the discreteness of entities that are continuous, which is one reason to pursue a reconceptualization of PDs in *DSM–5*.

A key issue confronting *DSM–5* is how best to conceptualize the PD domain and its inherent underlying continuities. With regard to domain conceptualization, normal range personality models such as the Five-factor model (FFM; see Costa & Widiger, 2002) provide a starting point for understanding the structure of pathological personality because they are based on data and on quantitative models that posit underlying continuous variation. This is only one potential starting point, and other approaches to conceptualizing clinically relevant personality variants have been described in the literature (e.g, Bornstein, 2010; Mischel & Shoda, 1995; Westen & Shedler, 2007). In addition, concerns have been raised regarding the acceptability of personality trait models such as the FFM to some clinicians (e.g., Rottman, Ahn, Sanislow, & Kim, 2009).

Nevertheless, personality trait models are, de facto, a major focus of the *DSM–5* process. Specifically, activities related to formulating PDs for *DSM–5* began with a meeting in December 2004 that took place at American Psychiatric Association headquarters. The specific focus of this meeting was on dimensional alternatives to categorical PDs, and the meeting was largely framed by research on dimensional models of human personality variation. The proceedings from this meeting were published in two successive issues of the *Journal of Personality Disorders* in 2005, as well as in an edited book (Widiger, Simonsen, Sirovatka, & Regier, 2006), and an overview of the meeting can be found in Widiger et al. (2005). This activity was followed by the formal appointment of persons with expertise in personality trait models to the *DSM–5* Personality and Personality Disorders Work Group (e.g., R. F. Krueger, among others), as well as the formal appointment of Work Group advisors with particular expertise in personality trait models (D. Watson and K. E. Markon).

A key challenge in the *DSM–5* process pertains to the integration and, ideally, the harmonization of personality trait models with models of personality stemming from other theoretical perspectives. How exactly these challenges will be met has not been resolved as of this writing, and these challenges are not the focus of this article. Moreover, no final decisions have been reached regarding the representation of personality and PDs in *DSM–5*. Hence, this article focuses on particular aspects of the *DSM–5* process that are in progress as of this writing, related to personality traits. Specifically, a personality trait model and measure are being developed as part of the *DSM–5* process, and there has been extensive discussion regarding how this model might intersect both with the conceptualization of PD, and with the overall "metastructure" of *DSM–5* (the organization of chapters and other broad classificatory rubrics).

DEVELOPING A CLINICALLY APPLICABLE DIMENSIONAL MODEL OF PERSONALITY FOR *DSM–5*

One challenge in implementing models such as the FFM is that they are largely operationalized in assessment tools that

were not designed specifically to capture pathological personality (Krueger, Eaton, et al., 2011; Widiger, 2007). Instruments such as the Big Five Inventory (John, Donahue, & Kentle, 1991) and the Revised NEO Personality Inventory (NEO PI–R; Costa & McCrae, 1992) capture important forms of personality variation but do not encompass fully the pathological range of trait variation (Krueger & Eaton, 2010; Morey et al., 2007). For example, psychotic-like experiences are often conceptualized as an aspect of the universe of PD variation (e.g., within Cluster A of *DSM–IV–TR*), but these experiences are not explicitly measured in typical five-factor inventories (e.g., Watson, Clark, & Chmielewski, 2008).

With this concern about range and breadth of psychopathological content in mind, Work Group members and consultants have been developing a self-report assessment tool targeting specific nonadaptive personality variants. This assessment instrument will be entirely in the public domain; as of this writing it can be obtained by writing to R. F. Krueger, and our aim is to make it widely available by posting it on the Web (e.g., it could be posted as a supplement on a journal Web site or on DSM5.org). Along these lines, an additional concern that this work is intended to address is the possible verbatim overlap between a trait model for *DSM–5* and published assessment instruments sold for profit. A potential conflict of interest exists if the *DSM–5* articulates a trait model that is isomorphic with a model assessed by a specific inventory sold by a specific test publisher. One intent of creating a public domain self-report personality inventory as part of the *DSM–5* process is to address this conflict of interest issue. This work is an official *DSM–5* activity and is supported under the *DSM–5* umbrella of activities.

With regard to the content of the inventory, our literature review of a variety of personality instruments designed to capture pathological personality (Krueger, Eaton, et al., 2011) identified six broad domains of content: emotional dysregulation/negative emotionality/neuroticism; detachment/low positive affectivity/introversion; disinhibition (encompassing elements of low FFM conscientiousness); antagonism (encompassing elements of low FFM agreeableness); compulsivity (which has some elements of excessive FFM conscientiousness, but also appears to encompass significant elements of negative affectivity); and schizotypy/oddity/peculiarity/psychoticism (which, although associated with openness, contains extensive variation not entirely encompassed by that normal-range domain; Harkness & McNulty, 1994; Krueger, Eaton, et al., 2011; Piedmont, Sherman, Sherman, Dy-Liacco, & Williams, 2009; Tackett, Silberschmidt, Krueger, & Sponheim, 2008; Watson et al., 2008).

As of this writing, preliminary analyses of data from this project suggest the presence of reliable facet-level personality dimensions in our provisional set of items. As additional data are gathered and analyzed, this list and the facet and domain names could change, so what we include here should be considered a "snapshot" of an ongoing endeavor. Nevertheless, with these caveats in mind, Table 1 presents a list of facets and domains that have emerged from our work to date. A formal report on this project has been submitted for publication (Krueger, Derringer, Markon, Watson, & Skodol, 2011); we provide some basic information regarding this project next.

Briefly, we began our work with self-report items designed to tap the 37 narrow-band constructs that were generated as a result of discussions in the *DSM–5* Personality and Personality Disorders Work Group, which were listed on the DSM5.org Web site. We conducted three rounds of data collection from

TABLE 1.—A provisional list of domains and core content criteria (facet traits) for describing pathological personality features in *DSM–5* and sample items.

	I. Negative Affectivity	
1.	Anxiousness:	I worry a lot about terrible things that might happen.
2.	Emotional lability:	I never know where my emotions will go from moment to moment.
3.	Hostility:	I'm nasty and short to anybody who deserves it.
4.	Perseveration:	I get fixated on certain things and can't stop.
5.	(Lack of) restricted affectivity:	I don't react much to things that seem to make others emotional.
6.	Separation insecurity:	I dread being without someone to love me.
7.	Submissiveness:	I do what other people tell me to do.
	II. Detachment	
8.	Anhedonia:	I almost never enjoy life.
9.	Depressivity:	The future looks really hopeless to me.
10.	Intimacy avoidance:	I steer clear of romantic relationships.
11.	Suspiciousness:	Plenty of people are out to get me.
12.	Withdrawal:	I don't like spending time with others.
	III. Antagonism	
13.	Attention seeking:	I do things to make sure people notice me.
14.	Callousness:	I don't care about other people's problems.
15.	Deceitfulness:	I don't hesitate to cheat if it gets me ahead.
16.	Grandiosity:	To be honest, I'm just more important than other people.
17.	Manipulativeness:	It is easy for me to take advantage of others.
	IV. Disinhibition	
18.	Distractibility:	I can't concentrate on anything.
19.	Impulsivity:	I always do things on the spur of the moment.
20.	Irresponsibility:	I make promises that I don't really intend to keep.
21.	(Lack of) rigid perfectionism:	If something I do isn't absolutely perfect, it's simply not acceptable.
22.	Risk taking:	I have no limits when it comes to doing dangerous things.
	V. Psychoticism	
23.	Eccentricity:	Other people seem to think my behavior is weird.
24.	Perceptual dysregulation:	Things around me often feel unreal, or more real than usual.
25.	Unusual beliefs and experiences:	Sometimes I can influence other people just by sending my thoughts to them.

Note. The instructions to respondents were, "This is a list of things different people might say about themselves. We are interested in how you would describe yourself. There are no right or wrong answers. So you can describe yourself as honestly as possible, we will keep your responses confidential. We'd like you to take your time and read each statement carefully, selecting the response that best describes you." The response format consisted of four options: "very false or often false," "sometimes or somewhat false," "sometimes or somewhat true," and "very true or often true."

representative community-dwelling samples of adult participants who reported in a previous survey that they had sought treatment from a psychiatrist or psychologist ($N = 1,128$); in the third round this inclusion criterion was not used to examine community norms on the instrument ($n = 264$). This research was designed to refine the ability to measure the constructs reliably across a range of individual differences in an iterative manner (via item response theory [IRT] modeling), and also to determine if some constructs could be combined, because they were

highly correlated. Analyses of these data as of this writing led us to reduce the 37 initial constructs to the list of 25 shown in Table 1. All 25 "restructured" constructs were measured reliably by the final round, as judged by both classical (Cronbach's alpha, range = .72–.96, median = .86) and modern (IRT) test theory approaches, and the current version of the instrument contains 220 items. In addition, the preliminary exploratory factor structure of the 25 facets corresponds with the five-domain structure portrayed in Table 1, based on placing facets into the domain where they had their strongest loading.

There are a number of fundamental limitations of these efforts to date. For example, this effort is limited to self-report and must ultimately be extended to reporters other than the self (cf. Oltmanns & Turkheimer, 2009), including both expert clinician and nonexpert collateral reporters; the effort was limited to adults, and assessment of these traits in different age groups would be an important extension of this work (cf. Shiner, 2005); the initial list of 37 traits was a result of Work Group discussion, and numerous additional facet-level traits could, in theory, be articulated. Consistent with the traditional focus of the *DSM,* the effort was limited to nonadaptive traits, whereas adaptive traits also have clinical utility (cf. Harkness & Lilienfeld, 1997). Nevertheless, work to date as an official part of the *DSM–5* process has resulted in a self-report instrument with 25 reliable scales measuring nonadaptive personality traits that appear to fall empirically into the five broad domains in Table 1.

APPLYING CORE ELEMENTS OF PERSONALITY DESCRIPTION TO SPECIFIC PATIENTS

The constructs in Table 1 cover a range of pathological content and, as such, one option under consideration in the *DSM–5* process is to conceptualize the Table 1 constructs as "core elements" of personality description. These core elements could potentially be thought of as a simplification and distillation of the criteria for PDs in *DSM–IV–TR* into a smaller number of reliable and narrow facet-level elements. Technically, if clinicians were to diagnose PD by following the *DSM–IV–TR* scheme, they would have to evaluate the 79 individual criteria for the 10 *DSM–IV–TR* PDs (or at least enough criteria to rule in or rule out the 10 PDs). This is rarely, if ever, done in clinical practice, which raises concerns about the clinical utility of the *DSM–IV–TR* approach to PD (cf. Bernstein et al., 2007). The current system, when formally and fully utilized, is rather complex, and it also includes a good deal of criterion overlap; for instance, both schizoid and schizotypal PD include criteria assessing a lack of close friends or confidants other than first-degree relatives. One potentially useful aspect of "core elements" or pathological personality facets could be the way they reduce the complex and overlapping *DSM–IV–TR* PD criteria to a streamlined set of reliable constructs. For example, there might be less of a need for a category of PD-not otherwise specified because of the wide variety of PD content that can be characterized using the core elements in Table 1.

A challenging issue under discussion pertains to merging a dimensional trait model with the clinical need to render specific PD diagnoses and to apply descriptive qualities such as traits to specific patients (for further discussion of this issue, see Strack & Millon, 2007). There are at least two aspects to this discussion. First, there is evidence that trait models and their associated instruments might not contain all the content of the PD construct (Verheul et al., 2008); PD is likely more than simply extreme temperament and brings other aspects of personality (e.g., representations of self and others) into play. Our perspective is that this understanding is relatively uncontroversial in the Work Group and we do not focus on this issue here because it is almost certain that a representation of the construct of PD will be part of *DSM–5* and that this representation will not be rendered solely via personality traits (cf. Skodol et al., 2011). Second, however, is the more controversial issue of how to organize and structure varieties of PD, and how this endeavor might dovetail with the constructs and structure portrayed in Table 1. All the options discussed in the following presume that general criteria for PD would be provided in *DSM–5,* and that, most likely, these criteria would include impairments in self-concept and interpersonal functioning (Bender & Skodol, 2007; Livesley, 2007; Parker et al., 2004).

One option under discussion is to focus the conceptualization of varieties of PD on combinations of traits that represent the "high poles" of empirically derived personality domains, such as those in Table 1. For example, the facet traits in the negative affectivity domain could be listed as criteria for "PD, negative affectivity type" and thresholds could be placed to justify a categorical diagnosis (e.g., four of the seven facets of negative affectivity in Table 1 elevated). Of note, an approach along these lines is being considered for ICD–11 (Tyrer, Crawford, & Mulder, in press; Tyrer et al., 2010). The upside of this approach is that the structure of the PD system would correspond with the structure of nonadaptive trait facets, at least those in Table 1, assessed by self-report. The downside is that the domains in Table 1 bear only a partial resemblance to the 10 PDs from *DSM–IV–TR,* constructs that are familiar to many in the field. For example, *DSM–IV* Borderline PD contains criteria that draw on multiple domains in Table 1, as well as features that pervade PDs (i.e., nonadaptive working models of self and others).

Along these lines, another option under discussion involves articulating trait combinations that correspond with the PDs described in *DSM–IV–TR.* For example, combining problems in establishing coherent representations of self and others (likely criteria for general PD) with traits from both the negative affectivity and disinhibition domains would provide reasonable coverage of the criteria for *DSM–IV–TR* Borderline PD. The upside of this approach is that it would create continuity from *DSM–IV–TR* to *DSM–5.* The downside of this approach is that there is little evidence that the PDs described in the *DSM–IV–TR,* taken as a whole, accurately parse the varieties of abnormal personality (see, however, Huprich, Schmitt, Richard, Chelminski, & Zimmerman, 2010, for a recent factor analytic study that recovered factors similar to *DSM–IV–TR* PDs).

A final option under discussion involves having separate personality "types" and personality "traits." For example, users of the *DSM–5* could choose to represent PDs in their own work based on correspondence with types, or in terms of the traits in Table 1. The upside to this approach is that clinicians unfamiliar with trait models would not have to become familiar with trait models. The downside is that two systems with overlapping content would exist side by side. For example, it is difficult to imagine a way of describing a "Borderline PD" type without using constructs such as those listed in Table 1—indeed, in many cases, using the same exact phrases, such as emotional lability (cf. Gunderson, 2010).

Importantly, all of these options are under discussion, and no decisions have been reached regarding personality and PDs in *DSM–5.* Nevertheless, the investment of the *DSM–5* leadership in personality traits suggests that these constructs likely will figure into the final *DSM–5* product. A key reason for this investment extends beyond the conceptualization of PD per se, and to the issue of the overall form and "metastructure" of *DSM–5,* a topic to which we now turn.

PERSONALITY TRAITS AND THE METASTRUCTURE OF *DSM–5*

The *DSM–5* revision endeavor is generally organized hierarchically. David Kupfer and Darrel Regier are the chairs of the *DSM–5* task force, which consists primarily of psychiatrists who are also the chairs of the specific Work Groups. Much of the *DSM–5* is thereby "prestructured" by the nature and composition of the Work Groups. However, Kupfer and Regier have been careful to create additional cross-cutting study groups focused on the "metastructure" of *DSM–5*; that is, the way in which specific disorders are sorted into particular chapters and classified in broader rubrics.

In addition to the activities of the individual Work Groups, various study groups have been formed to address these metastructural issues. Some initial ideas regarding the metastructure were published in a special section of *Psychological Medicine* (Andrews et al., 2009). More recently, a *DSM–5* study group formed in fall of 2010 focused on the difficult question of how to merge the PDs with the rest of *DSM–5* (R. F. Krueger and A. E. Skodol were members of this study group). The PDs are tricky in this regard because they are unified by the presence of personality pathology, but are also differentiated by the kinds of characteristics described in Table 1. Regardless of how PDs ultimately mesh with other aspects of *DSM–5,* one conclusion of the recent study group was that the metastructure of *DSM–5* is likely to reflect the fact that patterns of comorbidity among mental disorders are structured and systematic, in ways that relate to the structure of personality.

In *DSM–IV–TR,* disorders are organized into chapters to facilitate differential diagnosis. The idea behind the anxiety disorders chapter, for example, is that different kinds of anxiety disorders might be confused with each other, such that the clinician is encouraged to consider all of them and then pick the "best" or "primary" disorder. The problem with this approach is well known: Disorders rarely present singly and comorbid presentations are the norm, not the exception, in clinical settings (Clark, Watson, & Reynolds, 1995; Krueger & Markon, 2006; Zimmerman & Mattia, 1999). Recognizing this, the metastructure of *DSM–5* is likely to contain the traditional sorts of chapters seen in previous *DSMs,* but is also likely to contain broader rubrics that reflect robust patterns of comorbidity among mental disorders.

A potential metastructure that has been proposed in the *DSM–5* process is shown in Table 2. The 10-chapter arrangement results from the coding scheme of the ICD–10. Mental and behavioral disorders are one part of the ICD–10, and within that part there are 10 subdivisions. This 10-chapter convention might carry through to ICD–11 and might be adopted in *DSM–5* to facilitate harmonization between these two nosologies.

One intention of the metastructural proposal in Table 2 is to handle the comorbidity issue by proposing empirically derived

TABLE 2.—A potential metastructure for *DSM–5*

Chapter	Topic
0	Neurodevelomental disorders (e.g., autism spectrum disorders)
1	Late-onset cognitive disorders (e.g., dementia)
2	Disorders of self and interpersonal relations (i.e., personality disorders)
Psychosis metacluster	
3	Schizophrenia spectrum disorders (e.g., schizophrenia)
Emotional disorders (internalizing) metacluster	
4	Mood disorders (e.g., major depression)
5	Fear disorders (e.g., phobias)
6	Obsessive–compulsive disorders (e.g., obsessive–compulsive disorder)
7	Somatic and eating disorders (e.g., bulimia nervosa)
Disinhibitory disorders (externalizing) metacluster	
8	Antisocial disorders (e.g., conduct disorder)
9	Substance use disorders (e.g., alcohol disorder)

"metaclusters," reflecting core psychopathology spectra comprising multiple interrelated conditions. In this arrangement, broad emotional disorder (internalizing) and disinhibitory disorder (externalizing) spectra are recognized based on the way the chapters are arranged; within the emotion disorder spectrum, for instance, one would find unipolar mood and anxiety disorders. In addition, the text of *DSM–5* would reflect the move away from a primary focus on differential diagnosis within chapters, and toward recognizing that the disorders within these spectra have some shared features, as well as evidence for shared underlying pathophysiology (e.g., Iacono, Malone, & McGue, 2003) and etiology (e.g., disorders within spectra are genetically correlated; Kendler et al., 2008; Kendler et al., 2011), and the prospects for interventions targeting processes that unite disorders within spectra (Barlow et al., 2011).

In addition to recognizing comorbidity as a naturally occurring phenomenon to be accommodated, *DSM–5* could highlight the role of personality in the metastructural arrangement in Table 2 through an introductory chapter detailing how personality traits provide the core of the spectra in Table 2. For example, emotional dysregulation (also called neuroticism or negative affect in the literature) is linked to the emotional disorders (internalizing) spectrum, and trait disinhibition is linked to the disinhibitory disorders (externalizing) spectrum (e.g., Griffith et al., 2010; Krueger et al., 2002). Along these lines, parallels between the trait domains emerging from our structural work on the maladaptive traits in Table 1 and the structure of common mental disorders could be helpful in weaving together a coherent *DSM–5*. The parallels that appear to be emerging might help in creating a structural symmetry between personality psychopathology and psychopathology more generally.

Additional issues that arise in contemplating Table 2 also deserve careful consideration. In Table 2, neurodevelopmental and late-onset cognitive disorders are not linked to a metastructural rubric. This is primarily because they are not linked neatly with a coherent and broad underlying personality trait domain. Nevertheless, disorders such as autism and dementia are correlated with personality traits (e.g., Anckarsäter et al., 2006; Balsis, Carpenter, & Storandt, 2005), and this might be important to recognize in *DSM–5,* if the idea is to provide a comprehensive account of personality–psychopathology connections. In addi-

tion, neurodevelopmental and late-onset cognitive (neurocognitive) disorders could be thought of as two additional metastructural rubrics (cf. Andrews et al., 2009), akin to the way that the psychosis chapter constitutes its own metastructural group. Also, individual differences in cognitive ability, such as general intelligence, could be added to a model of personality in *DSM–5* to provide a more comprehensive dimensional account of human individual differences.

The PD chapter might be more the "odd man out" because of the way it contains entities that have both shared features, common to PD (cf. Verheul et al., 2008), and distinctive features, which are not shared among PDs but are shared with other disorders (Table 1). A question under discussion is this: Should different forms of PD be distributed throughout the *DSM–5*, based on features shared with other disorders, or should PD be in its own chapter because of features shared among various forms of PD? Distributing the forms of PD could be problematic, primarily because the PDs are united by problems related to, for instance, having a coherent working model of self and others, thus giving them a coherent core. Hence, an arrangement under discussion is to retain a PD chapter, perhaps even giving that chapter metastructural status as "disorders of self and interpersonal relations," acknowledging the features shared by PDs, and also detailing the content-related connections with other forms of psychopathology throughout *DSM–5*.

CONCLUSIONS

For those interested in PDs and psychiatric classification systems, we live in very interesting times. The *DSM–III* and its offspring (*DSM–III–R* and *DSM–IV*) served an important function in the zeitgeist in which they were created, by codifying definitions of mental disorders that were more reliable than previous definitions, thereby jumpstarting research into these debilitating and costly conditions. The limitations of the *DSM–III* paradigm, however, are also quite clear. In spite of extensive research, we do not have a good handle on the pathophysiology and etiology of psychopathology, and this is probably partly due to the fact that existing mental disorder categories suffer from problems such as within-category heterogeneity and comorbidity (Krueger & Markon, 2006). The process of questioning current diagnostic conventions can be unsettling, but if those conventions are not accurately parsing nature, then posing challenging questions is ultimately healthy for the field. We can successfully navigate this next phase in our field's development by sticking close to the data and incorporating formal quantitative models of individual differences in personality and psychopathological experiences into our nosological schemes.

REFERENCES

American Psychiatric Association. (2000). *Diagnostic and statistical manual of mental disorders* (4th ed., text revision). Washington, DC: Author.

Anckarsäter, H., Stahlberg, O., Larson, T., Hakansson, C., Jutblad, B., Niklasson, L., ... Rastam, M. (2006). The impact of ADHD and autism spectrum disorders on temperament, character, and personality development. *American Journal of Psychiatry, 163*, 1239–1244.

Andrews, G., Goldberg, D. P., Krueger, R. F., Carpenter, W. T., Jr., Hyman, S. E., Sachdev, P., & Pine, D. S. (2009). Exploring the feasibility of a meta-structure for *DSM–V* and ICD–11: Could it improve utility and validity? *Psychological Medicine, 39*, 1993–2000.

Balsis, S., Carpenter, B. D., & Storandt, M. (2005). Personality change precedes clinical diagnosis of dementia of the Alzheimer type. *Journals of Gerontology Series B: Psychological Sciences and Social Sciences, 60,* P98–P101.

Barlow, D. H., Farchione, T. J., Fairholme, C. P., Ellard, K. K., Boisseau, C. L., Allen, L. B., & Ehrenreich-May, J. (2011). *The unified protocol for transdiagnostic treatment of emotional disorders: Therapist guide.* New York, NY: Oxford University Press.

Bender, D. S., & Skodol, A. E. (2007). Borderline personality as a self–other representational disturbance. *Journal of Personality Disorders, 21,* 500–517.

Bernstein, D. P., Iscan, C., Maser, J., and the Boards of Directors of the Association for Research in Personality Disorder and the International Society for the Study of Personality Disorders. (2007). Opinions of personality disorder experts regarding the *DSM–IV* personality disorders classification system. *Journal of Personality Disorders, 21,* 536–551.

Bornstein, R. F. (2010). Psychoanalytic theory as a unifying framework for 21st century personality assessment. *Psychoanalytic Psychology, 27,* 133–152.

Clark, L. A. (2007). Assessment and diagnosis of personality disorder: Perennial issues and an emerging reconceptualization. *Annual Review of Psychology, 58,* 227–257.

Clark, L. A., Watson, D., & Reynolds, S. (1995). Diagnosis and classification of psychopathology: Challenges to the current system and future directions. *Annual Review of Psychology, 46,* 121–153.

Costa, P. T., Jr., & McCrae, R. R. (1992). *Revised NEO Personality Inventory NEO–PI–R and NEO Five-Factor Inventory NEO–FFI professional manual.* Odessa, FL: Psychological Assessment Resources.

Costa, P. T., Jr., & Widiger, T. A. (Eds.). (2002). *Personality disorders and the Five-factor model of personality* (2nd ed.). Washington, DC: American Psychological Association.

Eaton, N. R., Krueger, R. F., South, S. C., Simms, L. J., & Clark, L. A. (2011). Contrasting prototypes and dimensions in the classification of personality pathology: Evidence that dimensions, but not prototypes, are robust. *Psychological Medicine, 41,* 1151–1163.

Griffith, J. W., Zinbarg, R. E., Craske, M. G., Mineka, S., Rose, R. D., Waters, A. M., & Sutton, J. M. (2010). Neuroticism as a common dimension in the internalizing disorders. *Psychological Medicine, 40,* 1125–1136.

Gunderson, J. G. (2010). Revising the borderline diagnosis for *DSM–V*: An alternative proposal. *Journal of Personality Disorders, 24,* 694–708.

Harkness, A. R., & Lilienfeld, S. O. (1997). Individual differences science for treatment planning: Personality traits. *Psychological Assessment, 9,* 349–360.

Harkness, A. R., & McNulty, J. L. (1994). The personality psychopathology five (PSY-5): Issue from the pages of a diagnostic manual instead of a dictionary. In S. Strack & M. Lorr (Eds.), *Differentiating normal and abnormal personality* (pp. 291–315). New York, NY: Springer.

Haslam, N. (in press). The latent structure of personality and psychopathology: A review of trends in taxometric research. *Scientific Review of Mental Health Practice.*.

Huprich, S. K., & Bornstein, R. F. (2007). Categorical and dimensional assessment of personality disorders: A consideration of the issues. *Journal of Personality Assessment, 89,* 3–15.

Huprich, S. K., Schmitt, T. A., Richard, D. C. S., Chelminski, I., & Zimmerman, M. A. (2010). Comparing factor analytic models of the *DSM–IV* personality disorders. *Personality Disorders: Theory, Research, and Treatment, 1*(1), 22–37.

Iacono, W. G., Malone, S. M., & McGue, M. (2003). Substance use disorders, externalizing psychopathology, and P300 event-related potential amplitude. *International Journal of Psychophysiology, 48,* 147–178.

Insel, T. R., & Cuthbert, B. N. (2009). Endophenotypes: Bridging genomic complexity and disorder heterogeneity. *Biological Psychiatry, 66,* 988–989.

John, O. P., Donahue, E. M., & Kentle, R. L. (1991). *The Big Five Inventory-Versions 4a and 54.* Berkeley: University of California, Berkeley, Institute of Personality and Social Research.

Kendler, K. S., Aggen, S. H., Czajkowski, N., Røysamb, E., Tambs, K., Torgersen, S., & Reichborn-Kjennerud, T. (2008). The structure of genetic and environmental risk factors for *DSM–IV* personality disorders: A multivariate twin study. *Archives of General Psychiatry, 65,* 1438–1446.

Kendler, K. S., Aggen, S. H., Knudsen, G. P., Røysamb, E., Neale, M. C., & Reichborn-Kjennerud, T. (2011). The structure of genetic and environmental risk factors for syndromal and subsyndromal common *DSM–IV* Axis I and all Axis II disorders. *American Journal of Psychiatry, 168,* 29–39.

Krueger, R. F., Derringer, J., Markon, K. E., Watson, D., & Skodol, A. E. (2011). *Initial construction of a maladaptive personality trait model and inventory for* DSM–5. Manuscript submitted for publication.

Krueger, R. F., & Eaton, N. R. (2010). Personality traits and the classification of mental disorders: Toward a more complete integration in *DSM–5* and an empirical model of psychopathology. *Personality Disorders: Theory, Research, & Treatment, 1,* 97–118.

Krueger, R. F., Eaton, N. R., Clark, L. A., Watson, D., Markon, K. E., Derringer, J., ... Livesley, W. J. (2011). Deriving an empirical structure of personality pathology for *DSM–5*. *Journal of Personality Disorders, 25,* 170–191.

Krueger, R. F., Hicks, B. M., Patrick, C. J., Carlson, S. R., Iacono, W. G., & McGue, M. (2002). Etiologic connections among substance dependence, antisocial behavior, and personality: Modeling the externalizing spectrum. *Journal of Abnormal Psychology, 3,* 411–424.

Krueger, R. F., & Markon, K. E. (2006). Reinterpreting comorbidity: A model-based approach to understanding and classifying psychopathology. *Annual Review of Clinical Psychology, 2,* 111–133.

Livesley, W. J. (2007). A framework for integrating dimensional and categorical classifications of personality disorder. *Journal of Personality Disorders, 21,* 199–224.

Mischel, W., & Shoda, Y. (1995). A cognitive-affective system theory of personality Reconceptualizing situations, dispositions, dynamics, and invariance in personality structure. *Psychological Review, 102,* 246–268.

Morey, L. C., Hopwood, C. J., Gunderson, J. G., Skodol, A. E., Shea, M. T., Yen, S., & McGlashan, T. H. (2007). Comparison of alternative models for personality disorders. *Psychological Medicine, 37,* 983–994.

Oltmanns, T. F., & Turkheimer, E. (2009). Person perception and personality pathology. *Current Directions in Psychological Science, 18,* 32–36.

Parker, G., Hadzi-Pavlovic, D., Both, L., Kumar, S., Wilhelm, K., & Olley, A. (2004). Measuring disordered personality functioning: To love and to work reprised. *Acta Psychiatrica Scandinavica, 110,* 230–239.

Piedmont, R. L., Sherman, M. F., Sherman, N. C., Dy-Liacco, G. S., & Williams, J. E. (2009). Using the five-factor model to identify a new personality disorder domain: The case for experiential permeability. *Journal of Personality and Social Psychology, 96,* 1245–1258.

Rottman, B. M., Ahn, W., Sanislow, C. A., & Kim, N. S. (2009). Can clinicians recognize *DSM–IV* personality disorders from five-factor model descriptions of patient cases? *American Journal of Psychiatry, 166,* 427–433.

Shiner, R. L. (2005). A developmental perspective on personality disorders: Lessons from research on normal personality development in childhood and adolescence. *Journal of Personality Disorders, 19,* 202–210.

Skodol, A. E., Clark, L. A., Bender, D. S., Krueger, R. F., Livesley, W. J., Morey, L. C., ...Oldham, J. M. (2011). Proposed changes in personality and personality disorder assessment and diagnosis for *DSM–5* part I: Description and rationale. *Personality Disorders: Theory, Research, and Treatment, 2*(1), 4–22.

Strack, S., & Millon, T. (2007). Contributions to the dimensional assessment of personality disorders using Millon's model and the Millon Clinical Multiaxial Inventory (MCMI–III). *Journal of Personality Assessment, 89,* 56–69.

Tackett, J. L., Silberschmidt, A. L., Krueger, R. F., & Sponheim, S. R. (2008). A dimensional model of personality disorder: Incorporating *DSM* Cluster A characteristics. *Journal of Abnormal Psychology, 117,* 454–459.

Trull, T. J., & Durrett, C. A. (2005). Categorical and dimensional models of personality disorder. *Annual Review of Clinical Psychology, 1,* 355–380.

Tyrer, P., Crawford, M., & Mulder, R. (in press). Reclassifying personality disorders. *Lancet.*

Tyrer, P., Mulder, R., Crawford, M., Newton-Howes, G., Simonsen, E., Ndetei, D., & Barrett, B. (2010). Personality disorder: A new global perspective. *World Psychiatry, 9,* 56–60.

Verheul, R., Andrea, H., Berghout, C. C., Dolan, C., Busschbach, J. J. V., Van Der Kroft, P. J. A., & Fonagy, P. (2008). Severity indices of personality problems (SIPP-118): Development, factor structure, reliability, and validity. *Psychological Assessment, 20,* 23–34.

Watson, D., Clark, L. A., & Chmielewski, M. (2008). Structures of personality and their relevance to psychopathology: II. Further articulation of a comprehensive unified trait structure. *Journal of Personality, 76*, 1545–1585.

Westen, D., & Shedler, J. (2007). Personality diagnosis with the Shedler–Westen Assessment Procedure (SWAP): Integrating clinical and statistical measurement and prediction. *Journal of Abnormal Psychology, 116*, 810–822.

Widiger, T. A. (2007). Dimensional models of personality disorder. *World Psychiatry, 6*, 79–83.

Widiger, T. A., Simonsen, E., Krueger, R., Livesley, W., & Verheul, R. (2005). Personality disorder research agenda for *DSM–V*. *Journal of Personality Disorders, 19*, 315–338.

Widiger, T. A., Simonsen, E., Sirovatka, P. J., & Regier, D. A. (Eds.). (2006). *Dimensional models of personality disorders: Refining the research agenda for DSM–V*. Washington, DC: American Psychiatric Publishing.

Zimmerman, M., & Mattia, J. I. (1999). Psychiatric diagnosis in clinical practice: Is comorbidity being missed? *Comprehensive Psychiatry, 40*, 182–191.

Toward a Model for Assessing Level of Personality Functioning in *DSM–5*, Part I: A Review of Theory and Methods

Donna S. Bender,[1] Leslie C. Morey,[2] and Andrew E. Skodol[1]

[1]*Department of Psychiatry, University of Arizona College of Medicine*
[2]*Department of Psychology, Texas A & M University*

Personality disorders are associated with fundamental disturbances of self and interpersonal relations, problems that vary in severity within and across disorders. This review surveyed clinician-rated measures of personality psychopathology that focus on self–other dimensions to explore the feasibility and utility of constructing a scale of severity of impairment in personality functioning for *DSM–5*. Robust elements of the instruments were considered in creating a continuum of personality functioning based on aspects of identity, self-direction, empathy, and intimacy. Building on preliminary findings (Morey et al., 2011/this issue), the proposed Levels of Personality Functioning will be subjected to extensive empirical testing in the *DSM–5* field trials and elsewhere. The resulting version of this severity measure is expected to have clinical utility in identifying personality psychopathology, planning treatment, building the therapeutic alliance, and studying treatment course and outcome.

A recent study (Hopwood et al., 2011) of patients with personality disorders (PDs) participating in the Collaborative Longitudinal Personality Disorders Study (Gunderson et al., 2000) suggested that, in assessing personality psychopathology, "generalized severity is the most important single predictor of concurrent and prospective dysfunction." The authors concluded that PD might best be characterized by a generalized personality severity continuum with additional specification of stylistic elements. This recommendation is consistent with Tyrer's (2005) assertion that severity level must be part of any dimensionally specified system for assessing personality psychopathology. However, to this point there is little specific information about the optimum characterization of severity as related to personality problems.

In the Hopwood et al. (2011) analyses, the *Diagnostic and Statistical Manual of Mental Disorders* (4th ed. [*DSM–IV*]; American Psychiatric Association, 2000) PD items that loaded most highly on the severity dimension were preoccupation with social rejection, fear of social ineptness, feelings of inadequacy, anger, identity disturbance, and paranoid ideation. The importance of these elements is very much consistent with the notion that central disturbances of PDs of all types relate to how one views one's self and other people. Similarly, earlier analyses by Morey (2005) have demonstrated that difficulties in empathic capacity, at varying levels, can be found at the core of all types of personality psychopathology. This idea is consistent with Ronningstam's (2009) contention that narcissism—which involves problems with the self and views of others—is much more pervasive in various types of character pathology than is currently represented by *DSM–IV* PD diagnoses. In fact, the *DSM–IV* PD criteria are heavily oriented toward self and interpersonal difficulties. Considering these two issues together, the purpose of this review is to consider existing approaches to assessing personality psychopathology on self–other severity

dimensions, and to explore the utility of constructing a scale for *DSM–5* capturing levels of personality functioning, based on self–other problems.

Neither the *DSM–IV* general severity specifiers nor the Axis V GAF Scale, which confounds symptoms and maladaptive functioning, have sufficient specificity for personality psychopathology to be useful as personality functioning measures. The M-Axis Profile of Mental Functioning approach in the *Psychodynamic Diagnostic Manual* (*PDM*; PDM Task Force, 2006) is a useful model as it includes psychologically based dimensions such as capacity for relationships and quality of internal experience. However, there are nine separate dimensions that need to be rated, which is overly complex for incorporation into a single, integrated personality psychopathology continuum. Furthermore, the psychometric characteristics of the M-Axis have yet to be established. Nevertheless, it was determined by the Personality and Personality Disorders Work Group that psychological processes common to all PDs should make up a new personality functioning scale, as behavioral indicators can be vastly multidetermined and span both symptom and PDs. They subsequently proposed that a scale be developed for the updated *DSM* that would allow clinicians to denote not only the existence of personality psychopathology, but also its severity.

One important approach to characterizing severity in personality pathology has involved differentiating problems by assessing contrasts in characteristic patterns of thinking about self and self-in-relation-to-others (e.g., Blatt & Lerner, 1983; Dorpat, 1974; Kernberg, 1987; Lerner & St. Peter, 1984; Masterson, 1988). Kernberg (1970/1989) was one of the first contemporary writers to formulate a classification of character pathology that encompasses personality types arrayed along a severity continuum. A central component of Kernberg's system is the quality of an individual's mental representations of self and others (object relations). Livesley and Jang (2000) have conceptualized personality problems as difficulties in three self–other focused realms: (a) the adaptive self-system, allowing the individual to create and maintain integrated representations of self and others; (b) the capacity for intimacy; and (c) the ability to function effectively in society. Dimaggio, Semerari, Carcione,

Procacci, and Nicolo (2006) have asserted that individuals with personality disorders "possess problematical self-states, inadequate self-representations and restricted self-narratives, and poor self-reflection and self-regulatory strategies" (p. 610).

The deficits described by these authors are likely to result from processes of temperament, development, and environment that have been shown to influence how an individual typically views himself or herself and others. These processes have been characterized from a number of other perspectives. For example, Bowlby (1969), a pioneer in the area of development and attachment theory, posited that individuals develop their own "internal working models" to help them understand the external world, particularly interactions with other people. Although much exists in the literature concerning secure versus insecure styles of attachment, PDs are often associated with insecure status (e. g., Bender, Farber, & Geller, 1997; West, Keller, Links, & Patrick, 1993; West & Sheldon-Keller, 1994). Fonagy and Bateman (2009) elaborated on this model by describing four mental representational systems implicated in attachment:

1) expectations of interactive attributes of early caregivers created in the first year of life and subsequently elaborated; 2) event representations by which general and specific memories of attachment-related experiences are encoded and retrieved; 3) autobiographical memories by which specific events are conceptually connected because of their relationship to a continuing personal narrative and developing self-understanding; and 4) understanding of the psychological characteristics of other people and differentiating them from the characteristics of the self. (p. 211)

Thus, individuals function with a complex set of assumptions about the interpersonal world that have been shaped by early experiences with caregivers and are then generalized to relationships later in life.

Working from a social-cognitive perspective, Anderson and Cole (1990) explored the idea that individuals create social categories based on their preexisting mental models of significant others. Participants were given a series of cognitive tasks including listing features of four categories of people: significant other, nonsignificant other, stereotype, and type defined by a trait. Memory retrieval tests demonstrated that the significant other representations were more cognitively accessible and contained more distinctive information than the other categories. Participants were then exposed to descriptions of fictional individuals and asked to recall features after a brief distracter task. If the new figure triggered the significant other category, it was more likely assimilated into that category, with inappropriate attribution of preconceived features that were, in fact, quite inaccurate when compared to the original new figure description. This suggests that significant other representations have a much more powerful influence on perceptions of new people than categories based on other individuals or sets of factors.

Although such biases occur in individuals without PDs, studies suggest that these tendencies are even more pronounced in people with personality psychopathology. There is an extensive literature demonstrating that PDs are associated with distorted thinking about self and others. For example, Salvatore, Nicolo, and Dimaggio (2005) illustrated how patients with paranoid personality typically see themselves as weak and inadequate, while viewing others as hostile and deceitful. Patients with narcissistic PD have been found to have dominant states of mind that are

pervaded by distrust toward others and feelings of either being excluded or harmed (Dimaggio et al., 2008). Jovev and Jackson (2004) demonstrated that individuals with avoidant PD utilize maladaptive schemas centering on a self that is defective and shame-ridden, expecting to be abandoned because of their shortcomings, and persons with obsessive–compulsive PD were burdened by a schema of self-imposed, unrelenting standards. Several studies have found borderline patients' representations of self and others to be more elaborated and complicated than those of other types of patients, but also more distorted and biased toward hostile attributions (e.g., Blatt & Lerner, 1983; Lerner & St. Peter, 1984; Stuart et al., 1990, Westen, Ludolph, Lerner, Ruffins, & Wiss, 1990). Likewise, patients with borderline personality disorder (BPD) are significantly more likely to assign negative attributes and emotions to the picture of a face with a neutral expression (Donegan et al., 2003; Wagner & Linehan, 1999). Such representational styles are also evident in treatment: Patients with BPD show the most difficulty in creating a helpful mental image of treatment providers and the treatment relationship, compared with patients with other PDs or Axis I disorders only (Bender et al., 2003; Zeeck, Hartmann, & Orlinsky, 2006). These studies support the notion that maladaptive patterns of mentally representing self and others serve as the substrates for personality psychopathology common to a wide range of conceptualizations (e.g., psychodynamic, cognitive-behavioral, interpersonal, and trait) of core impairments (Bender & Skodol, 2007).

To be clear, we are not suggesting that a scale based on mental representations of self and others covers all domains of PD phenomena. What we do suggest is that such a scale can capture central functions common to all the disorders—common to all people, for that matter—and allow clinicians to identify the presence and severity of personality psychopathology, not a particular PD type. Additional specification of personality pathology phenomena such as disorder-characteristic behaviors and emotions will be elaborated in other parts of the model proposed for *DSM–5* by the Personality and Personality Disorders Work Group (Skodol et al., 2011).

REVIEW OF MEASURES

Our intention in this review is to consider a representative group of measures structured as continua to assess levels of functioning pertaining to mental representations of self and others. Because the *DSM* is used predominantly to assess information provided in clinical settings, we chose instruments that are typically applied to clinical interview information. More specifically, to guide our choice of relevant measures to review, we established a series of criteria. Each instrument should (a) contain salient mental functioning dimensions, rather than categories; (b) have a self–other focus; (c) have been employed in studies with general clinical samples, personality-disordered samples, or both; (d) feature central concepts and components useful to a broad range of clinicians; (e) be applicable to rating clinical interview material (self-reports were not included as clinical assessments utilizing the *DSM* are not typically self-report in nature); and (f) have published psychometric data on relevant domains of functioning. Table 1 summarizes the format, constituent dimensions, and scoring of the measures considered. Results of a number of studies demonstrating the clinical utility

PERSONALITY ASSESSMENT IN THE DSM-5

TABLE 1.—Summary of dimensional measures.

Measure	The Quality of Object Relations Scale (QORS; Azim, Piper, Segal, Nixon, & Duncan, 1991; Piper, McCallum, & Joyce, 1996)
Format	Four domains are assessed using data from two 1-hr interviews. Information in four domains is used to assign one of five levels of relations.
Dimensions	Assessment of four domains (behavioral manifestations, affect regulation, self-esteem regulation, antecedents) leading to one dimension rating quality of object relations: 9 = Mature, 7 = Triangular, 5 = Controlling, 3 = Searching, 1 = Primitive
Measure	Personality Organization Diagnostic Form, versions I and II (PODF–I & PODF–II; Diguer & Normandin, 1996; Diguer et al. 2001; Hebert et al., 2003; Gamache et al., 2009)
Format	Can be applied to a wide variety of clinical information, including intakes, therapy sessions, relationship narratives, and descriptions of self and other people. The latest version has five dimensions. Identity is rated on a 7-point scale, ranging from –3 (*identity diffusion*) to 3 (*identity integration*). The defenses and reality testing dimensions are rated on 4-point scales, ranging from 0 (*absence*) to 3 (*frequent*). The object relations dimension has five levels, four of which have subtypes.
Dimensions	Five dimensions comprised of 20 items: 1. Identity (.88), Experience of self (.78), Self-perceptions (.79), Experience in time (.78), Behavior-emotion integration (.86), Object perceptions (.80), Empathy 2. Primitive defenses, Denial (.75), Splitting, Omnipotence, Omnipotent control, Primitive devaluation 3. Mature defenses, Mature idealization, Mature devaluation, Isolation, Rationalization or intellectualization, Denigration or suppression 4. Reality testing, Self–other differentiation (.80), Hallucinations (.81), Evaluation of social norms, Inappropriateness 5. Object relations ratings on one item, Symbiotic with fear of annihilation, Low-level borderline, with fear of the object (subtypes: schizotypal, schizoid, and paranoid), Low-level borderline, with exploitation and control of object (subtypes: antisocial and malignant narcissist), High-level borderline with fear of abandonment and aloneness (subtypes: borderline, narcissistic, sadomasochistic, histrionic, dependent), Triadic with fear of retaliation (subtypes: depressive, obsessive–compulsive, hysterical)
Measure	Object Relations Inventory (ORI; Bers, Blatt, Sayward, & Johnston, 1993; Blatt et al., 1979; Diamond et al., 1991)
Format	Three measures are presented here that have predominantly been used with open-ended descriptions of self and significant others.
Dimensions	Three measures: A. Differentiation-Relatedness Scale (10 levels) (.86) ranging from: 1. Self/other boundary compromise 2. Self/other boundary confusion 3. Self/other mirroring 4. Self/other idealization/denigration 5. Semidifferentiated, tenuous consolidation of representations through splitting and/or by an emphasis on concrete part properties 6. Emergent, ambivalent constancy (cohesion) of self and an emergent sense of relatedness 7. Consolidated, constant (stable) self and other in unilateral relationships 8. Cohesive, individuated, empathically related self and others 9. Reciprocally related, integrated unfolding, self and others 10. Creative, integrated constructions of self and other in empathic, reciprocally attuned relationships B. Conceptual Level Scale (9 levels) (.80–.99) Sensorimotor-preoperational (Score 1) Concrete-perceptual (Score 3) External iconic (Score 5) Internal iconic (Score 7) Conceptual (Score 9) C. Self-Description Scales—Made up of four dimensions, each made up of several subdimensions 1. Sense of agency (weak–strong; striving; negative–positive self-regard) 2. Sense of relatedness (articulation of relationships [.96]; cold–warm to others; negative–positive view of others) 3. Cognitive-affective variables (depression, self-reflectivity, tolerance of contradictory aspects; differentiation and integration [.76]) 4. Use of dimensions (conceptual level; substantiality [.82])
Measure	Social Cognition and Object Relations Scale (SCORS; Hilsenroth, Stein, & Pinsker, 2004; Westen, Barends, Leigh, Mendel, & Silbert, 1990)
Format	Versions for use with Thematic Apperception Test stories and interview data, along with the latest, which is used with relational narratives and self-statements that are communicated to clinicians during treatment sessions. Eight dimensions scored on a 7-point scale.
Dimensions	Eight dimensions: 1. Complexity, 2. Affective quality (.81), 3. Emotional investment in relationships (.75), 4. Emotional investment in morals, 5. Social causality (.76), 6. Experience and management of aggression (.83), 7. Self-esteem (.80), 8. Identity
Measure	Reflective Functioning Scale (RFS; Fonagy et al., 1998)
Format	The RFS is applied to interview data obtained using the Adult Attachment Interview. One dimension is scored using an 11-point scale.
Dimensions	One dimension rating ability to self-reflect or mentalize (.86–.91): Negative reflective functioning (Score = –1), Absent reflective functioning (Score = 1), Questionable reflective functioning (Score = 3), Ordinary reflective functioning (Score = 5), Marked reflective functioning (Score = 7), Exceptional reflective functioning (Score = 9)

Note. Figures in parentheses indicate the reliability of dimensions with an intraclass correlation of .75 or better.

of each measure are summarized and illustrated with more detailed examples of the results of selected, representative studies.

The preceding criteria resulted in ruling out a number of instruments that might otherwise seem applicable (and are not listed in our review). For example, the McGill Object Relations Scale (Dymetryszyn, Bouchard, Bienvenu, de Carufel, & Gaston, 1997) specifies pertinent dimensions but demands extensive psychoanalytic knowledge (Huprich & Greenberg,

2003) and so was not included. Tyrer's (2005) proposed severity measure is tied to *DSM–IV* PD categorical diagnoses and does not reflect a self–other perspective. The Thematic Patterning Scale of Object Representations–II (Geller et al., 1992) is highly relevant but its psychometric attributes have never been adequately established in the literature. Further, there are a number of attachment measures available but most yield an attachment style category designation (the exception is the Reflective Functioning Scale, which is reviewed later).

The Quality of Object Relations Scale

The Quality of Object Relations Scale (QORS; Azim, Piper, Segal, Nixon, & Duncan, 1991; Piper, McCallum, & Joyce, 1996) was developed explicitly to evaluate both the level and quality of individuals' lifelong patterns of thinking about and forming relationships: "QOR is defined as a person's internal enduring tendency to establish certain types of relationships that range along an overall dimension from primitive to mature" (Piper, Ogrodniczuk, & Joyce, 2004, p. 348). To use the QORS two, 1-hr interviews are conducted 1 week apart and data are rated on four domains: behavioral manifestations (typical relationship patterns), affect regulation, self-esteem regulation, and antecedent (etiological) factors (past events or relationships that influence level of functioning). These four ratings are then weighted and aggregated into an overall dimensional score, a 5-point scale, with the following levels: primitive, searching, controlling, triangular and mature. Each is scored 1, 3, 5, 7, and 9, respectively, as the anchor points, and has criteria associated with the four domains. For example, two criteria associated with self-esteem regulation for the primitive level are: 1. Self-esteem dependent on idealization and/or devaluation of objects; and 2. Feelings of grandiosity and/or inferiority in relation to objects. On the other end of the continuum, a criterion for the mature level of self-esteem is: Self-esteem dependent on equitable receiving from and giving to objects (Piper et al., 2004).

The psychometric properties of the QORS include interclass correlation coefficients (ICCs) ranging from .50 to .72 for the overall level dimension (Piper & Duncan, 1999; Piper et al., 2004). The measure has been used extensively in psychotherapy research studies, and Piper and Duncan (1999) summarized evidence of concurrent and predictive validity. The primary research team has shown in a series of studies (Ogrodniczuk, Piper, Joyce & McCallum, 1999; Piper et al., 1991; Piper, Boroto, Joyce, McCallum, & Azim, 1995; Piper, Joyce, McCallum, & Azim, 1993, 1998; Piper, McCallum, Joyce, Rosie, & Ogrodniczuk, 2001; Piper et al., 2004) that quality of object relations as measured by the QORS is an important moderating variable in the development of a therapeutic alliance and for treatment outcome. For example, for patients with high QOR, analyses of the relationship among several alliance indicators (therapist-rated and patient-rated) and outcome variables (anxiety, depression, general symptomatic distress, and patient and therapist usefulness ratings) found that the average level of alliance was positively correlated with good treatment outcome (e.g., patient-rated alliance was highly correlated with patient-rated treatment usefulness [$r = .82$] and therapist-rated reflective alliance was associated with patient-rated usefulness [$r = .60$; Piper et al., 1995]. Experience of improvement in the alliance, rather than average alliance, was more important for achieving positive outcomes for low QOR patients (e.g., hi-

erarchical linear modeling change analyses revealed a significant relationship between change in therapist-rated, reflective alliance and patient-rated usefulness). Another study comparing QOR and other functioning measures assessing the areas of interpersonal functioning, psychiatric symptoms, self-esteem, and life satisfaction, found that QOR was the best predictor of both patient- and therapist-rated alliance, as well as general and target-specific improvement as a result of treatment (e.g., patient-rated alliance was inversely related to posttherapy outcome assessment of achievement of individualized objectives; $r = -.52$, $p < .001$; Piper et al., 1991). Several other studies showed that high and low QOR patients reacted differently to the same kinds of therapeutic interventions (Ogrodniczuk et al., 1999; Piper et al., 1991; Piper et al., 1993, Piper et al., 1998; Piper et al., 2001). These findings support the idea that it is important to have an understanding of the nature of a patient's ways of thinking about self and others to address alliance issues that shape treatment outcome.

A review paper by Piper and Duncan (1999) demonstrated that low-QOR patients were more likely to have a PD diagnosis. A recent study (Loffler-Stastka, Ponocny-Seliger, Fischer-Kern, & Leithner, 2005) conducted canonical correlation analyses relating QORS with PD diagnoses, which yielded a solution with two canonical variates or factors (F_1: $R = .637$, $p < .001$; F_2: $R = .553$, $p = .010$, redundancy $= 12.9\%$). The first canonical variate was associated with a positive loading for mature QORS ratings (.61) and negatively correlated with primitive level QOR (−.75), and also demonstrated inverse relationships with borderline (−.87), schizotypal (−.51), and antisocial PD (−.50). The second variate was positively associated with higher obsessive–compulsive PD scores (.47) and with lower histrionic PD scores (−.69), as well as negatively associated with controlling level QORS (−.61) designation and triangular QORS (−.70) level.

The requirement of two 1-hr interviews limits this measure's utility for use by a broad range of clinicians doing a *DSM–5* assessment. However, its usefulness for this review lies in its characterizations of various levels of impairment in the self and other realm. Furthermore, researchers using this measure have demonstrated that the qualities of self–other representations—object relations—are strongly related to therapeutic alliance and to outcome, and that different PDs are associated with different levels of the QORS.

Personality Organization Diagnostic Form, versions I and II

The original Personality Organization Diagnostic Form (PODF–I; Diguer & Normandin, 1996) was constructed to operationalize Kernberg's model of personality organization, which includes three levels: psychotic (PPO; including schizoid, schizotypal, and paranoid types), borderline (BPO; including antisocial, narcissistic, borderline, passive-aggressive, dependent, and histrionic types), and neurotic (NPO; including depressive-masochistic, obsessive–compulsive, and hysterical subtypes; Hebert et al., 2003). The PODF can be applied to a wide variety of clinical information, including intake evaluations, therapy sessions, relationship narratives, and descriptions of self and other people. In the original version, there were 16 items on four dimensions: identity diffusion, primitive defenses, lack of reality testing, and object relations (the object relations dimension is synonymous with the item assessing it). A global personality organization (GPO) level—psychotic, borderline, or neurotic—is assigned, based on the scoring of the four dimensions.

To improve differential diagnosis and validity, Gamache et al. (2009) made a number of changes to the PODF–II, including the addition of 11 NPO and normal personality items, and adjustments to previously poor-performing or ambiguous items. This resulted in a model with five dimensions rather than four and the renaming of several dimensions: identity, primitive defenses, mature defenses, reality testing, and object relations (more details each of the domains are presented in Table 1). Identity is rated on a 7-point scale, ranging from –3 (*identity diffusion*) to 3 (*identity integration*). The defenses and reality testing dimensions are rated on 4-point scales: 0 = absence, 1 = rare but clear identifiable occurrences of a given item, 2 = moderate occurrence of a given item, 3 = frequent occurrence of a given item. The object relations dimension has five levels, four of which have subtypes: symbiotic with fear of annihilation; low-level borderline, with fear of the object (subtypes: schizotypal, schizoid, and paranoid); low-level borderline, with exploitation and control of object (subtypes: antisocial and malignant narcissist); high-level borderline with fear of abandonment and aloneness (subtypes: borderline, narcissistic, sadomasochistic, histrionic, dependent); and triadic with fear of retaliation (subtypes: depressive, obsessive–compulsive, hysterical). Mean ICCs for the five dimensions range from good (.68 for mature defenses) to excellent (.88 for identity), and the ICC for GPO was .81. The identity items had good to excellent ICCs (.69–.86), fair to good for primitive defenses (.61–.75), poor to fair for mature defenses (.21–.55), and fair to excellent for reality testing items (.63–.81; Gamache et al., 2009).

To explore the PODF–II's construct validity, Gamache et al. (2009) conducted a factor analysis yielding two factors: a borderline–neurotic continuum, and a psychotic factor. Concurrent validity was tested by comparing PODF–II scores with therapists' personality organization diagnoses. The ICCs ranged from moderate (.56) for the reality testing dimension to excellent (.82) for the object relations dimension. Convergent validity with mental health and psychiatric severity was shown to be good, using the Health-Sickness Rating Scale (HSRS; Luborsky, 1975) and a psychiatric severity measure (PS) based on the presence of *DSM–IV* Axis I and Axis II disorders. Correlations between the HSRS global score and PODF–II dimensions and GPO were moderate to high, ranging from –.41 for reality testing to –.71 for primitive defenses, reflecting a large effect size. PODF–II dimensions and PS score correlated at moderate levels, ranging from –.48 for identity (higher identity score is related to lower psychiatric severity) to .53 for primitive defenses (indicating more primitive defenses are associated with greater psychiatric disturbance).

The original PODF was used in a study investigating the hypothesis that progressing from the lowest level of personality organization to the highest would be associated with increasing differentiation between self and other representations, along with greater integration of good and bad elements of representations (Diguer et al., 2004). Results found an increasing level of object differentiation (as represented by conceptual level, see next section) moving from PPO (lowest level) to BPO to NPO (highest level; r = .26). Similarly, the NPO group had more positive self-representations (measured by an affective valence

factor) than the others (r = .39). An additional finding was that psychiatric severity was more strongly related to object dimensions, whereas personality organization was more significantly related to self-dimensions.

Considering the utility of the PODF for *DSM–5*, the use of the measure itself is impractical as it requires extensive training. The value of considering the PODF is the empirical confirmation it has provided that personality psychopathology exists on a continuum as Kernberg suggested. Furthermore, the good reliability and convergent validity of its dimensions, which include a number of self–other attributes, suggest the consideration of these concepts in the development of a new *DSM–5* assessment tool.

Object Relations Inventory

Using cognitive developmental concepts and object relations theory, Blatt and his colleagues constructed an interview protocol and a series of scales for assessing qualities of patients' mental representations of self and other: the Object Relations Inventory (ORI; Bers, Blatt, Sayward, & Johnston, 1993; Blatt & Auerbach, 2003; Blatt, Wein, Chevron, & Quinlan, 1979; Diamond, Blatt, Stayner, & Kaslow, 1991). We consider three of the scales from the ORI. The first is the Conceptual Level of Descriptions of Self and Other (CLS; Blatt, Bers, & Schaffer, 1992; Blatt, Chevron, Quinlan, Schaffer, & Wein, 1992; Blatt et al., 1979), a measure, based on both object relations and Piagetian theoretical concepts, for assessing levels of differentiation, integration, and accuracy in open-ended descriptions of significant others. The lowest level of this 9-point scale (see Table 1 for all levels) is Level 1, sensorimotor preoperational, which is defined as "Persons are described primarily in terms of the gratification or frustration they provide. There is little sense that others exist as entities separate and independent of their direct effect on the individual's pleasure or pain" (Blatt, Auerbach, & Levy, 1997, p. 360). The highest Level 9, conceptual level, is defined as "Using a range of levels, the description integrates external appearances and activities (behavior) with internal dimensions (feelings, thoughts, and values). Apparent contradictions are resolved in an integrated, complex, coherent synthesis" (Blatt et al., 1997, p. 360). The manual (Blatt, Chevron, et al., 1992) has reported interrater reliability of .88 for CLS scores, and selected other studies (Blatt, Stayner, Auerbach, & Behrends, 1996; Blatt, Wiseman, Prince-Gibson, & Gatt, 1991) have shown interrater reliabilities of .80 to .99. Construct and convergent validity have been demonstrated (Blatt & Auerbach, 2003; Bornstein & O'Neill, 1992).

Another measure that is part of this system is the Differentiation-Relatedness Scale (D–RS; Diamond et al., 1991), which addresses the degree to which a person possesses an individuated sense of self and maturity of interpersonal relatedness. This scale has been described as being "based on the assumption that psychological development moves toward the emergence of (a) a consolidated, integrated, and individuated sense of self-definition and (b) empathically attuned, mutual relatedness with significant others" (Blatt & Auerbach, 2003, p. 275). The D–RS is a 10-point scale (all points shown in Table 1) ranging from the lowest level of 1—"self/other boundary compromise"—to Level 10, which is described as "creative, integrated constructions of self and other in empathic, reciprocally attuned relationships." Interrater reliability has been reported as .86 (Blatt et al., 1996; Diamond, Kaslow, Coonerty, & Blatt,

1990), and several studies support convergent and construct validity of this measure in assessing differentiation-relatedness (e.g., Blatt et al., 1996; Diamond et al., 1990).

The CLS and the D–RS have been used in a number of studies over the course of three decades to study psychopathology and therapy process. Selected examples will be presented here. Gruen and Blatt (1990) qualitatively analyzed patient descriptions of mother, father, self, and therapist at intake and every 6 months until termination for psychiatrically hospitalized patients using responses obtained with the ORI interview procedure. They found that by 6 months, there were already shifts in the descriptions indicating increased differentiation and ambivalence and less polarized views. For instance, at admission, one patient described her mother in completely negative terms: "worried, aggressive, unhappy, and lonely." By 6 months, the patient had progressed to a more ambivalent view of her mother, able to add "caring" to the negative attributes. Another assessment by Blatt et al. (1991) relating Global Assessment of Functioning Scale (GAS) scores to attributes of mother, father, and therapist descriptions concluded that change in clinical functioning from admission to discharge is significantly correlated with changes in the conceptual level (CL; representing degree of differentiation and articulation) associated with mental representations of parents (partial correlation between GAS and a combined mother and father score and CL: $r = .76$. Similarly, using the CLS, D-RS, or both, several other studies demonstrated improvements in degree of differentiation and integration of significant other representations over the course of treatment, and as related to symptom improvement (Bender et al., 1997; Blatt & Auerbach, 2001; Diamond et al., 1990; Lindgren, Werbart, & Philips, 2010; Vermote et al., 2010). Changes on the D–RS and CLS have also been shown to correlate with functioning improvements in adolescent populations (Besser & Blatt, 2007; Blatt et al., 1996; Harpaz-Rotem & Blatt, 2009).

Bers et al. (1993) developed a companion instrument to the self scale of the CLS with the intent of capturing richer characterizations of self-descriptions beyond CL. This instrument—Self-Description Scales (S-DS)—is made up of four dimensions, each made up of several subdimensions: (a) sense of agency (weak–strong; striving; negative–positive self-regard); (b) sense of relatedness (articulation of relationships; cold–warm to others; negative–positive view of others); (c) cognitive-affective variables (depression, self-reflectivity, tolerance of contradictory aspects; differentiation and integration); and (d) use of dimensions (conceptual level; substantiality). Interrater reliabilities of .62 to .96 have been reported for the subdimensions of the scale (Bers, Blatt, & Dolinsky, 2004; Bers et al., 1993; Docherty, Cutting, & Bers, 1998).

One example of the application of the S-DS is a study comparing psychiatric inpatients (many of whom had PDs) with nonpatients (Bers et al., 1993). Patients' self-descriptions had more negative self-regard ($d = .85$), expressed more depressive feelings ($d = -.78$) and expressed a lack of effectiveness as measured by the weak–strong dimension ($d = .75$), and were less differentiated and integrated ($d = 1.06$), compared with the self-descriptions of nonpatients. Over the course of treatment, patients' self-descriptions became more positive and effective, more differentiated, with more references to relatedness and agency; these changes were consistent with improvements in clinical functioning.

The CLS, D–RS, and the S-DS have been employed extensively in studies of psychopathology and treatment process and outcome, and have consistently shown clinical utility. Although the scales themselves require training that is likely beyond the scope of what *DSM–5* could accommodate, the empirical evidence suggests that the concepts measured should be considered in the development of a new scale. In addition, most of the studies already mentioned used brief written or verbal descriptions of self and significant others as the clinical assessment material to which the scales were applied. This type of information is easily obtained in the course of a clinical interview and suggests that routinely asking patients to describe themselves and others could be easily incorporated into standard *DSM–5* assessment practice.

Social Cognition and Object Relations Scale

One frequently used measure is the Social Cognition and Object Relations Scale (SCORS; Hilsenroth, Stein, & Pinsker, 2004; Westen, Barends, Leigh, Mendel, & Silbert, 1990), which has several different versions designed to score narrative material such as clinical interviews, Thematic Apperception Test (TAT) stories, and psychotherapy transcripts (Westen, Barends, et al., 1990; Westen, Lohr, Silk, Gold, & Kerber, 1990). There are several versions of this measure and the characteristics and psychometrics of the two most used in PD research will be mentioned here. The earlier version of SCORS (Westen, 1991; Westen et al., 1990) integrated social cognition and object relations theory and assesses four dimensions: (a) complexity of representations of people; (b) affect-tone of relationship paradigms; (c) capacity for emotional investment in relationships and moral standards; and (d) understanding of social causality. These dimensions are rated on 5-point scales, with the lowest level of 1 representing developmentally immature or pathological representations that are poorly differentiated, malevolent, self-preoccupied, and illogical to mature Level 5, where representations are complex, predominantly positive, with an autonomous self in committed relationships with others and an appreciation for a range of mental processes in self and others. Porcerelli et al. (2006) demonstrated the convergent validity of SCORS for performance-based data, as well as its utility as an outcome measure in assessing clinical treatment. Interrater reliability was reported as an ICC of .75. A study by Porcerelli, Cogan, and Hibbard (1998) utilized the interview version (Westen, Berends, et al., 1990) of SCORS. Pearson interrater reliability was reported for each of the four dimensions: complexity, .71; affect tone, .96; emotional investment, .95; social causality, .93.

A more recent version of SCORS has been developed (Hilsenroth et al., 2004) that is applicable to relational narratives and self-statements that are communicated to clinicians during treatment sessions. This version consists of eight dimensions: complexity (richness of self–other representations and integration of positive and negative attributes); affective quality (assesses positive/negative expectations from others and how patient describes relationships); emotional investment in relationships (level of commitment and emotional sharing); emotional investment in morals (distinguishes between showing no remorse for selfish actions and genuine thoughtfulness about moral questions); social causality (extent of understanding about why people behave the way they do); experience and management of aggression (degree and quality of expressed aggression); self-esteem (affective quality of self-representation); and identity (level of identity integration and goal-directed behavior). Each dimension is scored on a 7-point anchored scale, with lower scores indicating greater psychopathology and higher scores greater psychological health (Peters, Hilsenroth, Eudell-Simmons, Blagys, & Handler, 2006). A study by Peters et al. (2006) of the SCORS–II reliability and validity reported ICCs of .61 to .83, and demonstrated the convergent validity of SCORS as a measure of psychiatric, social-occupational, and interpersonal functioning, as well as personality psychopathology when applied to clinical material produced by patients in treatment.

The SCORS has been utilized extensively over the past two decades in psychopathology and treatment research; several pertinent studies are summarized here. For example, Westen, Lohr, et al. (1990) found that borderline patients scored significantly lower on all four SCORS dimensions, compared with normal participants, and had lower ratings on affect-tone and capacity for emotional investment than patients with major depression and no BPD. In another study of an adolescent population (Westen, Ludolph, et al., 1990), borderline patients were compared to normals and other nonborderline psychiatric patients. Results indicated that patients with BPD, although having complex object representations, were significantly different than the other two groups in having more malevolence in representations of others, difficulty in seeing other people beyond their ability to be need-gratifying, and illogical attributions of motivations to others.

Tramantano, Javier, and Colon (2003) identified three possible subtypes of borderline personality using the SCORS that were based on differing interpersonal styles—moving away, against, or toward others. They demonstrated that patients with BPD have more malevolent views of others compared with non-BPD patients. Greater malevolence was evident, for example, in the finding that the BPD groups differed from the non-BPD control group on the SCORS Affect-Tone scale (computed effect size $r = .57$). Another study showed significant differences among normal, sociopathic, and psychotic groups on the SCORS capacity for emotional investment in relationships and moral standards dimension, where normal controls scored higher ($d = 1.31$) than a sociopathic group, who in turn scored higher ($d = 0.82$) than a psychotic group (Porcerelli, Hill, & Dauphin, 1995).

The SCORS has also been shown to have utility in understanding affective elements across a spectrum of personality psychopathology. Hibbard, Hilsenroth, Hibbard, and Nash (1995) studied patients with a wide range of PD pathology. Those with more severe personality pathology scored lower than those with less severe personality pathology on the SCORS Affect-Tone scale (computed effect size $r = .28$) indicating greater malevolence associated with more severe PD pathology. Similarly, Peters et al. (2006) showed that a composite score of all eight SCORS (the more recent SCORS clinical version) dimensions and the identity dimension predicted level of PD functioning, and SCORS dimensions also predicted GAF, global relational functioning, and social and occupational functioning.

In a treatment outcome study of PTSD patients, Ford, Fisher, and Larson (1997) found that higher scores on a SCORS composite variable were associated with more favorable treatment outcomes (e. g., Quality of Life Inventory ($r = .62$) and Self-Control Schedule ($r = .43$). Ackerman, Hilsenroth, Clemence,

Weatherill, and Fowler (2000) evaluated how the SCORS was related to PD patients' continuation in group psychopathology. A greater likelihood of continuing in treatment was associated with more disturbed representations of others and expectations of negative experiences or painful affect, accompanied by a higher score on emotional investment in relationships (indicating a desire or capacity for interpersonal engagement).

The SCORS has extensive clinical utility in differentiating among levels and types of psychopathology, and in treatment research. The latest version (Peters et al., 2006) has established that the SCORS is reliable and valid in predicting various types of psychosocial functioning, including levels of personality functioning, using self and interpersonal information produced by patients in the normal course of treatment. These findings support the feasibility of developing a scale for *DSM–5* that would include multifaceted level descriptions of personality functioning that are meaningful for use by practicing clinicians and researchers alike.

Reflective Functioning Scale

The Reflective Functioning Scale (RFS; Fonagy, Target, Steele, & Steele, 1998) assesses the ability to "mentalize"—that is, to understand and interpret one's own and others' mental states and operationalizes mental processes related to attachment described earlier (Fonagy & Bateman, 2009). Although this instrument assesses only one capacity, we believe that the ability to mentalize is important in the assessment of levels of personality functioning. Specifically, impairments in mentalizing function make it difficult to create, maintain, and use stable internal representations of self and other. Furthermore, mentalization assists with modulating affective states, and more fundamentally, it is linked to regulation of the self, including the inhibition of impulsive responses to distress (Fonagy & Target, 2006). Problems with the ability to mentalize might be particularly relevant to narcissistic and borderline difficulties, given the association of these types of pathology with difficulties in considering or integrating multiple perspectives from self and other (Bender, 2009). Research using the reflective functioning (RF) construct is becoming increasingly common, and it has also been suggested that RF should be considered as one mechanism of change in treatment outcome studies (Levy, Clarkin, et al., 2006). Furthermore, it is very similar conceptually to a number of other dimensions in the measures we have reviewed.

The RFS is applied to data obtained from the Adult Attachment Interview (Main & Goldwyn, 1998), a semistructured interview that includes multiple questions about memories of experiences with parents and caregivers. Interviews are recorded and transcribed, and this material is used for the assessment by the RFS. The RFS is an anchored 11-point scale ranging from –1 (*negative reflective functioning;* responses distinctively antireflective, hostile, bizarre, or inappropriate) to 9 (*exceptional reflective functioning;* sophisticated, complex regard to mental states across contexts). Table 1 presents all anchor points. Selected reports of interrater reliability include Pearson correlations of .91 (Fonagy et al., 1996), and .86 (Bouchard et al., 2008), and an ICC of .86 (Levy, Meehan, et al., 2006). Convergent and discriminant validity were demonstrated by Bouchard et al. (2008).

Although the RFS has also been used in child–parent attachment studies, we focus on examples of applications to adult mentalizing and psychopathology here. Pertaining to self and interpersonal functioning in general, a recent study showed a significant positive relationship between RF and dimensions of self-perception ($r = .54$) and communication ($r = .52$) from an operationalized psychodynamic diagnostic structure (Muller, Kaufhold, Overbeck, & Grabhorn, 2006). In the PD realm, Fonagy et al. (1996) found lower RF in patients with BPD compared to patients with other types of PD pathology (computed effect size $r = .38$), and Bouchard et al. (2008) demonstrated that level of RF is significantly inversely ($r = -.29$) related to the number of PDs diagnosed for a given patient.

The RFS has also been utilized in treatment studies. For instance, RF for patients with BPD was shown to significantly improve after 1 year of transference-focused psychotherapy (Levy, Meehan, et al., 2006). Diamond, Stovall-McClough, Clarkin, and Levy (2003) studied RF in both patients and therapists and found that there can be reciprocal influence of level of RF within the treatment dyad (e.g., a therapist who normally has a high level of RF might have a decrement in function when working with certain patients who have low-level RF). Indeed, Bateman and Fonagy (2008) developed a mentalization-based treatment for BPD and demonstrated that patients who had received this treatment for 18 months in a day treatment setting, with 18 months of outpatient follow-up, improved significantly in global functioning (GAF, $d = 75$), treatment utilization (e. g., number of psychiatric hospital days, $d = 1.5$, and number of emergency room visits, $d = 1.4$), vocational functioning (length of employment, $d = .94$), and suicidality (number of suicide attempts, $d = 1.4$), compared to BPD patients in treatment as usual. Further, the patients who received the mentalization-based treatment retained their gains 5 years posttermination.

PROPOSAL OF A SELF–OTHER DIMENSION FOR *DSM–5*

We have reviewed a number of reliable and valid measures that assess personality functioning and psychopathology, and have demonstrated that a self–other dimensional perspective is of significant utility, both clinically and empirically. Numerous studies using these measures have shown that a self–other approach is informative in understanding mental processes associated with personality psychopathology phenomenology, in planning treatment interventions, in anticipating treatment course and outcome, and in measuring change in treatment. Most of the measures evaluated, however, were designed for use by researchers and require extensive training to implement. Thus, it is not practical to simply adopt any individual measure for clinical use in *DSM–5*. At the same time, because many of the concepts measured by these instruments have validity and utility in characterizing levels of personality psychopathology, they serve as the foundation for creating a new scale.

To this end, we synthesized the various concepts across models to form a foundation for rating personality functioning on a continuum. The Personality and Personality Disorder Work Group members reviewed a proposed continuum definition based on this synthesis, leading to a preliminary structure with three broad dimensions in each of the self and interpersonal domains (Skodol et al., 2011):

Self:
1. Identity integration: Regulation of self-states; coherence of sense of time and personal history; ability to experience a

unique self and to identify clear boundaries between self and others; capacity for self-reflection.
2. Integrity of self-concept: Regulation of self-esteem and self-respect; sense of autonomous agency; accuracy of self-appraisal; quality of self-representation (e.g., degrees of complexity, differentiation, and integration).
3. Self-directedness: Establishment of internal standards for one's behavior; coherence and meaningfulness of both short-term and life goals.

Interpersonal:

1. Empathy: Ability to mentalize (create an accurate model of another's thoughts and emotions); capacity for appreciating others' experiences; attention to range of others' perspectives; understanding of social causality.
2. Intimacy: Depth and duration of connection with others; tolerance and desire for closeness; reciprocity of regard and support and its reflection in interpersonal/social behavior.
3. Complexity and integration of representations of others: Cohesiveness, complexity, and integration of mental representations of others; use of other representations to regulate self.

Table 2 suggests an approximation of the correspondence of these domains and their accompanying facets to various elements represented in the measures reviewed earlier. More precise relationships between the domains and facets and the existing research instruments will need to be tested empirically.

REFINEMENT OF THE PROPOSED LEVELS OF PERSONALITY FUNCTIONING

To both validate the dimensional approach of the proposed Levels of Personality Functioning, and to make the continuum more readily usable by clinicians of various disciplines, three subsequent steps were taken to refine the levels: (a) a secondary data analysis; (b) a reduction of elements by retaining only the psychometrically strongest aspects of the various measures surveyed for the levels development; and (c) a synthesis of a and b into a final proposed Levels of Personality Functioning.

Secondary Data Analysis

To explore empirically the validity of a core dimension of personality pathology based on deficits in representations of self and others, Morey et al. (2011/this issue) conducted analyses using specific items from the Severity Indices of Personality Problems (SIPP–118: Verheul et al., 2008) and the General Assessment of Personality Disorder (GAPD: Livesley, 2006) measures that were identified as reliable and discriminating markers of the dimensions identified previously in the preliminary Levels of Personality Functioning. The results of these analyses demonstrated that it is, indeed, possible to delineate a global coherent dimension of personality pathology that is clearly related to the likelihood of receiving any PD diagnosis, as well as to the likelihood of receiving multiple personality diagnoses. Morey and colleagues concluded that, "indicators of this dimension involve important functions related to self (e.g., identity integration, integrity of self-concept) and interpersonal relatedness (e.g., capacity for empathy and intimacy)."

TABLE 2.—Evaluation of measure dimensions

	QORS	PODF	D–RS	CLS	S-DS	SCORS	RFS
Self: Identity integration	X	X	X			X	
Regulation of self-states	X	X	X			X	X
Boundary delineation (self–other differentiation)		X	X	X	X	X	X
Meaningful sense of time and personal history		X					X
Ability to differentiate a unique self from representation of other people		X	X	X		X	X
Self-reflectiveness			X		X	X	X
Self: Integrity of self-concept	X	X	X	X		X	
Self-esteem regulation	X	X			X	X	
Self-respect	X	X				X	
Autonomous agency			X			X	X
Realistic self-appraisal		X				X	
Complex and multifaceted self-representation		X	X	X		X	X
Self: Self-directedness					X	X	
Establishment of reasonable standards		X				X	
Goal-directedness			X			X	X
Interpersonal: Empathy		X	X	X			
Ability to mentalize		X	X	X		X	X
Capacity for identifying with others' experiences		X	X	X			X
Attention to range of others' perspectives	X		X	X			X
Understanding of social causality	X	X	X		X	X	X
Interpersonal: Intimacy	X					X	
Depth and duration of connection with others	X					X	
Tolerance and desire for closeness	X					X	
Reciprocity of regard and support	X		X			X	
Interpersonal: Complexity and integration of representations of others	X		X	X	X	X	
Cohesiveness, complexity, and integration of mental representations of others			X	X	X	X	X
Use of other representations to regulate self	X	X	X	X	X	X	

Note. QORS = Quality of Object Relations Scale; PODF = Personality Organization Diagnostic Form; D–RS = Differentiation-Relatedness Scale; CLS = Conceptual Level of Descriptions of Self and Other; S-DS = Self-Description Scales; SCORS = Social Cognition and Object Relations Scale; RFS = Reflective Functioning Scale.

Simplification Using Most Reliable Elements of Measures

A second step in refining the model involved identifying the most reliable dimensions among those found in the eight measures considered in this review. A criterion ICC threshold of .75 or better was established. Table 1 shows the dimensions that met this criterion and their respective reliabilities.

Synthesis

Using as guidance the example scale set forth by Morey et al. (2011/this issue) and the dimensions retained for use as presented in Table 1, as well as input received from experts during the *DSM–5* public comment process, the Work Group undertook a revision of the levels. It was determined that certain language, such as "mentalize" and "complexity of representations" might be too unfamiliar or rely excessively on a particular theoretical jargon, so adjustments of this sort were also made to the original levels version. Identity integration and integrity of self-concept were seen as greatly overlapping concepts and so were combined to form one facet called identity. The following components were eliminated based on the considerations previously mentioned—regulation of self-states, sense of autonomous agency and quality of self-representation—and the capacity for a range of emotional experience and its regulation was added to the identity domain to capture an affect component that was deemed important. For the interpersonal domain, the complexity and integration of representations of others facet was eliminated, and the term *mentalize* was deleted as well. The resulting revised proposal for the definition of the Levels of Personality Functioning is as follows.

Self:

Identity: Experience of oneself as unique, with boundaries between self and others; coherent sense of time and personal history; stability and accuracy of self-appraisal and self-esteem; capacity for a range of emotional experience and its regulation.

Self-direction: Pursuit of coherent and meaningful short-term and life goals; utilization of constructive and prosocial internal standards of behavior; ability to productively self-reflect.

Interpersonal:

Empathy: Comprehension and appreciation of others' experiences and motivations; tolerance of differing perspectives; understanding of social causality.

Intimacy: Depth and duration of connection with others; desire and capacity for closeness; mutuality of regard reflected in interpersonal behavior.

A complete presentation of the revised Levels of Personality Functioning, including a rating scale with a detailed definition of each level, is included in the Appendix.

DISCUSSION

DSM–IV had no provision for delineating severity of impairment specific to personality functioning. This review has shown that there is considerable evidence that dimensional measures of personality psychopathology based on representations of self and interpersonal relations hold significant clinical utility, particularly in (a) identifying the presence and extent of personality psychopathology, (b) planning treatment, (c) building the thera-peutic alliance, and (d) studying treatment course and outcome. Two of the measures, ORI and SCORS, demonstrate that mean-ingful and multifaceted information regarding views of self and others can be easily and quickly obtained during patient in-terviews. Various core concepts from the reviewed measures serve as the foundation of the Levels of Personality Functioning continuum, derived for consideration in assessing personality functioning in *DSM–5*. Secondary data analyses have provided empirical support for this continuum. This continuum is meant to capture core personality psychopathology common to all PDs, and different types of variation among disorders, such as behav-ioral inhibition and disinhibition, will be elaborated in other parts of the PD model proposed by the *DSM–5* Personality and Personality Disorders Work Group (Skodol et al., 2011).

Impairment in self and interpersonal functioning has been recognized by reviewers of the proposed *DSM–5* model to be consistent with multiple theories of PD and their research bases, including cognitive-behavioral, interpersonal, psychodynamic, attachment, developmental, social cognitive, and evolutionary theories, and to be key aspects of personality pathology in need of clinical attention (Clarkin & Huprich, 2011; Pincus, 2011). A factor-analytic study of existing measures of psychosocial functioning found "self-mastery" and "interpersonal and so-cial relationships" to be two of four major factors measured (Ro & Clark, 2009). Furthermore, the Levels of Personality Functioning constructs align well with the National Institute for Mental Health Research Domain Criterion (RDoC) of "social processes" (Sanislow et al., 2010). The interpersonal dimen-sion of personality pathology has been related to attachment and affiliative systems regulated by neuropeptides (Stanley & Siever, 2010), and variation in the encoding of receptors for these neuropeptides could contribute to variation in complex human social behavior and social cognition, such as trust, altru-ism, social bonding, and the ability to infer the emotional state of others (Donaldson & Young, 2008). Neural instantiations of the "self" and of empathy for others have also been linked to the me-dial prefrontal cortex and other cortical midline structures—the sites of the brain's so-called default network (Fair et al., 2008; Northoff et al., 2006; Preston et al., 2007).

Further empirical work investigating the validity, reliability, and utility of the new Levels of Personality Functioning, as well as of the other elements of the proposed PD assessment, is needed. Of primary importance will be testing the reliability of the new Levels of Personality Functioning Scale as admin-istered by clinicians to patients during conventional diagnostic evaluations. A formal test–retest reliability study is underway in Phase I of the official *DSM–5* Field Trials in 11 large academic settings in the United States and Canada, where two independent clinicians are evaluating patients with and without PDs within a 2-week time frame (Kraemer, Kupfer, Narrow, Clarke, & Regier, 2010). In addition, in these large clinical settings videotapes of patient interviews are being made for review by the Personality and Personality Disorders Work Group to provide expert con-sensus diagnoses and other dimensional ratings against which the validity of the clinician-made diagnoses and other assess-ments will be assessed. All five specific PDs currently proposed for retention in *DSM–5* (i. e., antisocial/psychopathic, avoidant, borderline, obsessive–compulsive, and schizotypal) will be rep-resented in substantial numbers (e.g., $N = 50$) in this field trial, so that the specificity of the levels' ratings for PDs as opposed

to other types of psychopathology and the calibration of the levels' ratings against PDs with varying degrees of severity can be assessed. The feasibility and perceived clinical utility of the levels' ratings will also be assessed at the large academic sites, as well as in a representative sample of U.S. psychiatrists and other volunteer mental health clinicians in "clinical practice" field trials supported by the American Psychiatric Association (Kraemer et al., 2010). Relationship of the levels' ratings to other general measures of adaptive functioning, to *DSM–IV* and *DSM–5* PD diagnoses, and to clinical decision making and prog-nosis is planned for a clinician survey designed by Work Group members. Other types of validity research should also be con-ducted in other geographic, cultural, and clinical settings and with other types of subjects (e.g., nontreatment seeking) to in-crease the generalizability of the levels' rating.

CONCLUSION

This review of existing clinician-rated measures of personal-ity pathology that focus on self–other dimensions suggests that core constructs of personality functioning can be assessed reli-ably using information readily obtainable in a clinical interview. The Levels of Personality Functioning continuum has been de-veloped and proposed for inclusion in the *DSM–5* personality and PDs assessment model, and reliability, validity and clinical utility will be tested extensively in the *DSM–5* field trials and elsewhere. It is expected that the final version of the Levels of Personality Functioning will offer a means of assessing the severity of personality psychopathology, which was heretofore lacking in the *DSM*.

REFERENCES

Ackerman, S. J., Hilsenroth, M. J., Clemence, A. J., Weatherill, R., & Fowler, J. C. (2000). The effects of social cognition and object representation on psychotherapy continuation. *Bulletin of the Menninger Clinic, 64*, 386–408.

American Psychiatric Association. (2000). *Diagnostic and statistical manual of mental disorders* (4th ed.). Washington, DC: Author.

Anderson, S. M., & Cole, S. W. (1990). "Do I know you?": The role of signif-icant others in general social perception. *Journal of Personality and Social Psychology, 59*, 384–399.

Azim, H. F. A., Piper, W. E., Segal, P. M., Nixon, G. W. H., & Duncan, S. (1991). The quality of object relations scale. *Bulletin of the Menninger Clinic, 55*, 323–343.

Bateman, A., & Fonagy, P. (2008). 8-year follow-up of patients treated for bor-derline personality disorder: Mentalization-based treatment versus treatment as usual. *American Journal of Psychiatry, 165*, 631–638.

Bender, D. S. (2009). Therapeutic alliance. In J. M. Oldham, A. E. Skodol, & D. S. Bender (Eds.), *Essentials of personality disorders* (pp. 289–308). Washington, DC: American Psychiatric Publishing.

Bender, D. S., Farber, B. A., & Geller, J. D. (1997). Cluster B personality traits and attachment. *Journal of the American Academy of Psychoanalysis, 29*, 551–563.

Bender, D. S., Farber, B. A., Sanislow, C. A., Dyck, I. R., Geller, J. D., & Skodol, A. E. (2003). Representations of therapists by patients with person-ality disorders. *American Journal of Psychotherapy, 57*, 219–236.

Bender, D. S., & Skodol, A. E. (2007). Borderline personality as a self–other representational disturbance. *Journal of Personality Disorders, 21*, 500–517.

Bers, S. A., Blatt, S. J., & Dolinsky, A. (2004). The sense of self in anorexia-nervosa patients: A psychoanalytically informed method for studying self-representation. *Psychoanalytic Study of the Child, 59*, 294–316.

Bers, S. A., Blatt, S. J., Sayward, H. K., & Johnston, R. S. (1993). Normal and pathological aspects of self-descriptions and their change over long-term treatment. *Psychoanalytic Psychology, 10*, 17–37.

Besser, A., & Blatt, S. J. (2007). Identity consolidation and internalizing and externalizing problem behaviors in early adolescence. *Psychoanalytic Psychology, 24*, 126–149.

Blatt, S. J., & Auerbach, J. S. (2001). Mental representations, severe psychopathology, and the therapeutic process. *Journal of the American Psychoanalytic Association, 49*, 113–159.

Blatt, S. J., & Auerbach, J. S. (2003). Psychodynamic measures of therapeutic change. *Psychoanalytic Inquiry, 23*, 268–307.

Blatt, S. J., Auerbach, J. S., & Levy, K. N. (1997). Mental representations in personality development, psychopathology, and the therapeutic process. *Review of General Psychology, 1*, 351–374.

Blatt, S. J., Bers, A. B., & Schaffer, C. E. (1992). *The assessment of self description*. Unpublished manuscript, Yale University, New Haven, CT.

Blatt, S. J., Chevron, E. S., Quinlan, D. M., Schaffer, C. E., & Wein, S. (1992). *The assessment of qualitative and structural dimensions of object representations*. Unpublished manuscript, Yale University, New Haven, CT.

Blatt, S. J., & Lerner, H. (1983). The psychological assessment of object representation. *Journal of Personality Assessment, 47*, 7–28.

Blatt, S. J., Stayner, D. A., Auerbach, J. S., & Behrends, R. S. (1996). Change in object and self-representations in long-term, intensive, inpatient treatment of seriously disturbed adolescents and young adults. *Psychiatry, 59*, 82–107.

Blatt, S. J., Wein, S., Chevron, E. S., & Quinlan, D. M. (1979). Parental representations and depression in normal young adults. *Journal of Abnormal Psychology, 78*, 388–397.

Blatt, S. J., Wiseman, H., Prince-Gibson, E., & Gatt, C. (1991). Object representations and change in clinical functioning. *Psychotherapy, 28*, 273–283.

Bornstein, R. F., & O'Neill, R. M. (1992). Parental perceptions and psychopathology. *The Journal of Nervous and Mental Disease, 180*, 475–483.

Bouchard, M.-A., Target, M., Lecours, S., Fonagy, P., Tremblay, L.-M., Schachter, A., & Stein, H. (2008). Mentalization in adult attachment narratives: Reflective functioning, mental states, and affect elaboration compared. *Psychoanalytic Psychology, 25*, 47–66.

Bowlby, J. (1969). *Attachment and loss: Vol. IAttachment and loss: Vol.* New York, NY: Basic Books.

Clarkin, J. F., & Huprich, S. K. (2011). Do *DSM–5* personality disorder proposals meet criteria for clinical utility? *Journal of Personality Disorders, 25*, 192–205.

Diamond, D., Blatt, S., Stayner, D., & Kaslow, N. (1991). *The Differentiation-Relatedness Scale of Self and Object Representations*. Unpublished research manual, Yale University, New Haven, CT.

Diamond, D., Kaslow, N., Coonerty, S., & Blatt, S. J. (1990). Changes in separation-individuation and intersubjectivity in long-term treatment. *Psychoanalytic Psychology, 7*, 363–397.

Diamond, D., Stovall-McClough, C., Clarkin, J. F., & Levy, K. N. (2003). Patient–therapist attachment in the treatment of borderline personality disorder. *Bulletin of the Menninger Clinic, 67*, 227–259.

Diguer, L., & Normandin, L. (1996). *The Personality Organization Diagnostic Form (PODF)*. Unpublished manuscript, Universite Laval, Laval, PQ, Canada.

Diguer, L., Pelletier, S., Hebert, E., Descoteaux, J., Rousseau, P., & Daoust, J.-P. (2004). Personality organizations, psychiatric severity, and self and object representations. *Psychoanalytic Psychology, 21*, 259–275.

Dimaggio, G., Nicolo, A., Fiore, D., Centenero, E., Semerari, A., Carcione, A., & Pedone, R. (2008). States of minds in narcissistic personality disorder: Three psychotherapies analyzed using the grid of problematic states. *Psychotherapy Research 18*, 466–480.

Dimaggio, G., Semerari, A., Carcione, A., Procacci, M., & Nicolo, G. (2006). Toward a model of self pathology underlying personality disorders: Narratives, metacognition, interpersonal cycles and decision making processes. *Journal of Personality Disorders, 20*, 597–617.

Docherty, N. M., Cutting, L. P., & Bers, S. A. (1998) Expressed emotion and differentiation of self in the relatives of stable schizophrenic patients. *Psychiatry: Interpersonal and Biological Process, 61*, 269–278.

Donaldson, Z. R., & Young, L. J. (2008). Oxytocin, vasopressin, and the neurogenetics of sociality. *Science, 322*, 900–904.

Donegan, N. H., Sanislow, C. A., Blumberg, H. P., Fulbright, R. K., Lacadie, C., Skudlarski, P., & Wexler, B. E. (2003). Amygdala hyperreactivity in borderline personality disorder: Implications for emotional dysregulation. *Biological Psychiatry, 54*, 1284–1293.

Dorpat, T. L. (1974). Internalization of the patient–analyst relationship in patients with narcissistic disorders. *International Journal of Psycho-Analysis, 55*, 183–188.

Dymetryszyn, H., Bouchard, M. A., Bienvenu, J. P., de Carufel, F., & Gaston, L. (1997). Overall maturity of object relations as assessed by the McGill Object Relations Scale. *Bulletin of the Menninger Clinic, 61*, 44–72.

Fair, D. A., Cohen, A. L., Dosenbach, N. U. F., Church, J. A., Miezen, F. M., Barch, D. M., . . . Schlaggar, B. L. (2008). The maturing architecture of the brain's default network. *PNAS, 105*, 4028–4032.

Fonagy, P., & Bateman, A. W. (2009). Mentalization-based treatment of borderline personality disorder. In J. M. Oldham, A. E. Skodol, & D. S. Bender (Eds.), *Essentials of personality disorders* (pp. 209–233). Washington, DC: American Psychiatric Publishing.

Fonagy, P., Leigh, T., Steele, M., Steele, H., Kennedy, R., Mattoon, G., & Gerber, A. (1996). The relation of attachment status, psychiatric classification, and response to psychotherapy. *Journal of Consulting and Clinical Psychology, 64*, 22–31.

Fonagy, P., & Target, M. (2006). The mentalization-focused approach to self pathology. *Journal of Personality Disorders, 20*, 544–576.

Fonagy, P., Target, M., Steele, H., & Steele, M. (1998). *Reflective-functioning manual, version 5.0, forapplication to adult attachment interviews*. London, UK: University College London.

Ford, J. D., Fisher, P., & Larson, L. (1997). Object relations as a predictor of treatment outcome with chronic posttraumatic stress disorder. *Journal of Consulting and Clinical Psychology, 65*, 547–559.

Gamache, D., Laverdiere, O., Diguer, L., Hebert, E., Larochelle, S., & Descoteaux, J. (2009). The Personality Organization Diagnostic Form: Development of a revised version. *The Journal of Nervous and Mental Disease, 197*, 368–377.

Geller, J. D., Hartley, D., Behrends, R., Farber, B., Andrews, C., Marciano, P., & Brownlow, A. (1992). *Thematic patterning scale of object representations: II*. Unpublished manuscript, Yale University, New Haven, CT.

Gruen, R. J., & Blatt, S. J. (1990). Change in self and object representation during long-term dynamically oriented treatment. *Psychoanalytic Psychology, 7*, 399–422.

Gunderson, J. G., Shea, M. T., Skodol, A. E., McGlashan, T. H., Morey, L. C., Stout, R. L., & Keller, M. B. (2000). The Collaborative Longitudinal Personality Disorders Study: Development, aims, design, and sample characteristics. *Journal of Personality Disorders, 14*, 300–315.

Harpaz-Rotem, I., & Blatt, S. J. (2009). A pathway to therapeutic change: Changes in self-representation in the treatment of adolescents and young adults. *Psychiatry, 72*, 32–49.

Hebert, E., Diguer, L., Descoteaux, J., Daoust, J-P., Rousseau, J-P., Normandin, L., & Scullion, M. (2003). The Personality Organization Diagnostic Form (PODF): A preliminary report on its validity and interrater reliability. *Psychotherapy Research, 13*, 243–254.

Hibbard, S., Hilsenroth, M. J., Hibbard, J. K., & Nash, M.R. (1995). A validity study of two projective object representations measures. *Psychological Assessment, 7*, 432–439.

Hilsenroth, M., Stein, M., & Pinsker, J. (2004). *Social Cognition and Object Relations Scale: Global Method (SCORS–G)*. Unpublished manuscript, The Derner Institute of Advanced Psychological Studies, Adelphi University, Garden City, NY.

Hopwood, C. J., Malone, J. C., Ansell, E. B., Sanislow, C. A., Grilo, C. M., McGlashan, T. H., . . . Morey, L. C. (2011). Personality assessment in *DSM–V*: Empirical support for rating severity, style, and traits. *Journal of Personality Disorders, 25*, 305–320.

Huprich, S. K., & Greenberg, R. P. (2003). Advances in the assessment of object relations in the 1990s. *Clinical Psychology Review, 23*, 665–698.

Jovev, M., & Jackson, H. J. (2004). Early maladaptive schemas in personality disordered individuals. *Journal of Personality Disorders, 18*, 467–478.

Kernberg, O. (1987). An ego psychology–object relations theory approach to the transference. *Psychoanalytic Quarterly, 56*, 197–221.

Kernberg, O. F. (1989). A psychoanalytic classification of character pathology. In R. Lax (Ed.), *Essential papers on character neurosis and treatment* (pp. 191–210). New York, NY: New York University Press. (Original work published 1970)

Kraemer, H. C., Kupfer, D. J., Narrow, W. E., Clarke, D. E., & Regier, D. A. (2010). Moving toward *DSM–5*: The field trials. *American Journal of Psychiatry, 167*, 1158–1160.

Lerner, H. D., & St. Peter, S. (1984). Patterns of object relations in neurotic, borderline, and schizophrenic patients. *Psychiatry, 47*, 77–92.

Levy, K. N., Clarkin, J. F., Yeomans, F. E., Scott, L. N., Wasserman, R. H., & Kernberg, O. F. (2006). The mechanisms of change in the treatment of borderline personality disorder with transference focused psychotherapy. *Journal of Clinical Psychology, 62*, 481–501.

Levy, K. N., Meehan, K. B., Kelly, K. M., Reynoso, J. S., Weber, M., Clarkin, J. F., & Kernberg, O. F. (2006). Change in attachment patterns and reflective function in a randomized control trial of transference-focused psychotherapy for borderline personality disorder. *Journal of Consulting and Clinical Psychology, 74*, 1027–1040.

Lindgren, A., Werbart, A., & Philips, B. (2010). Long-term outcome and posttreatment effects of psychoanalytic psychotherapy with young adults. *Psychology & Psychotherapy: Theory, Research & Practice, 83*, 27–43.

Livesley, W. J. (2006). *General Assessment of Personality Disorder (GAPD)*. Unpublished manuscript, Department of Psychiatry, University of British Columbia, Vancouver, Canada.

Livesley, W. J., & Jang, K. L. (2000). Toward an empirically based classification of personality disorder. *Journal of Personality Disorders, 14*, 137–151.

Loffler-Stastka, H., Ponocny-Seliger, E., Fischer-Kern, M., & Leithner, K. (2005). Utilization of psychotherapy in patients with personality disorder: The impact of gender, character traits, affect regulation, and quality of object-relations. *Psychology and Psychotherapy: Theory, Research and Practice, 78*, 531–548.

Luborsky, L. (1975). Clinician's judgments of mental health: Specimen case descriptions and forms for the Health-Sickness Rating Scale. *Bulletin of the Menninger Clinic, 39*, 448–480.

Main, M., & Goldwyn, R. (1998). *Adult attachment scoring and classification system*. Unpublished manuscript, Department of Psychology, University of California, Berkeley, CA.

Masterson, J. F. (1988). *The search for the real self: Unmasking the personality disorders of our age*. New York, NY: The Free Press.

Morey, L. C. (2005). Personality pathology as pathological narcissism. In M. Maj, H. S. Aklskal, J. E. Mezzich, & A. Okasha (Eds.), *World Psychiatric Association series: Evidence and experience in psychiatry* (pp. 328–331). New York, NY: Wiley.

Morey, L. C., Berghuis, H., Bender, D. S., Verheul, R., Krueger, R. F., & Skodol, A. E. (2011/this issue). Toward a model for assessing level of personality functioning in *DSM–5*, Part II: Empirical articulation of a core dimension of personality pathology. *Journal of Personality Assessment, 93*, 347–353.

Muller, C., Kaufhold, J., Overbeck, G., & Grabhorn, R. (2006). The importance of reflective functioning to the diagnosis of psychic structure. *Psychology and Psychotherapy: Theory, Research and Practice, 79*, 485–494.

Northoff, G., Heinzel, A., de Greck, M., Bermpohl, F., Dobrowolny, H., & Panksepp, J. (2006). Self-referential processing in our brain: A meta-analysis of imaging studies on the self. *Neuroimage, 31*, 440–457.

Ogrodniczuk, J. S., Piper, W. E., Joyce, A. S., & McCallum, M. (1999). Transference interpretations in short-term dynamic psychotherapy. *Journal of Nervous and Mental Disease, 187*, 572–579.

PDM Task Force. (2006). *Psychodynamic diagnostic manual*. Silver Spring, MD: Alliance of Psychoanalytic Organizations.

Peters, E. J., Hilsenroth, M. J., Eudell-Simmons, E. M., Blagys, M. D., & Handler, L. (2006). Reliability and validity of the Social Cognition and Object Relations Scale in clinical use. *Psychotherapy Research, 16*, 617–626.

Pincus, A. L. (2011). Some comments on nomology, diagnostic process, and narcissistic personality disorder in the *DSM–5* proposal for personality and personality disorders. *Personality Disorders: Theory, Research, and Treatment, 2*, 41–53.

Piper, W. E., Azim, H. F. A., Joyce, A. S., McCallum, M., Nixon, G. W. H., & Segal, P. S. (1991). Quality of object relations vs. interpersonal functioning

as predictors of therapeutic alliance and psychotherapy outcome. *Journal of Nervous and Mental Disease, 179*, 432–438.

Piper, W. E., Boroto, D. R., Joyce, A. S., McCallum, M., & Azim, H. F. A. (1995). Pattern of alliance and outcome in short-term individual psychotherapy. *Psychotherapy, 32*, 639–647.

Piper, W. E., & Duncan, S. C. (1999). Object relations theory and short-term dynamic psychotherapy: Findings from the quality of object relations scale. *Clinical Psychology Review, 19*, 669–685.

Piper, W. E., Joyce, A. S., McCallum, M., & Azim, H. F. A. (1993). Concentration and correspondence of transference interpretations in short-term psychotherapy. *Journal of Consulting and Clinical Psychology, 61*, 586–595.

Piper, W. E., Joyce, A. S., McCallum, M., &Azim, H. F. A. (1998). Interpretive and supportive forms of psychotherapy and patient personality variables. *Journal of Consulting and Clinical Psychology, 66*, 558–567.

Piper, W. E., McCallum, M., & Joyce, A. S. (1996). *Manual for assessment of quality of object relations*. Unpublished manuscript, Department of Psychiatry, University of British Columbia, Vancouver, Canada.

Piper, W. E., McCallum, M., Joyce, A. S., Rosie, J. S., & Ogrodniczuk, J. S. (2001). Patient personality and time-limited group psychotherapy for complicated grief. *International Journal of Group Psychotherapy, 51*, 525–552.

Piper, W. E., Ogrodniczuk, J. S., & Joyce, A. S. (2004). Quality of object relations as a moderator of the relationship between pattern of alliance and outcome in short-term individual psychotherapy. *Journal of Personality Assessment, 83*, 345–356.

Porcerelli, J., Cogan, R., & Hibbard, S. (1998). Cognitive and affective representations of people: MCMI–II personality psychopathology. *Journal of Personality Assessment, 70*, 535–540.

Porcerelli, J. H., Hill, K. A., & Dauphin, V. B. (1995). Need-gratifying object relations and psychopathology. *Bulletin of the Menninger Clinic, 59*, 99–104.

Porcerelli, J. H., Shahar, G., Blatt, S. J., Ford, R. Q., Mezza, J. A., & Greenlee, L. M. (2006). Social cognition and object relations scale: Convergent validity and changes following intensive inpatient treatment. *Personality and Individual Differences, 41*, 407–417.

Preston, S. D., Bechara, A., Damascio, H., Grabowski, T. J., Stansfield, R. B., Mehta, S., & Damascio, A. R. (2007). The neural substrates of cognitive empathy. *Social Neuroscience, 2*, 254–275.

Ro, E., & Clark, L. A. (2009). Psychosocial functioning in the context of diagnosis: Assessment and theoretical issues. *Psychological Assessment, 21*, 313–324.

Ronningstam, E. (2009). Narcissistic personality disorder: Facing *DSM–V*. *Psychiatric Annals, 39*, 111–121.

Salvatore, G., Nicolo, G., & Dimaggio, G. (2005). Impoverished dialogical relationship patterns in paranoid personality disorder. *American Journal of Psychotherapy, 59*, 247–265.

Sanislow, C. A., Pine, D. S., Quinn, K. J., Kozak, M. J., Garvey, M. A., Heinssen, R. K., & Cuthbert, B. N. (2010). Developing constructs for psychopathology research: Research domain criteria. *Journal of Abnormal Psychology, 119*, 631–639.

Skodol, A. E., Bender, D. S., Oldham, J. M., Clark, L. A., Morey, L. C., Verheul, R., & Siever, L. J. (2011). Proposed changes in personality and personality disorder assessment and diagnosis for *DSM–5*. Part II: Clinical application. *Personality Disorders: Theory, Research, and Treatment, 2*, 23–40.

Stanley, B., & Siever, L. J. (2010). The interpersonal dimension of borderline personality disorder: Toward a neuropeptide model. *American Journal of Psychiatry, 167*, 24–39.

Stuart, J., Westen, D., Lohr, N., Silk, K., Benjamin, J., Becker, S., & Vorus, N. (1990). Object relations in borderlines, major depressives, and normals: Analysis of Rorschach human figure responses. *Journal of Personality Assessment, 55*, 296–318.

Tramantano, G., Javier, R. A., & Colon, M. (2003). Discriminating among subgroups of borderline personality disorder: An assessment of object representations. *American Journal of Psychoanalysis, 63*, 149–162.

Tyrer, P. (2005). The problem of severity in the classification of personality disorders. *Journal of Personality Disorders, 19*, 309–314.

Verheul, R., Andrea, H., Berghout, C. C., Dolan, C., Busschbach, J. J., Van Der Kroft, P. J. A., & Fonagy, P. (2008). Severity Indices of Personality

Problems (SIPP–118): Development, factor structure, reliability and validity. *Psychological Assessments, 20,* 23–34.

Vermote, R., Lowyck, B., Luyten, P., Vertommen, H., Corveleyn, J., Verhaest, Y., & Peuskens, J. (2010). Process and outcome in psychodynamic hospitalization-based treatment for patients with a personality disorder. *Journal of Nervous & Mental Disease, 198,* 110–115.

Wagner, A. W., & Linehan, M. M. (1999). Facial expression recognition ability among women with borderline personality disorder: Implications for emotion regulation? *Journal of Personality Disorders, 13,* 329–344.

West, M., Keller, A., Links, P., & Patrick, J. (1993). Borderline disorder and attachment pathology. *Canadian Journal of Psychiatry, 18,* 16–22.

West, M. L., & Sheldon-Keller, A. E. (1994). *Patterns of relating: An adult attachment perspective.* New York, NY: Guilford.

Westen, D. (1991). Social cognition and object relations. *Psychological Bulletin, 109,* 429–455.

Westen, D., Barends, A., Leigh, J., Mendel, M., & Silbert, D. (1990). *Social Cognition and Object Relations Scales (SCORS).* Unpublished manuscript, Department of Psychology, University of Michigan, Ann Arbor, MI.

Westen, D., Lohr, N., Silk, K., Gold, L., & Kerber, K. (1990). Object relations and social cognition in borderlines, major depressives, and normals: A Thematic Apperception Test analysis. *Psychological Assessment: A Journal of Consulting and Clinical Psychology, 2,* 355–364.

Westen, D., Ludolph, P., Lerner, H., Ruffins, S., & Wiss, F. C. (1990). Object relations in borderline adolescents. *Journal of the American Academy of Child and Adolescent Psychiatry, 29,* 338–348.

Zeeck, A., Hartmann, A., & Orlinsky, D. E. (2006). Internalization of the therapeutic process: Differences between borderline and neurotic patients. *Journal of Personality Disorders, 20,* 22–41.

APPENDIX

PROPOSED LEVELS OF PERSONALITY FUNCTIONING

Levels of Personality Functioning

Human beings are fundamentally social creatures whose development from birth encompasses adaptation in an interpersonal world. People create mental models of self and others that shape their patterns of emotional, cognitive, and affiliative engagement. Biologically based temperament and environmental factors act to influence how individuals typically view themselves and others. These mental representations reciprocally interact with emotional, cognitive, and behavioral propensities—which together comprise personality. Biological and environmental problems and their interactions can lead to maladaptive mental models of self and others, and to maladaptive patterns of emotional experience and expression, cognition, and behavior. These, in turn, may lead to the development of psychopathology in general and personality pathology in particular.

Like most human tendencies, personality functioning is distributed across a continuum. An optimally functioning person has a complex, fully elaborated, and well-integrated psychological world that includes a mostly positive, volitional, and effective self-concept; a rich, broad, and appropriately regulated emotional life; and the capacity to behave as a well-related, productive member of a society. At the opposite end of the continuum, an individual with severe personality pathology has an impoverished, disorganized, and/or conflicted psychological world that includes a weak, unclear, and ineffective self-concept; a propensity to negative, dysregulated emotions; and a deficient capacity for adaptive interpersonal functioning and social behavior.

Self and Interpersonal Functioning Dimensional Definition

This review of the empirical literature on the dimensional models pertinent to individuals' mental representations of self and others, and subsequent empirical analyses (Morey et al., 2011/this issue), suggest that the following components are most central in comprising a personality functioning continuum:

Self:
Identity: Experience of oneself as unique, with boundaries between self and others; coherent sense of time and personal history; stability and accuracy of self-appraisal and self-esteem; capacity for a range of emotional experience and its regulation
Self-direction: Pursuit of coherent and meaningful short-term and life goals; utilization of constructive and prosocial internal standards of behavior; ability to productively self-reflect

Interpersonal:
Empathy: Comprehension and appreciation of others' experiences and motivations; tolerance of differing perspectives; understanding of social causality
Intimacy: Depth and duration of connection with others; desire and capacity for closeness; mutuality of regard reflected in interpersonal behavior

In applying these dimensions, self and interpersonal difficulties should not be better understood as a norm within an individual's dominant culture.

Self and Interpersonal Functioning Continuum

Although the degree of disturbance of the self and interpersonal domains is continuously distributed, in practice it is useful to consider levels of impairment in functioning for efficient clinical characterization and for treatment planning and prognosis. Patients' conceptualization of self and others affects the nature of interaction with mental health professionals and can have a significant impact on treatment efficacy and outcome. The following continuum uses each of the dimensions just listed to differentiate five levels of self-interpersonal functioning impairment: No, Mild, Moderate, Serious, and Extreme.

Please indicate the level that most closely characterizes the patient's functioning in the self and interpersonal realms:
—— No Impairment
—— Mild Impairment
—— Moderate Impairment
—— Serious Impairment
—— Extreme Impairment

Definitions of Levels

No Impairment:
Self:
Identity: Has ongoing awareness of a unique, volitional self, integrated into past and ongoing personal history. Sense of individuality is not compromised in relationships. Able to recognize and maintain role-appropriate boundaries. Relatively consistent and self-regulated level of positive self-esteem. Accurate or slightly positively biased self-appraisal.

Capable of experiencing, tolerating, and regulating a range of emotions.

Self-direction: Able to set and aspire to reasonable goals based on a realistic assessment of personal capacities. Utilizes appropriate and effective standards of behavior, and able to attain fulfillment in multiple realms. Can reflect on, and make constructive meaning of, internal experience.

Interpersonal:

Empathy: Capable of accurately understanding the full range of others' experiences in most situations. Comprehends and appreciates others' perspectives, even if disagreeing. Is aware of the effect of own actions on others.

Intimacy: Desires and engages in multiple caring, close and reciprocal relationships in personal and community life. Flexibly responds to a range of others' ideas, emotions, and behaviors, striving for cooperation and mutual benefit.

Mild Impairment:
Self:

Identity: Relatively intact sense of self that is unique and grounded in personal history, with some decrease in effectiveness and clarity of interpersonal boundaries when strong emotions and mental conflict are experienced. Self-esteem is somewhat well-regulated, although self-appraisal may be overly or insufficiently self-critical. Emotional experience may be inhibited or restricted in range, and strong emotions may be distressing.

Self-direction: Goal-directed, but may be excessively or somewhat maladaptively so, somewhat goal-inhibited, or conflicted. May have an unrealistic or socially inappropriate set of personal standards, limiting some aspects of fulfillment. Able to reflect upon internal experiences, but may overemphasize a single (e.g., intellectual, emotional) type of self-knowledge rather than integrate all types.

Interpersonal:

Empathy: Somewhat compromised in ability to appreciate and understand others' experiences and differing perspectives. May tend to see others as having unreasonable expectations or a wish for control. Inconsistent in awareness of effect of own behavior on others.

Intimacy: Capacity and desire to form intimate and reciprocal relationships, but may be inhibited in meaningful expression and sometimes constrained by any intense emotion or conflict. Ability to cooperate may be constrained by unrealistic standards. Somewhat limited in ability to respect or respond to the full range of others' ideas, emotions and behaviors.

Moderate Impairment:
Self:

Identity: Excessive other-dependent identity definition, with somewhat compromised boundary delineation, a less differentiated sense of uniqueness, and inconsistency in sense of personal history. Vulnerable self-esteem controlled by exaggerated attunement to external evaluation, with a wish for approval and admiration from other people. Sense of incompleteness or inferiority, with inflated or deflated self-appraisal. Emotional regulation is predicated on the avail-

ability of others in specific ways and/or success in situations that bring external positive appraisal. Threats to self-esteem may engender strong emotions such as rage and shame.

Self-direction: Goals are more often a means of gaining external approval than self-generated, and thus may lack coherence and/or stability. Personal standards may be unreasonably high (e.g., a need to be special or please others) or too low (e.g., not consonant with prevailing social values). Fulfillment is compromised by a sense of lack of authenticity. Impaired capacity to reflect upon internal experience.

Interpersonal:

Empathy: Compromised ability to consider alternative perspectives; hyper-attuned to the experience of others, but only with respect to perceived relevance to self. Generally unaware of or unconcerned about effect of own behavior on others, or unrealistic appraisal of own effect.

Intimacy: Capacity and desire to form relationships, but connections may be superficial and limited to meeting self-regulatory and self-esteem needs. Compromised in ability to respond appropriately to others; conversely has unrealistic expectation of being magically and perfectly understood by others. Tends not to view relationships in reciprocal terms, and cooperates predominantly for personal gain.

Serious Impairment:
Self:

Identity: Sense of unique personal attributes is dysregulated, accompanied by confusion or lack of continuity in personal history. Weak sense of autonomy/agency, and may experience a lack of identity, or emptiness. Boundary definition is poor or rigid; may be overidentification with others, overemphasis on independence from others, or vacillation between these. Fragile self-concept, easily influenced by events and circumstances, and lacking coherence. Self-appraisal is un-nuanced: self-loathing, self-aggrandizing, or an illogical, unrealistic combination. Emotions may be rapidly shifting or a chronic, unwavering feeling of despair.

Self-direction: Difficulty establishing and/or achieving personal goals. Internal standards for behavior are unclear, contradictory, and/or circumstantial. Life is experienced as meaningless or dangerous. Compromised ability to reflect upon and understand one's mental processes.

Interpersonal:

Empathy: Ability to consider and understand the thoughts, feelings and behavior of other people is significantly limited. May discern very specific aspects of others' experience, particularly vulnerabilities and suffering, and destructive motivations are often misattributed to others. Generally unable to consider alternative perspectives, or threatened by a different perspective. Confusion or unawareness of social causality, including the impact of one's actions on others.

Intimacy: Relationships are based on a strong belief in the absolute need for the intimate other(s), and/or expectations of instability, abandonment, and/or abuse. Feelings about intimate involvement with others are unstable, alternating between fear/ rejection and desperate desire for connection. Little mutuality: others are conceptualized primarily

48

in terms of how they affect the self (negatively or positively); focused on what (negative or positive) others have to offer. Cooperative efforts are often disrupted due to the perception of slights from others.

Extreme Impairment:

Self:

Identity: Experience of a unique self is virtually absent as is any sense of continuity of personal history. A sense of agency/autonomy is virtually absent, or is organized around perceived external persecution. Boundaries with others are confused or lacking. Diffuse self-concept, prone to significant distortions in self-appraisal. Personal motivations may be unrecognized and/or experienced as external to self. Hatred and aggression may be dominant affects, are disorganizing and often disavowed and projected.

Self-direction: Poor differentiation of thoughts from actions, so goal-setting ability is severely compromised, goals often are unrealistic, and goal-setting is incoherent. Internal standards for behavior are virtually lacking. Genuine fulfillment is elusive and virtually inconceivable. Profound inability to constructively reflect upon one's experience.

Interpersonal:

Empathy: Pronounced inability to consider and understand others' experience and motivation. Attention to others' perspectives virtually absent (attention is hypervigilant, focused on need-fulfillment and harm avoidance). Social interactions can be confusing and disorienting.

Intimacy: Desire for affiliation is limited because of profound disinterest or expectation of harm. Engagement with others is detached, disorganized or consistently negative. Relationships are conceptualized primarily as power based, and considered in terms of their ability to provide comfort or inflict pain and suffering. Social/ interpersonal behavior is not reciprocal; rather, it represents fundamental approach (e.g., fulfillment of basic needs) and avoidance (e.g., escape from pain) tendencies.

Toward a Model for Assessing Level of Personality Functioning in *DSM–5*, Part II: Empirical Articulation of a Core Dimension of Personality Pathology

LESLIE C. MOREY,[1] HAN BERGHUIS,[2] DONNA S. BENDER,[3] ROEL VERHEUL,[4,5] ROBERT F. KRUEGER,[6] AND ANDREW E. SKODOL[3]

[1]*Department of Psychology, Texas A&M University*
[2]*Symfora Groep Psychiatric Center, Amersfoort, The Netherlands*
[3]*Department of Psychiatry, University of Arizona College of Medicine*
[4]*Faculty of Social and Behavioural Sciences–Clinical Psychology, University of Amsterdam, The Netherlands*
[5]*Viersprong Institute for Studies on Personality Disorders, Amsterdam, The Netherlands*
[6]*Psychology Department, University of Minnesota*

The extensive comorbidity among *Diagnostic and Statistical Manual of Mental Disorders* (4th ed. [*DSM–IV*]; American Psychiatric Association, 1994) personality disorders might be compelling evidence of essential commonalities among these disorders reflective of a general level of personality functioning that in itself is highly relevant to clinical decision making. This study sought to identify key markers of such a level, thought to reflect a core dimension of personality pathology involving impairments in the capacities of self and interpersonal functioning, and to empirically articulate a continuum of severity of these problems for *DSM–5*. Using measures of hypothesized core dimensions of personality pathology, a description of a continuum of severity of personality pathology was developed. Potential markers at various levels of severity of personality pathology were identified using item response theory (IRT) in 2 samples of psychiatric patients. IRT-based estimates of participants' standings on a latent dimension of personality pathology were significantly related to the diagnosis of *DSM–IV* personality disorder, as well as to personality disorder comorbidity. Further analyses indicated that this continuum could be used to capture the distribution of pathology severity across the range of *DSM–IV* personality disorders. The identification of a continuum of personality pathology consisting of impairments in self and interpersonal functioning provides an empirical foundation for a "levels of personality functioning" rating proposed as part of a *DSM–5* personality disorder diagnostic formulation.

Although the *Diagnostic and Statistical Manual of Mental Disorders* (4th ed. [*DSM–IV*]; American Psychiatric Association, 1994) characterized personality disorders (PDs) as 10 discrete categories of personality problems, one of the most consistent findings in the PD literature is that of comorbidity; it is far more common for individuals to receive cooccurring rather than single PD diagnoses. Comorbidity has been cited as an important weakness of the *DSM–IV*, and as a rationale for a dimensional personality pathology system (Widiger, Simonsen, Sirovatka, & Regier, 2006). However, individuals with PDs often tend to lie within similar "regions" of the space defined by dimensional systems, even across dimensional approaches. For example, within the Five-factor personality trait model, a number of different *DSM–IV* PDs demonstrate similar configurations involving high neuroticism, low agreeableness, and low conscientiousness (Morey, Gunderson, Quigley, & Lyons, 2000; Morey et al., 2002; Saulsman & Page, 2004; Zweig-Frank & Paris, 1995). Although often understood as a problem with discriminant validity, comorbidity might also be compelling evidence of essential commonalities among PDs (Krueger & Markon, 2006; Morey, 2005), with presumably distinct criteria sets or personality dimensions tapping into these commonalities.

The *DSM–IV* conceptualization of PD is largely uninformative on PD commonalities. The general criteria for PD involve (a) manifestations in two domains of functioning; (b) enduring inflexibility; (c) clinically significant distress or impairment; (d) temporal stability, and diagnostic primacy relative to (e) other psychiatric or (f) medical conditions. Difficult to operationalize effectively (Livesley, 1998), this definition is nonspecific regarding to the nature of the personality dysfunctions. Furthermore, discontinuity between those with PDs and those without such disorders is implied, when there is an increasing consensus that PD is a dimensional rather than categorical phenomenon, manifesting at different levels of severity (Tyrer & Johnson, 1996).

In light of the shortcomings of the *DSM–IV* conceptualization of PD, the *DSM–5* Personality and Personality Disorders Work Group has proposed an approach that describes core features of personality psychopathology at different levels of severity (Skodol et al., 2011). As noted in the accompanying review by Bender, Morey, and Skodol (2011/this issue), there is considerable convergence in theoretical accounts and empirical research on measures of core personality pathology (e.g., Blatt & Auerbach, 2003; Diguer et al., 2004; Dimaggio, Semerari, Carcione, Procacci, & Nicolo, 2006; Fonagy & Target, 2006; Huprich & Greenberg, 2003; Kernberg & Caligor, 2005; Levy et al., 2006; Piper, Ogrodniczuk, & Joyce, 2004), and each of these formulations discusses the potential clinical utility of a severity dimension of personality pathology. Such a dimension can be viewed as conceptually independent of specific personality traits, instead representing a more general adaptive failure or delayed development of an intrapsychic system needed to fulfill adult life tasks (Livesley, 2003). As noted by Bornstein (1998), "the best predictor of the therapeutic outcome for PD patients is severity—not type—of personality pathology" (p. 337). This conclusion is also supported by the findings of Hopwood et al. (in press), who found that general severity of personality pathology was the single best predictor of prospectively assessed functional impairment in patients with PD after 10 years of follow-up. Furthermore, such a severity dimension can be modeled independently from various trait dimensional systems of personality that have been proposed (Berghuis, Kamphuis, & Verheul, in press; Hopwood et al., in press). An influential mapping of various *DSM–IV* PD concepts onto a core continuum of "personality organization" is provided by Kernberg and Caligor (2005), who organized the various specific disorders into a conceptual scheme that described the range of severity of personality organization from the more severe (e.g., schizoid, borderline) to less severe (e.g., obsessive–compulsive, avoidant, dependent) PD phenomena.

Bender et al. (2011/this issue) describe a severity continuum consisting of impairment in identity, self-direction, empathy, and intimacy. The purpose of this article was to provide an empirically based articulation of this global continuum, with the aim of characterizing its manifestations at different levels of severity. It was hypothesized that a core dimension of personality pathology, involving impairments in self and interpersonal functioning, can be extracted from symptomatic and phenomenological measures of personality problems, with key markers identified to anchor dimensional ratings of severity of personality pathology and to help establish "caseness" in personality pathology. The study sought to identify these markers at different levels of this continuum, using item response theory (IRT; Lord, 1980). Articulation of this dimension is critical both as a basis for defining the core features of personality pathology, as well as representing differences in personality functioning within and among different PDs.

METHOD

Participants

Two samples involving participants from the Netherlands were examined. The Berghuis et al. (in press) sample included 424 psychiatric patients: a mixture of outpatients (87.3%) and inpatients (12.7%), ranging in age from 17 to 66 years old ($M = 33.9$, $SD = 11.3$), and 72.4% women. Among participants 33.1% had a specific *DSM–IV* PD diagnosis (i.e., assigned by their treating clinician); 39.0% received a PD not otherwise specified (PD-NOS) diagnosis, and 27.9% received no or deferred PD diagnosis. Study diagnoses were assigned with the Structured Clinical Interview for *DSM–IV* Axis II Personality Disorders (SCID–II), as described later: 43.9% met criteria for at least one *DSM–IV* PD, and 11.3% met criteria for more than one. The most common SCID–II diagnoses were borderline PD (21.2%) and avoidant PD (20.5%). Most patients met criteria for one or more comorbid Axis I disorders (clinical diagnosis), most often a mood disorder (42%) or an anxiety disorder (13.7%). IRT models and parameter estimates were derived from this sample.

A second sample, from Verheul et al. (2008) came from multiple sites and included a total of 2,730 participants (2,252 psy-

chiatric patients from treatment centers in the Netherlands and 478 from the general population). A total of 1,759 participants who provided complete data were included in the analyses. Study diagnoses were assigned with the Structured Interview for *DSM–IV* Personality (SIDP–IV), as described later; 52.1% met criteria for at least one *DSM–IV* PD, and 23.3% met criteria for more than one. The most common SIDP–IV diagnoses were avoidant PD (24.6%) and PD-NOS (19.5%). This sample was used to test the generalization of results from the Berghuis et al. (24) sample and to examine the relationship of the empirically derived markers to specific *DSM–IV* PDs in more detail.

Instruments

Study instruments included two self-report instruments, the Severity Indices of Personality Problems (SIPP–118; Verheul et al., 2008), and the General Assessment of Personality Disorder (GAPD; Livesley, 2006), to measure markers of global personality pathology, and two semistructured interviews, the SCID–II (First, Spitzer, Gibbon, & Williams, 1997) and the SIDP–IV (Pfohl, Blum, & Zimmerman, 1997), from which *DSM–IV* PD diagnoses and associated criteria were obtained. Data on the SIPP–118, GAPD, and SCID–II were collected in the Berghuis et al. (in press) sample, whereas data on the SIPP–118 and SIDP–IV were gathered for the Verheul et al. (2008) study.

GAPD (Livesley, 2006). The GAPD is a recently developed questionnaire measuring hypothesized core components of personality pathology according to Livesley's (2003) adaptive failure model. The GAPD version used in this study consists of 142 items rated on a 5-point Likert scale, ranging from 1 (*very unlike me*) to 5 (*very like me*), and made up of two main scales: Self-Pathology and Interpersonal Problems, and 19 subscales. Self-Pathology covers items regarding the structure of personality (e.g., problems of differentiation and integration) and agency (e.g., conative pathology). The Interpersonal Problems scale includes items measuring various impairments in social functioning. This study utilized the authorized Dutch translation by Berghuis (2007). In this sample, the internal consistency (coefficient alpha) reliability for the Self-Pathology scale was .87, and for the Interpersonal Problems scale was .89. However, it is important to note that for this project all analyses of GAPD were at the level of individual items rather than scales.

SIPP–118 (Verheul et al., 2008). The SIPP–118 is a dimensional self-report measure of the severity and core components of personality pathology. The SIPP–118 consists of 118 4-point Likert scale items (time frame of last 3 months), covering 16 facets of personality functioning, clustering in five higher order domains: self-control, identity integration, relational functioning, social concordance, and responsibility. Good psychometric properties, including (cross-national) validity, have been reported (Arnevik, Wilberg, Monsen, Andrea, & Karterud, 2009; Verheul et al., 2008). The median internal consistency (coefficient alpha) reliability of the 16 facets as measured in this sample was .77. As with the GAPD, all analyses of SIPP–118 data were at the level of individual items rather than scales.

SCID–II. The SCID–II (First et al., 1997; Weertman, Arntz, & Kerkhofs, 2000) is a widely used 119-item semistructured interview for the assessment of personality disorders. Each item is scored as 1 (*absent*), 2 (*subthreshold*), or 3 (*threshold*). In the Berghuis et al. (in press) sample, dimensional scores were obtained by summing raw scores of the criteria for each PD category and cluster. Master's-level psychologists conducted the interviews, but no formal assessment of interrater reliability was conducted.

SIDP–IV (Pfohl et al., 1997). The Verheul et al. (2008) study measured PDs using the SIDP–IV (Dutch version) administered by master's-level psychologists. Verheul et al. reported a median interrater reliability of 95% agreement (ranging from 84%–100%) on diagnosis, with a median intraclass correlation coefficient of .74 (ranging from .60–.92) for the sum of *DSM–IV* PD traits present.

Analyses

Specific items from the SIPP–118 and GAPD questionnaires were selected based on markers of global personality pathology identified in the Bender et al. (2011/this issue) literature review, using a Situational Judgment Test (Motowidlo, Dunnette, & Carter, 1990) strategy. Two expert Work Group members (D. Bender and A. Skodol) independently rated every item on the SIPP–118 and GAPD questionnaires, specifying the level of personality pathology expected to be associated with each potential response on the Likert-type scales of these items. Consensual agreement on ratings was used to identify a set of items to discriminate across different levels of personality pathology. This set of items was examined using internal consistency analyses, made up of coefficient alpha, item–total correlations, and principal components analyses. The goal was to isolate a unidimensional set of items, consistent with the assumptions of IRT and with developing a single coherent index of overall personality pathology. Items demonstrating low item–total correlations or factorial complexity were eliminated.

The final step in the analysis involved constructing a two-parameter IRT model of the remaining items. The SIPP–118 and GAPD both use Likert-type scales, but the number of response alternatives differ (four vs. five alternatives). Because the goal of the study was to relate item content to severity of global personality pathology rather than to scale responses from particular options, scoring was dichotomized to facilitate interpretation (for the SIPP–118, *fully agree* and *agree* responses were combined and contrasted with other responses, whereas for the GAPD *completely applicable* and *more applicable than not* item scores were combined). Threshold parameters of these items were used to identify items characterizing the types of problems associated with different levels of severity on the latent trait of personality pathology, whereas discrimination parameters provided an estimate of the ability of the item to distinguish individuals at this level of the trait from those at lower levels of pathology. Analyses were performed with the MULTILOG 7.0 (Scientific Software International, 2003) program. Estimates of the score for each individual in the sample on this latent trait (i.e., the maximum likelihood estimate of theta, or estimated theta) were retained for additional analyses examining the relationship of this trait to *DSM–IV* PD diagnoses.

RESULTS

The first step in selecting items from the two self-report instruments was based on the situational judgment ratings of individual items from the instruments, as provided by the two expert

raters. There was reasonable interrater reliability for these ratings of the SIPP–118 and GAPD items (interrater correlation on the *fully agree* ratings on the SIPP–118 was .76; and .74 on *completely applicable to me* ratings on GAPD items). Items on these two instruments that demonstrated high agreement across the two expert raters were selected if the raters agreed that a particular item was discriminating for the theoretical construct. Agreement between the raters was calculated as the squared Euclidean distance between the ratings for each response option across the two raters. Based on their agreement and differentiation properties, a total of 49 (of 118) potential SIPP–118 markers and 57 (of 142) GAPD items were retained as potential indicators of the global personality pathology dimension. Subsequent analyses were then conducted to empirically refine this subset of items in preparation for the IRT analyses, using patient data from the Berghuis et al. sample. Internal consistency analyses for patient responses in the Berghuis et al. sample yielded an alpha for the 49-item SIPP–118 scale of .93, with a mean interitem correlation of .22; the alpha for the 57-item GAPD scale was .96, with a mean interitem correlation of .30. One item from the GAPD was eliminated as it demonstrated a moderate (i.e., neither extremely high nor low) mean and low item–total correlation (below .25). Remaining items were factor analyzed to further assess the unidimensionality of these constructed scales and their suitability for IRT analyses (Hambleton, Swaminathan, & Rogers, 1991). For both the SIPP and the GAPD, there were large first components (representing 17.8% and 27.1% of the variance, respectively) and two other components (on both instruments) with eigenvalues above what would be predicted from parallel analyses (O'Connor, 2000), but each accounting for 6% of the variance or less. On both the SIPP–118 and the GAPD, six items were identified with potentially problematic cross-loadings on secondary components, factors that appeared to tap aggressive behaviors and anhedonia. The factor scores from the first principal component of the SIPP–118 correlated .80 with the first principal component of the GAPD, supporting the conclusion that the primary factors from both sets of items were measuring the same construct.

After eliminating items from the SIPP–118 and GAPD that had low item–total correlations or problematic factor loadings, the two scales were combined to form a single 93-item scale (43 from the SIPP–118 and 50 from the GAPD) that demonstrated considerable internal consistency (coefficient alpha = .96). This 93-item scale was then analyzed using a two-parameter IRT model. Items achieving a discrimination parameter > 1 were retained (a total of 65 items); a summed binary scoring of these items yielded a score that correlated .98 with the theta estimate from the IRT analyses. This scale also correlated above .90 with both the earlier GAPD and SIPP–118 separate versions, as well as .51 with the sum of the total *DSM–IV* PD criteria as assessed by the SCID–II. A sampling of items providing information at various levels of the latent trait is presented in Table 1, with estimated threshold and discrimination parameters for these items. Items are listed in order of threshold values; higher (positive) threshold scores indicate items that tend to discriminate at milder levels of personality pathology, whereas lower (negative) threshold scores indicate items informative around more severe pathology.

For each patient in the sample, the estimated theta score was computed as an estimate of the patient's score on the latent trait of global personality pathology. It was hypothesized that

TABLE 1.—Item response theory parameters for example GAPD/SIPP–118 items discriminating at different levels of a core personality pathology continuum.

Item	Discrimination	SE	Threshold	SE
I believe that it does not help to try to work together with people.	1.15	0.24	−1.28	0.2
I can hardly remember what kind of person I was only a few months ago.	1.61	0.24	−0.53	0.12
I can't make close ties with people.	1.29	0.22	−0.47	0.14
My feelings about people change a great deal from day to day.	2.01	0.31	−0.23	0.09
Sometimes I think that I am a fake or a sham.	1.91	0.26	−0.16	0.09
I worry that I will lose my sense of who I really am.	2.40	0.33	0.02	0.08
My feelings about other people are very confused.	1.61	0.24	0.29	0.11
I drift through life without a clear sense of direction.	2.76	0.41	0.48	0.08
I have very contradictory feelings about myself.	2.23	0.32	0.95	0.11
I mostly have the feeling that my true self is hidden.	2.05	0.33	0.96	0.11

Note. GAPD = General Assessment of Personality Disorder; SIPP–118 = Severity Indices of Personality Problems.

this score would prove to be a predictor of the assignment of a *DSM–IV* PD diagnosis, as well as predicting comorbidity among PDs. Table 2 provides the estimated theta means for study participants who received none, one, or two or more specific *DSM–IV* PD diagnoses as determined by the SCID–II. One-way analysis of variance followed by Bonferroni post-hoc tests revealed that these three diagnostic groupings all differed significantly, $F(2, 421) = 54.18$, $p < .001$. These results demonstrate that lower (i.e., more severe) theta scores were associated with assignment of a specific PD diagnosis and were also associated with assignment of multiple PD diagnoses. The area under the receiver operating characteristic (ROC) curve of .756 ($SE = .023$; asymptotic significance $< .001$) reveals that the theta score was a significant predictor of being assigned a specific PD diagnosis; a cutting score of zero (the theoretical mean of theta in a clinical sample) demonstrated a 73% sensitivity and 63% specificity for identifying individuals diagnosed with at least one of the 10 specific PDs in the Berghuis et al. sample.

To relate this latent trait dimension to specific *DSM–IV* PD criteria, a regression function (using a stepwise procedure with

TABLE 2.—Predicted theta means by number of personality disorder diagnoses in two study samples.

Number of Personality Disorder Diagnoses	Berghuis et al. (in press)			Verheul et al. (2008)		
	M	SD	N	M	SD	N
0	.3802	.9231	238	.3874	.7449	842
1	−.3416	.7297	138	.0613	.6733	507
2+	−.7120	.5673	48	−.2263	.6624	410

Note. All three groups significantly different within each sample, $p < .001$.

TABLE 3.—Coefficients for predicting estimated theta from SCID–II *DSM–IV* criteria.

Model	Unstandardized Coefficients		Standardized Coefficients		
	B	Std. Error	Beta	t	Sig.
(Constant)	2.398	.255		9.418	.000
Identity disturbance (BPD3)	−.291	.053	−.262	−5.478	.000
Views self as inept (AVD7)	−.143	.048	−.140	−2.955	.003
Impulsivity (BPD4)	−.204	.050	−.194	−4.068	.000
Unwilling to get involved (AVD2)	−.231	.054	−.195	−4.274	.000
Reads hidden threat (PAR4)	−.176	.060	−.138	−2.932	.004
Emptiness (BPD7)	−.134	.048	−.129	−2.799	.005
Overconscientious (OCPD4)	.227	.074	.133	3.085	.002
Deceitfulness (ANT2)	−.218	.112	−.084	−1.958	.051
Reckless (ANT5)	−.302	.121	−.108	−2.490	.013
Seductive (HIS2)	.221	.097	.100	2.288	.023
Reluctant to confide (PAR3)	−.110	.055	−.090	−1.997	.047
Bears grudges (PAR5)	−.113	.057	−.092	−1.983	.048

Note. Dependent variable: theta; multiple $r = .679$. 1 = absent, 2 = subclinical, 3 = present; SCID–II = Structured Clinical Interview for *DSM–IV* Axis II Personality Disorders.

backward elimination) was calculated to estimate the obtained theta score for each patient, using all specific SCID–II criteria (see Table 3). Twelve *DSM–IV* PD criteria were retained in this function, sampled from across 6 of the 10 PD categories. The estimates provided by this function demonstrated a multiple correlation of .68 with the calculated theta score for participants.

To extend these findings into a second patient sample, estimated theta scores were also derived for participants in the Verheul et al. (2008) sample using only the SIPP–118 items. To estimate corresponding theta scores in this second sample, a regression model was constructed from the sum of the 43 SIPP–118 items included in the original IRT scaling. The fit of this model was quite high (multiple $r = .97$) and as such should provide a reasonable estimate of theta in this new sample.

As was the case in the derivation sample, the estimated theta score in this cross-validation sample was significantly correlated with the total dimensional PD symptom score from the SIPD–IV (−.52, as compared to −.51 in the derivation sample). As with the Berghuis et al. data, the mean score on the predicted theta score was compared for patients from the Verheul et al. sample who received no specific PD diagnosis (for this sample, this included those receiving a PD-NOS designation), those receiving a single specific *DSM–IV* PD diagnosis, and those receiving multiple PD diagnoses. These means are shown in Table 2; one-way analysis of variance followed by Bonferroni post-hoc tests revealed that these three diagnostic groupings all differed significantly, $F(2, 1756) = 54.75$, $p < .001$. Results were similar to those noted in the Berghuis et al. sample, in that lower (i.e., more severe) theta scores were associated with assignment of a specific PD diagnosis, although there were also higher levels of personality pathology in those receiving multiple PD diagnoses. ROC analyses to determine the diagnostic efficiency of the theta estimate to predict a SIPD–IV personality diagnosis in the Verheul et al. (2008) data resulted in a significant but somewhat lower (relative to the original sample) estimated area under the curve of .673 ($SE = .015$; asymptotic significance $< .001$). As with the Berghuis et al. sample, in the Verheul et al. data, a theta

TABLE 4.—Mean theta estimates for personality disorder categories: Verheul et al. (2008) data.

SIDP–IV Diagnosis	N	M	SD
Paranoid	86	−.4116	.6762
Schizoid	18	−.1130	.7435
Schizotypal	16	−.2942	.7950
Antisocial	55	−.3086	.7675
Borderline	314	−.3692	.6439
Histrionic	41	−.1764	.6000
Narcissistic	89	.0035	.6131
Avoidant	432	−.1427	.6395
Dependent	165	−.2410	.7436
Obsessive–compulsive	316	.0544	.7044
PD NOS	343	.2517	.6597
No PD	499	.4807	.7854

Note. SIDP–IV = Structured Interview for *DSM–IV* Personality; PD = personality disorder; NOS = not otherwise specified.

cutting score of zero demonstrated reasonable diagnostic efficiency for identifying individuals diagnosed with at least one of the 10 specific PDs by the SIDP–IV, with 72% sensitivity and 82% specificity.

The large size of the Verheul et al. (2008) sample also allowed for examining mean estimated theta scores for each of the specific PDs; in addition, the SIDP–IV provides for scoring of PD-NOS (which includes the three PDs found in the *DSM–IV* appendix), which allows an exploration as to how this concept fits within a dimension of general personality pathology. The mean theta values for the specific PD diagnostic groups (note that, because of PD comorbidity, these groups are not independent) and the PD-NOS group are presented in Table 4. As might be expected theoretically, the most pathological scores (i.e., the greatest level of personality pathology) were found in the borderline, schizotypal, antisocial, and paranoid groups. The least pathological specific *DSM–IV* PDs appeared to be narcissistic and obsessive–compulsive. Those receiving a PD-NOS diagnosis from the SIDP–IV had mean theta scores indicative of appreciably less personality pathology than those meeting criteria for one of the specific PDs, whereas those with no indication of PD had theta scores that were consistent with low personality pathology.

DISCUSSION

The results presented here indicate that it is possible to identify a global dimension of personality pathology that is significantly associated with (a) the probability of being assigned any *DSM–IV* PD diagnosis, (b) the total number of *DSM–IV* PD features manifested, and (c) the probability of being assigned multiple *DSM–IV* PD diagnoses. Indicators of this dimension involve important functions related to self (e.g., identity integration, integrity of self-concept) and interpersonal (e.g., capacity for empathy and intimacy) relatedness—features that, as reviewed earlier (Bender et al., 2011/this issue) play a prominent role in influential theoretical conceptualizations of core personality pathology (Livesley, 2003; Kernberg & Caligor, 2005; Kohut, 1971). Such results support the feasibility and potential utility of establishing a global PD severity scale in *DSM–5* to capture this dimension, in doing so helping to clarify the continuum that distinguishes PD from non-PD patients, unlike more global measures such as the GAF scale (Axis V) in *DSM–IV.*

TABLE 5.—Example of a clinician rating scale for levels of personality pathology.

Level of Personality Pathology	GAPD/SIPP–118 Item Indicators
Level 5 (item IRT thresholds in the +0.75 and greater range)	Some uncertainty and indecision around values and goals; occasional lapses in self-directedness; periodic self-doubt
Level 4 (item IRT thresholds in the +0.25 to +0.75 range)	Feelings of emptiness, insincerity, or lack of authenticity around identity; low frustration tolerance; consistent feelings of worthlessness
Level 3 (item IRT thresholds in the −0.25 to +0.25 range)	Little sense of direction or meaning in life; marked instability in perception and evaluation of others
Level 2 (item IRT thresholds in the −0.55 to −0.25 range)	Alienation from others and from own feelings; poorly integrated and contradictory aspects of personality
Level 1 (item IRT thresholds in the −0.75 and lower range)	Marked shifts in identity and goals; fragmentary and defective sense of self; poor boundaries between self and other; little or no capacity for cooperative relationships

Note. GAPD = General Assessment of Personality Disorder; SIPP–118 = Severity Indices of Personality Problems.

As an example, total number of *DSM–IV* PD criteria present (which demonstrated significant correlations with the continuum described here) have been found to predict longer term personological and functional outcomes, differentiating the PDs from Axis I disorders such as major depression (Morey et al., 2010). Future research should be directed at a more detailed examination of the specificity of these self–other issues to the PD with respect to other psychiatric disorders.

The nature of the items presented in Table 1 reveals that this continuum reflects variations in degree of self–other pathology. Certain items proved to be good indicators of personality function at various points on this continuum. However, these are self-report items; ultimately, the challenge is to try to turn these self-reported experiences into a clinical rating scale, using the identified items as guidelines to markers of level of personality pathology. Table 5 represents an approximation of what such a rating scale might involve, drawing directly from the content of SIPP–118 and GAPD that are maximally informative at various points on this personality pathology continuum. It will be important for future studies to evaluate the reliability and validity of a clinician-based rating scale that incorporates such concepts.

The ordinal patterning of severity described in Table 5 has a number of interesting features. Various features such as identity issues, interpersonal relatedness deficits, low self-worth, and low self-direction appeared to differentiate levels of personality pathology. In most instances, these indicators tended to vary quantitatively more than qualitatively at different levels of severity. However, as shown in Table 5, the markers that differentiated milder forms of personality pathology addressed primarily self and identity issues, whereas interpersonal issues (in addition to self-pathology) become discriminating at the more severe levels of personality pathology. Such a finding is consistent with the view of Kernberg (e.g., 1984, 1996) and others that identity issues play a foundational role in driving the characteristic interpersonal dysfunction noted in PDs. However, this observation needs replication using markers independent of the particular set of items examined in this study.

As a statistical manual, the *DSM–5* will ultimately identify a threshold necessary to describe an individual as having a "personality disorder." In *DSM–IV,* there was considerable ambiguity around the nature and placement of this threshold, particularly with respect to the PD-NOS category (Pagan, Oltmanns, Whitmore, & Turkheimer, 2005; Trull, 2005; Verheul, Bartak, & Widiger, 2007). It was also unclear whether the boundary was to be drawn along some continuum, and if so, what the rationale for that cutting point might have been. The analyses described here provide both a foundation for articulating this continuum, as well as some information about the relationship of *DSM–IV* PD concepts to this latent continuum. It is worth noting that the ordering of *DSM–IV* disorders along this continuum shown in Table 4 bears considerable correspondence to the comparable ordering of personality organization severity described in Kernberg and Caligor's (2005) characterization; in fact, the ordinal association between the two orderings was moderately strong (Spearman's rho = .57). Perhaps the largest difference between these two conceptualizations involved the placement of narcissistic personality, which was described by Kernberg and Caligor in the moderate to severe range, whereas in our analyses it appeared to characterize milder forms of personality impairment. This difference might reflect differences between the *DSM–IV* characterization of narcissism as primarily involving inflated self-esteem, as compared to a broader description of narcissistic pathology described by Kernberg and other authors. These latter theoretical accounts of the narcissism construct tend to resemble the core dimension described here—suggesting that narcissistic impairments can be found across a broad range of personality functioning. Such a view is corroborated by the characterization of the severity of narcissistic personality described in Kernberg and Caligor's (2005) conceptual scheme, which indicated that narcissism and malignant narcissism spans the full range of personality organization. It is worth noting that a proposal to exclude narcissistic personality as a specific PD type has proven to be controversial; for this construct to be useful, it will be important to clarify with greater precision how this concept relates to personality severity.

Although this study represents an important step in describing a global dimension of personality pathology, future research is needed to address a number of questions. As noted previously, important questions remain regarding whether such a rating scale reflecting this dimension can be assessed by clinicians with reasonable interrater reliability, and whether such ratings will also be related to *DSM–IV* PD diagnoses (as were the self-reported characteristics examined in this study), as well as to adaptive functioning and outcome. It should also be noted that this continuum needs to be examined in additional samples. For example, the treatment-seeking nature of the samples examined here both limits the inclusion of some forms of PD (e.g., antisocial) that might not seek treatment, and it also limits the study of the "healthier" end of this continuum, which could be accomplished through the use of community samples. Furthermore, the use of European samples of patients bears replication in North American samples, as well as in other cultures, to determine whether the descriptors of general personality pathology generalize across such cultures. Finally, given the variability in theta estimates for patients with PD diagnoses observed across the two samples (noted in Table 2), additional samples would be particularly useful for calibrating diagnostic thresholds for PD as referenced against the *DSM–IV.*

Although our data indicate clear differences between individuals manifesting *DSM–IV* PDs and those without such disorders on a latent variable reflecting general personality pathology, we conceptualize it as a continuous dimension, analogous to intelligence, and that like the concept of mental retardation superimposed on this intelligence continuum, any threshold for diagnosis will be arbitrary, in that individuals slightly above and below this threshold can be quite similar. It appears that there is considerable variability in severity on the personality pathology dimension among the *DSM–IV* disorders, with some (e.g., paranoid, borderline) representing particularly severe variants, whereas others—in particular, PD-NOS, but also obsessive–compulsive—appreciably less severe. Although a threshold for PD diagnosis could be calibrated against the *DSM–IV,* ultimately it will be important to examine other validators—such as functional impairment or disability—for optimal placement of a diagnostic boundary. Regardless, increasing efforts to describe and understand this core dimension of personality pathology will provide critical information about essential commonalities in these conditions, with significant implications for their etiology and treatment.

ACKNOWLEDGMENT

This project was supported by a *DSM–5* Research Group Data Analysis proposal grant.

REFERENCES

American Psychiatric Association. (1994). *Diagnostic and statistical manual of mental disorders* (4th ed.). Washington, DC: Author.

Arnevik, E., Wilberg, T., Monsen, J. T., Andrea, H., & Karterud, S. (2009). A cross-national validity study of the Severity Indices of Personality Problems (SIPP–118). *Personality and Mental Health, 3,* 41–55.

Bender, D. S., Morey, L. C., & Skodol, A. E. (2011/this issue). Toward a model for assessing level of personality functioning in *DSM–5,* Part I: A review of theory and methods. *Journal of Personality Assessment, 93,* 332–346.

Berghuis, H. (2007). *Assessment of General Personality Disorder (AGPD): Translation.* Amersfoort, The Netherlands: Symfora Groep.

Berghuis, H., Kamphuis, J. H., & Verheul, R. (in press). Core features of personality disorder: Differentiating general personality dysfunctioning from personality traits. *Journal of Personality Disorders.*

Blatt, S. J., & Auerbach, J. S. (2003). Psychodynamic measures of therapeutic change. *Psychoanalytic Inquiry, 23,* 268–307.

Bornstein, R. F. (1998). Reconceptualizing personality disorder diagnosis in the *DSM–V:* The discriminant validity challenge. *Clinical Psychology: Science and Practice, 5,* 333–343.

Diguer, L., Pelletier, S., Hebert, E., Descoteaux, J., Rousseau, P., & Daoust, J.-P. (2004). Personality organizations, psychiatric severity, and self and object representations. *Psychoanalytic Psychology, 21,* 259–275.

Dimaggio, G., Semerari, A., Carcione, A., Procacci, M., & Nicolo, G. (2006). Toward a model of self-pathology underlying personality disorders: Narratives, metacognition, interpersonal cycles and decision making processes. *Journal of Personality Disorders, 20,* 597–617.

First, M. B., Spitzer, R. L., Gibbon, M., & Williams, J. B. W. (1997). *Structured Clinical Interview for DSM–IV personality disorders (SCID–II).* Washington, DC: American Psychiatric Press.

Fonagy, P., & Target, M. (2006). The mentalization-focused approach to self-pathology. *Journal of Personality Disorders, 20,* 544–576.

Hambleton, R. K., Swaminathan, H., & Rogers, H. J. (1991). *Fundamentals of item response theory.* Newbury Park, CA: Sage.

Hopwood, C. J., Malone, J. C., Ansell, E. B., Sanislow, C. A., Grilo, C. M., McGlashan, T. H., ... Morey, L. C. (in press). Personality assessment in *DSM–V:* Empirical support for rating severity, style, and traits. *Journal of Personality Disorders.*

Huprich, S. K., & Greenberg, R. P. (2003). Advances in the assessment of object relations in the 1990s. *Clinical Psychology Review*, *23*, 665–698.

Kernberg, O. F. (1984). *Severe personality disorders*. New Haven, CT: Yale University Press.

Kernberg, O. F. (1996). A psychoanalytic model for the classification of personality disorders. In M. Achenheil, B. Bondy, E. Engle, M. Ermann, & N. Nedopil (Eds.), *Implications of psychopharmacology to psychiatry* (pp. 66–78). New York, NY: Springer.

Kernberg, O. F., & Caligor, E. (2005). A psychoanalytic theory of personality disorders. In J. F. Clarkin & M. F. Lenzenweger (Eds.), *Major theories of personality disorder* (pp. 114–156). New York, NY: Guilford.

Kohut, H. (1971). *The analysis of the self*. New York, NY: International Universities Press.

Krueger, R. F., & Markon, K. E. (2006). Reinterpreting comorbidity: A model-based approach to understanding and classifying psychopathology. *Annual Review of Clinical Psychology*, *2*, 111–133.

Levy, K. N., Clarkin, J. F., Yeomans, F. E., Scott, L. N., Wasserman, R. H., & Kernberg, O. F. (2006). The mechanisms of change in the treatment of borderline personality disorder with transference focused psychotherapy. *Journal of Clinical Psychology*, *62*, 481–501.

Livesley, W. J. (1998). Suggestions for a framework for an empirically based classification of personality disorder. *Canadian Journal of Psychiatry*, *43*, 137–147.

Livesley, W. J. (2003). *Practical management of personality disorders*. New York, NY: Guilford.

Livesley, W. J. (2006). *General Assessment of Personality Disorder (GAPD)*. Unpublished manuscript, Department of Psychiatry, University of British Columbia, Vancouver, BC, Canada.

Lord, F. M. (1980). *Applications of item response theory to practical testing problems*. Hillsdale, NJ: Erlbaum.

Morey, L. C. (2005). Personality pathology as pathological narcissism. In M. Maj, H. S. Akiskal, J. E. Mezzich, & A. Okasha, *World Psychiatric Association series: Evidence and experience in psychiatry* (pp. 328–331). New York, NY: Wiley.

Morey, L. C., Gunderson, J. G., Quigley, B. A., & Lyons, M. (2000). Dimensions and categories: The "big five" factors and the *DSM* personality disorders. *Assessment*, *7*, 203–216.

Morey, L. C., Gunderson, J. G., Quigley, B. D., Shea, M. T., Skodol, A. E., McGlashan, T. H., . . . Zanarini, M. C. (2002). The representation of borderline, avoidant, obsessive–compulsive and schizotypal personality disorders by the Five-factor model. *Journal of Personality Disorders*, *16*, 215–234.

Morey, L. C., Shea, M. T., Markowitz, J. C., Stout, R. L., Hopwood, C. J., Gunderson, J. G., . . . Skodol, A. E. (2010). State effects of Major Depression on the assessment of personality and personality disorder. *American Journal of Psychiatry*, *167*, 528–535.

Motowidlo, S. J., Dunnette, M. D., & Carter, G. W. (1990). An alternative selection procedure: The low-fidelity simulation. *Journal of Applied Psychology*, *75*, 640–647.

O'Connor, B. P. (2000). SPSS and SAS programs for determining the number of components using parallel analysis and Velicer's MAP test. *Behavior Research Methods, Instrumentation, and Computers*, *32*, 396–402.

Pagan, J. L., Oltmanns, T. F., Whitmore, M. J., & Turkheimer, E. (2005). Personality disorder not otherwise specified: Searching for an empirically-defined diagnostic threshold. *Journal of Personality Disorder*, *19*, 674–689.

Pfohl, B., Blum, N., & Zimmerman, M. (1997). *Structured Interview for DSM–IV Personality: SIDP–IV*. Washington, DC: American Psychiatric Press.

Piper, W. E., Ogrodniczuk, J. S., & Joyce, A. S. (2004). Quality of object relations as a moderator of the relationship between pattern of alliance and outcome in short-term individual psychotherapy. *Journal of Personality Assessment*, *83*, 345–356.

Saulsman, L. M., & Page, A. C. (2004). The five-factor model and personality disorder empirical literature: A meta-analytic review. *Clinical Psychology Review*, *23*, 1055–1085.

Scientific Software International. (2003). Multilog 7.0 [Software]. Available from http://www.ssicentral.com/

Skodol, A. E., Clark, L. A., Bender, D. S., Krueger, R. F., Livesley, W. J., Morey, L. C., . . . Bell, C. C. (2011). Proposed changes in personality and personality disorder assessment and diagnosis for *DSM–5*: Part I: Description and rationale. *Personality Disorders: Theory, Research and Treatment*, *2*(1), 4–22.

Trull, T. J. (2005). Dimensional model of personality disorder: Coverage and cutoffs. *Journal of Personality Disorder*, *19*, 262–282.

Tyrer, P., & Johnson, T. (1996). Establishing the severity of personality disorder. *American Journal of Psychiatry*, *153*, 1593–1597.

Verheul, R., Andrea, H., Berghout, C., Dolan, C. C., van Busschbach, J. J., Van Der Kroft, P. J. A., . . . Fonagy, P. (2008). Severity Indices of Personality Problems (SIPP–118): Development, factor structure, reliability, and validity. *Psychological Assessment*, *20*, 23–34.

Verheul, R., Bartak, A., & Widiger, T. A. (2007). Prevalence and construct validity of personality disorder not otherwise specified (PDNOS). *Journal of Personality Disorder*, *21*, 359–370.

Weertman, A., Arntz, A., & Kerkhofs, M. L. M. (2000). *SCID-II: Gestructureerd Klinisch Interview* DSM–IV *As-II Persoonlijkheidsstoornissen* [Structured Clinical Interview for *DSM–IV* Axis II Personality Disorders]. Amsterdam: Pearson.

Widiger, T. A., Simonsen, E., Sirovatka, P. J., & Regier, D. A. (2006). *Dimensional models of personality disorders: Refining the research agenda for DSM–V*. Washington, DC: American Psychiatric Press.

Zweig-Frank, H., & Paris, J. (1995). The five-factor model of personality in borderline and nonborderline personality disorders. *Canadian Journal of Psychiatry*, *40*, 523–526.

Assessing Personality in the *DSM–5*: The Utility of Bipolar Constructs

Douglas B. Samuel[1, 2]

[1]*Department of Psychiatry, Yale School of Medicine*
[2]*VA New England MIRECC, West Haven, Connecticut*

All previous editions of the American Psychiatric Association's *Diagnostic and Statistical Manual of Mental Disorders* (*DSM*) have described and assessed personality solely in terms of pathological categories. Nonetheless, there is compelling evidence that normal-range personality traits also provide clinically useful information, emphasizing the importance of thoroughly assessing both adaptive and maladaptive aspects of personality within a clinical context. The proposed inclusion of a dimensional trait model in the upcoming *DSM–5* represents an important shift in the understanding of personality pathology and provides an ideal opportunity to integrate the assessment of normal personality into clinical practice. Building on research conceptualizing personality disorders as maladaptive, extreme variants of general personality traits, it is proposed that both normal and abnormal personality can be assessed within the same dimensional model using bipolar constructs. The inclusion of bipolar traits, such as a continuum ranging from introversion to extraversion, would hold numerous advantages for a dimensional model. These benefits include a strong foundation of existing validity research, comprehensive coverage of personality pathology, and the ability to provide useful information about all individuals. Despite potential complexities, the adoption of bipolar constructs within *DSM–5*'s dimensional model presents the greatest opportunity to maximize efficiency, validity, and clinical utility.

Despite dramatic changes in their assessment and diagnosis, personality disorders (PDs) have been defined as categorical constructs since the American Psychiatric Association published the first *Diagnostic and Statistical Manual of Mental Disorders* in 1952. The diagnostic labels associated with these categorical constructs provide relatively straightforward and rapid communication about a person (Frances, 1993). Additionally, many of the categorical constructs have relatively lengthy histories and are quite familiar to clinicians. Another potential advantage of diagnostic categories is stimulating research and generating specific treatment recommendations. Although this has not occurred for a majority of the disorders (Blashfield & Intoccia, 2000), there are certain PD categories (e.g., borderline, antisocial, schizotypal, narcissistic, and dependent) that are being actively studied.

Nonetheless, there are also numerous disadvantages to the current categorical approach including excessive diagnostic cooccurrence, inadequate coverage, excessive heterogeneity within categories, lack of a meaningful or well-validated boundary between normal and disordered personality, and dissatisfaction among the clinicians who use it (Clark, 2007; Trull & Durrett, 2005; Widiger & Samuel, 2005). Based in part on these limitations, there is increasing consensus among researchers that a dimensional trait model can more validly represent personality pathology (Widiger & Simonsen, 2005). Accordingly, the *DSM–5* Personality and Personality Disorders Work Group (2010) proposed the inclusion of such a model in the upcoming revision of the diagnostic manual.

The trait model proposed by the *DSM–5* Personality and Personality Disorders Work Group (2010) includes six domains labeled negative emotionality, introversion, antagonism, compulsivity, disinhibition, and schizotypy. Four to 10 subtraits, or facets, that provide further description and differentiation, underlie these higher order constructs. The inclusion of a dimensional trait model is an important step in clarifying our understanding of personality pathology. However, it also presents a momentous opportunity to translate basic science into clinical practice by integrating well-established findings from normal personality research into the psychiatric nomenclature. Unfortunately, this opportunity is not realized as the current *DSM–5* proposal indicates that the "traits will be unipolar, with definitions indicating maladaptive functioning" (Skodol, 2009). In other words, they will focus on only one tail of the underlying latent trait distribution. Practically this means that an elevated score for introversion indicates that an individual has a pathological level of this trait, whereas a low score will simply indicate the absence of maladaptive introversion.

The proposal to adopt a unipolar trait paradigm fails to capitalize on the promise of a dimensional system and has three important consequences that might limit the ultimate validity and utility of the model. These include (a) producing a factor structure that is inconsistent with previously published research, (b) failing to capture comprehensively the range of personality pathology, and (c) eliminating the ability to integrate normal and adaptive personality traits. I detail each of these concerns and contend that altering this model to include bipolar traits would greatly increase the utility and efficiency of the resulting system. Specifically, I propose the adoption of a model that would encompass the full range of both normal and abnormal personality functioning. Like others (Clark, 2005; Trull & Durrett, 2005; Widiger & Trull, 2007), I argue that both adaptive personality traits and PD pathology can be effectively and efficiently assessed within the same integrative model through the use of bipolar constructs that acknowledge the possibility of maladaptivity at both ends of a trait.

PITFALLS OF UNIPOLARITY

Factor Structure Inconsistent with Previous Research

A central question for any dimensional model of personality pathology is how many higher order domains it should include. Fortunately, a great deal of research has examined the factor structure that underlies personality disorder (e.g., Clark, 1993; Clark, Livesley, Schroeder, & Irish, 1996; Livesley & Jackson, 2009; O'Connor, 2005). Markon, Krueger, and Watson (2005) nicely summarized and extended this research in a seminal analysis that concluded five factors best captured the variation and that this was the "crucial level of analysis" for psychopathology research (p. 154).

In this respect, perhaps the most noticeable aspect of the proposed *DSM–5* trait model is the inclusion of six higher order domains rather than the five dimensions of personality pathology indicated by previous research (e.g., Clark et al., 1996; Markon et al., 2005). Nonetheless, the model does share many similarities with other dimensional models of PD (Widiger & Simonsen, 2005). In particular, the proposed *DSM–5* domains of emotional dysregulation, introversion, and antagonism are largely equivalent to domains that have emerged from reviews of the literature (e.g., Trull & Durrett, 2005; Widiger & Simonsen, 2005). For example, negative emotionality is quite similar to the domain Trull and Durrett (2005) labeled negative affectivity/neuroticism/emotional dysregulation; *DSM–5* introversion is equivalent to low extraversion/positive emotionality; and *DSM–5* antagonism is comparable to dissocial/antagonism behavior. Additionally, although some have argued that *DSM–5* schizotypy is unrelated to other trait models (i.e., Watson, Clark, & Chmielewski, 2008), there is evidence to suggest that the cognitive-perceptual aberrations, magical thinking, and eccentricity associated with schizotypy are maladaptively high variants of a domain identified as openness to experience (e.g., Haigler & Widiger, 2001; Kwapil, Barrantes-Vidal, & Silvia, 2008; Lynam & Widiger, 2001; Piedmont, Sherman, Sherman, Dy-Liacco, & Williams, 2009; Ross, Lutz, & Bailey, 2002; Samuel & Widiger, 2004; Tackett, Silberschmidt, Krueger, & Sponheim, 2008; Wiggins & Pincus, 1989). Thus, it appears that despite semantic differences, four of the six domains proposed for *DSM–5* have obvious counterparts in existing trait models.

However, a primary divergence from the previous research is that the proposed *DSM–5* model separates the domains of compulsivity (encompassing traits such as perfectionism, perseveration, rigidity, orderliness, and risk aversion) and disinhibition (encompassing traits such as impulsivity, distractibility, recklessness, and irresponsibility). Within existing frameworks, compulsivity and disinhibition typically define opposite poles of a single latent dimension. In fact, Widiger and Simonsen's (2005) review of 13 dimensional trait models concluded that "all but a couple of the models also include a domain concerned with the control and regulation of behavior, referred to as constraint, compulsivity, or conscientiousness, or, when keyed in the opposite direction, impulsivity or disinhibition" (p. 116). Although Clark and Krueger (2010) did provide a brief rationale for the proposed six-factor model, justification for the separation of these traits is notably absent.

Indeed, quite the opposite conclusion appears warranted as a substantial empirical literature supports the conceptualization of compulsivity and disinhibition as contrasting poles of the same latent trait. In fact, two predominant dimensional measures of personality pathology are the Schedule for Nonadaptive and Adaptive Personality (SNAP; Clark, 1993) and the Dimensional Assessment of Personality Pathology–Basic Questionnaire (DAPP–BQ; Livesley & Jackson, 2009), which explicitly contain scales labeled disinhibition and compulsivity, respectively. Both instruments are authored by members of the *DSM–5* Work Group and correlational studies routinely demonstrate that these scales correlate negatively with one another (e.g., −.51 from Pryor, Miller, & Gaughn, 2009) and relate in opposite directions with the related trait of conscientiousness. For example, the Revised NEO Personality Inventory (NEO PI–R; Costa & McCrae, 1992) Conscientiousness scale correlated −.59 with SNAP disinhibition (Clark, 1993) and .63 with DAPP–BQ compulsivity (Samuel & Widiger, in press).

Perhaps even more compelling support is provided by numerous factor analyses that suggest these traits fall at opposite ends of a common construct. For instance, Clark and colleagues (1996) conducted a joint factor analysis of the DAPP–BQ and SNAP and found that one factor was "most strongly marked by SNAP Impulsivity and Disinhibition, versus DAPP–BQ Compulsivity" and "can be identified with (low) conscientiousness" (p. 297). Additionally, a factor identified by Markon and colleagues (2005) was defined by positive loadings for Five-factor model (FFM) conscientiousness and SNAP workaholism as well as negative loadings for SNAP disinhibition and impulsivity. In fact, similar findings have been repeated throughout the factor analytic literature (e.g., Clark, 1993; O'Connor, 2005; Watson et al., 2008) and there does not appear to be a single published study that would support disinhibition and compulsivity as separate dimensions.

Failure to Capture Adequately the Range of Personality Pathology

Another potential hazard of a unipolar model is the failure to appreciate the potential for maladaptivity at the "opposite" end of a given trait. For example, the proposed *DSM–5* trait model includes a domain of introversion that contains a reasonably comprehensive set of subtraits (e.g., social withdrawal and intimacy avoidance) that elaborate the more specific problematic aspects associated with this domain. Nonetheless, such a domain is limited in that a low standing indicates only the absence of introversion and does not provide information about the equally problematic aspects associated with the opposite end of the trait (e.g., extraversion). Maladaptive expressions of high extraversion have lengthy precedents within the psychiatric nomenclature, as Millon's (1981) original description of histrionic PD was the "gregarious pattern" (p. 131). Aspects of excessive extraversion continue to appear in dimensional models of personality disorder, such as the Exhibitionism scale from the SNAP, which falls beneath the domain of positive emotionality and loads opposite of a trait labeled detachment (Clark, 1993).

Similar arguments can also be made for other domains. For instance, the failure to include a maladaptive variant of low antagonism (i.e., compliance or agreeableness) reduces the proposed model's ability to account for traits such as excessive gullibility and self-sacrifice. Indeed, high agreeableness can be maladaptive as others can routinely victimize an individual who is overly agreeable (Pincus, 2002).

In this sense, one might actually argue that the inclusion of both compulsivity and disinhibition is a strength of the proposed *DSM–5* model because it allows a more thorough assessment of what research indicates are opposite poles of the same construct. It is the only one of the five domains identified by Markon and colleagues (2005) for which the proposed *DSM–5* trait model acknowledges both maladaptively high and low standings. It is conceivable that one could similarly divide the other constructs, such as including separate assessments of introversion and a domain that could be labeled exhibitionism or extraversion. Of course, this solution would be particularly inefficient, as it would require the separate assessment of highly negatively correlated traits, unnecessarily doubling the time needed for an assessment and creating an unwieldy model with up to 10 dimensions.

In addition, even if such a model were adopted, much time would be spent assessing specific traits that will be largely irrelevant to a given person. For example, it is unlikely that any individual could be considered to have high standings on all facets of both introversion and extraversion. This is, of course, not to suggest that individuals will never behave in ways that are at odds with their overall level of a trait. Indeed, even someone with particularly high levels on the trait of exhibitionism will be likely to sit quietly and keep to himself or herself during a lecture or religious service. In addition, some persons can be elevated on certain facets of introversion and elevated on other facets of extraversion. This will not happen frequently, but can occur. However, a model that includes all of the relevant facets of introversion and extraversion in a unipolar format would require a clinician to assess both poles for all of the facets in all persons, which would typically involve a considerable waste of time. For example, it is rather inefficient to assess an individual for the trait of exhibitionism after already ascertaining him or her to be high on the trait of social withdrawal. It seems likely that similarly strange situations might emerge for the assessments of compulsivity and disinhibition with the proposed *DSM–5* trait model.

Eliminates the Assessment of Normal or Adaptive Personality

As indicated by its title, the *DSM–5* Personality and Personality Disorders Work Group appears to have been designed with the intention of including normative, or adaptive, personality traits as well as defining personality pathology. Such a goal is a notable shift from previous editions of the *DSM* and highlights the increasing recognition that personality traits have profound public health significance (e.g., Lahey, 2009) and meaningfully relate to numerous clinically relevant outcomes (e.g., Hopwood et al., 2009; Ozer & Benet-Martinez, 2006). Unfortunately, the current proposal, which is confined to maladaptive functioning, does not realize this goal.

The inclusion of a method for assessing normal or adaptive personality would be quite valuable. Ozer and Benet-Martinez (2006) systematically reviewed the literature and concluded that personality traits are linked to a wide variety of important life outcomes, including subjective well-being, supportive family and peer relationships, and successful romantic relationships. In a clinical context, these traits can be highly informative both

for their ability to predict dysfunction in a variety of life arenas (e.g., Hopwood et al., 2009) and to identify an individual's strengths that might be adaptive within the therapeutic setting (Costa, 2008). For example, an adaptive standing on a trait such as conscientiousness would be quite advantageous for an individual engaged in cognitive behavioral therapy, which requires the completion of tracking sheets and other weekly homework assignments. Likewise, traits such as extraversion and agreeableness might facilitate entry and engagement in a group therapy modality (Sanderson & Clarkin, 2002). The inclusion of adaptive traits within a clinical assessment can also hold benefits, as this feedback might be more acceptable to the client, aid his or her self-understanding, or provide clues for coping with maladaptive traits. Finally, the formal recognition of one's strengths or beneficial characteristics by a therapist could also increase rapport.

It does appear that the committee considered the inclusion of adaptive or normal traits, but as a separate list rather than as an integrated component of the model (Skodol, 2009). Ultimately, however, no such list of adaptive traits appears in the official proposal and one must assume this effort was abandoned. This is perhaps understandable as it might be unreasonably cumbersome for clinicians to first assess 37 maladaptive traits and then another 20 or so adaptive traits. Not only would this create an additional burden on clinicians, making a thorough assessment unlikely, but it would amplify the concerns that the currently proposed model is already too complex (First, 2010).

One might also question whether any traits are purely adaptive. The progress report from the Work Group (Skodol, 2009) provides the example of optimism as an adaptive trait. There is certainly ample evidence to suggest that optimism is quite beneficial (Carver, Scheier, & Segerstrom, 2010); however, research has also indicated that extremely high levels relate to negative consequences (Dillard, Midboe, & Klein, 2009). Indeed, it seems possible to have "too much of a good thing" and that almost any trait or characteristic can be maladaptive at certain levels. As such, rather than specifying a priori which traits are adaptive and which are maladaptive, it might be more fruitful to identify a comprehensive list of important personality traits and then determine empirically at which levels, and in which situational contexts, these traits lead to impaired functioning.

BENEFITS OF BIPOLARITY

In light of these potential limitations of a model including unipolar traits, it is important to acknowledge that the model currently presented on the *DSM–5* Web site is only a proposal and not the final decision. It is formally noted, "The proposed trait set is provisional, and currently is being tested for its structural validity before finalizing the *DSM–V* proposal" (Clark & Krueger, 2010). In this sense, the committee members are commended for their openness in inviting comment on an unfinished product. Given the concerns I have presented, it is my sincere hope that there will be notable changes to the current model before it is finalized and that the Work Group is receptive to constructive suggestions for improvement.

One alternative to these potentially problematic consequences of unipolar traits would be the adoption of a model that encompasses the full range of personality variability and acknowledges the possibility of maladaptivity at either end of the spectrums. This type of system might be described as bipolar, in contrast to the unipolar description of the current *DSM–5* proposal. Such a bipolar model, based on the dimensions that are common to both personality pathology and normal personality functioning, would have appreciable benefits. It would yield a cohesive model with a factor structure that extends comfortably and strongly from the existing research literature. Not only would this provide a more empirically sound foundation for the diagnostic nomenclature, but it also would embrace a factor structure that would be more replicable across future studies. For instance, it appears likely that further testing of the structural validity of the currently proposed model would evidence substantial overlap and covariance between disinhibition and compulsivity. Additionally, a bipolar model would comprehensively cover the range of possible personality pathology, including even those aspects not currently identified within the *Diagnostic and Statistical Manual of Mental Disorders* (4th ed. [*DSM–IV*]; American Psychiatric Society, 1994) system (e.g., Piedmont et al., 2009). Finally, and perhaps most important, it would provide an efficient method of incorporating the assessment of normal personality traits into clinical practice.

A dimensional trait model that endorsed a bipolar perspective would likely resemble the FFM of general personality functioning (McCrae & Costa, 2008). The FFM is made up of five bipolar domains that have been labeled surgency or extraversion (vs. introversion), agreeableness (vs. antagonism), conscientiousness (vs. disinhibition), neuroticism (vs. emotional stability), and intellect or openness (vs. closedness to experience). Although alternative models of normal range personality exist, such as the HEXACO of Ashton and Lee (2007) or Cloninger's (2008) psychobiological theory, the FFM has succeeded well in integrating diverse personality models into a commonly understood framework and is considered the consensus model of normal personality (John, Naumann, & Soto, 2008). There is a substantial research literature supporting the validity of the FFM as it pertains to general personality functioning. This includes evidence concerning behavioral genetics (Krueger & Johnson, 2008; Yamagata et al., 2006), developmental antecedents (Caspi, Roberts, & Shiner, 2005; Widiger, De Clercq, & De Fruyt, 2009), universality across cultures (Allik, 2005; McCrae et al., 2005), and temporal stability (Roberts & DelVecchio, 2000).

In addition to FFM being considered the predominant model of general personality functioning, there have been two decades of research since the seminal paper by Wiggins and Pincus (1989) studying its links with personality pathology. Reviews, meta-analyses, and statistical evaluations of this literature have all converged on the conclusion that the *DSM–IV* PDs can be understood as maladaptive variants of the FFM (Clark, 2007; Samuel & Widiger, 2008). In other words, the difference between FFM neuroticism and the emotional dysregulation that characterizes borderline personality disorder is one of degree, rather than of kind (Samuel, Simms, Clark, Livesley, & Widiger, 2010).

Support for this viewpoint has been provided by Livesley (2001), who reviewed the literature and concluded that "multiple studies provide convincing evidence that the *DSM* personality disorder diagnoses show a systematic relationship to the five factors and that all categorical diagnoses of *DSM* can be accommodated within the five-factor framework" (p. 24). More recently, Clark (2007) agreed, "The five-factor model of personality is widely accepted as representing the higher-order structure of both normal and abnormal personality traits"

(p. 246). Systematic meta-analyses of correlations between FFM and PD measures have also reached similar conclusions. Saulsman and Page (2004) reviewed 12 published studies and determined that PDs obtained consistent and predictable relationships with the FFM. For example, the mean weighted correlation between borderline and neuroticism was .49. Samuel and Widiger (2008) later replicated these findings with a meta-analysis of an additional 15 studies. Finally, the link between adaptive and maladaptive personality has also been supported by studies suggesting that they share a common latent structure (Markon et al., 2005; O'Connor, 2005). Markon et al. (2005) combined 77 independent samples that studied the structural relationships between normal and abnormal personality instruments and factor analyzed the resultant meta-analyzed correlation matrix. From this procedure they concluded that "Our results reinforce the position that the Big Five represent a crucial level of analysis for normal personality research and extend this position to include psychopathology research as well" (p. 154). In sum, the FFM is not only the predominant model for describing normal personality, but it also has well-established links to the *DSM–IV* PD categories, making it an attractive choice should the *DSM–5* committee adopt a bipolar approach.

COMPLEXITIES OF BIPOLARITY

In addition to the benefits already discussed, there are complexities associated with the assessment and scoring of bipolar constructs. One assessment challenge is providing a comprehensive coverage of the relevant traits. Whereas unipolar constructs make fine distinctions within a narrow range of relatively specific traits, bipolar constructs discriminate among individuals across the full spectrum. Additionally, unipolar constructs are relatively uncomplicated in that they tend to maintain convenient linear relationships with indicators of dysfunction. However, on a conceptual level, bipolar constructs can be somewhat more complex in that they do not presume purely linear relationships with indicators of pathology. This can be illustrated by the example of body mass index (BMI), which is the ratio of one's weight to height.

Higher BMIs are diagnostic of obesity and are associated with negative health outcomes, including heart failure (Lavie, Milani, & Ventura, 2009). However, the World Health Organization (WHO) also classifies those with a BMI under a certain threshold as "underweight," which indicates that the lower end of this dimension is also potentially problematic in terms of one's health. Because both ends of this dimension are maladaptive, a correlation between BMI and pathology might not provide a complete picture. Nearly 70% of adult Americans are considered "overweight" or "obese" (Flegal, Carroll, Ogden, & Johnson, 2002) by the World Health Organization standards, and accordingly BMI correlates negatively with a variety of health outcomes at the population level.

It is important to note that although the overall relationship between BMI and health is negative, this relationship is reversed when considering only those individuals at the lowest extremes of the BMI distribution. Indeed, having a low BMI is often used to make psychiatric treatment decisions, including hospitalization, among individuals being treated for eating disorders (Golden, Jacobson, Sterling, & Hertz, 2008). In addition, Tesfaye and colleagues (2007) showed that among Ethiopian men (a country in which malnutrition is more prevalent than obesity) the risk for hypertension was higher for men at the lowest levels of BMI than for those closer to the mean. Thus, the overall relationship between BMI and physical health might theoretically look something like an inverted U. In short, although BMI correlates negatively with health outcomes at the population level in the United States, this does not indicate that decreasing scores are universally adaptive for all individuals.

It seems likely that similar logic applies to personality, such that although certain traits relate to adaptive functioning across the population, particularly high scores are not necessarily adaptive. This becomes even more complicated for personality traits in that their assessment is based on instruments with limited bandwidth to cover the full range of the possible trait. Whereas BMI has a potentially unlimited distribution, personality traits are limited by the range of scores possible on a given measure.

Conscientiousness, for example, relates to a variety of positive life outcomes including familial satisfaction, career success, reduction of risky behavior, and longevity (Ozer & Benet-Martinez, 2006). Given the strong associations with positive outcomes, it is somewhat difficult for the same measures to evince correlations with impairment. Perhaps then, it is not surprising that the relationship between conscientiousness and obsessive–compulsive personality disorder (OCPD) has been among the least consistent relationships in studies correlating measures of the FFM with the *DSM–IV* PDs. For example, two meta-analyses have estimated that the correlation between these constructs is .23 (Saulsman & Page, 2004) and .24 (Samuel & Widiger, 2008). Although notable, this correlation is lower in magnitude that those between other PDs and domains of normal personality functioning.

This is likely attributable to the fact that instruments used to assess conscientiousness are generally restricted to the low to normal range of the trait. In fact, only a fraction of the items on most personality instruments assess the range of conscientiousness that can be problematically high. Haigler and Widiger (2001), for example, found that only 10% of the conscientiousness items from the NEO PI–R (Costa & McCrae, 1992) were coded such that low scores were more adaptive than high scores. Haigler and Widiger then experimentally manipulated those items to ensure that they assessed the more maladaptive aspects of high conscientiousness, such as by including the words *excessively* or *too much*. After doing so, they found the resulting scale obtained much higher correlations (e.g., median of .69) with three measures of OCPD. This suggested that just as the range of BMIs studied dictates its relationship with health outcomes such as hypertension, the range of conscientiousness being studied also dictates the relationship with OCPD.

Overcoming this measurement challenge is not necessarily difficult, as what is needed is an assessment that comprehensively covers the entire range of the trait distribution. Similar to BMI, personality scientists should develop assessments that capture all possible variability on the trait from the lowest to the highest levels (i.e., minimal floor or ceiling effects). Modern assessments of intellectual functioning, which provide reliable IQ estimates across quite a large range of the population, provide an example of this approach. More important, intellectual assessments are required for making discriminations and diagnostic decisions at the lowest levels of the trait (e.g., mental retardation), but are equally adept at identifying individuals at the uppermost levels (e.g., giftedness). Similarly, a dimensional

model of personality requires a complete assessment of the complete range of traits.

Given an instrument with the requisite bandwidth, research should determine at which points problematic functioning becomes more likely. Accordingly, the assessment should provide the greatest fidelity for assessing those levels of the traits where differentiation among individuals is most crucial for specific purposes. In the case of personality pathology, it seems likely this would be at either extreme of the distribution as the ability to discriminate among individuals within normal ranges of traits would not be particularly important for most clinical purposes. Fine distinctions, however, would be necessary at those points along the distribution where diagnostic decisions are relevant.

A PROPOSAL FOR BIPOLAR CONSTRUCTS

There have been several proposals as to how one might effectively implement a diagnostic system with traits that acknowledge maladaptivity associated with high or low standings (e.g., Widiger, Costa, & McCrae, 2002; Widiger, Livesley, & Clark, 2009), and it is beyond the scope of this article to repeat these suggestions in detail. However, at the broad level, such a system would involve a series of iterative steps. The first of these is the assessment of broad domains that are common to normal and abnormal personality functioning. When individuals fall within the normal/adaptive range, the assessment ends and the clinician then records a descriptor (e.g., low conscientiousness). However, scores beyond certain cutpoints (determined empirically) in either direction would prompt the assessment of several narrow traits that more clearly define the specific and maladaptive aspects of that pole. For example, a low score on a trait labeled conscientiousness might elicit an assessment of the traits that define the disinhibition domain of the current *DSM–5* proposal (i.e., impulsivity, distractibility, recklessness, and irresponsibility). Similarly, a high score on the general domain of conscientiousness would prompt the assessment of the compulsivity pole (e.g., perfectionism, rigidity, and orderliness). In this way, a detailed assessment of the specific lower order traits is provided only for those individuals for whom it is relevant. This is based on the understanding that an individual who is high on conscientiousness (e.g., organized, methodical, and punctual) is unlikely to exhibit maladaptive levels of traits such impulsivity, recklessness, or irresponsibility. Nonetheless, the assessment of the domain of conscientiousness would include the assessment of individual facets and could then accommodate individuals who are low on some facets but high on others.

The "tailored" testing approach that characterizes these steps could be implemented efficiently in a computerized adaptive testing (CAT) format. Using advances from item response theory, items and or diagnostic indicators could be written that effectively discriminate across the range of the personality traits and help pinpoint an individual's standing much more efficiently. Such an approach is now widely used within educational and achievement testing (e.g., the Graduate Record Examination) and has already been applied to measures of personality pathology (Simms & Clark, 2005). Simms and Clark (2005) demonstrated that a CAT version of the SNAP (Clark, 1993) obtained psychometric properties roughly equivalent to the traditional version, yet the administration was nearly 60% faster. A CAT approach holds great promise for providing a similarly efficient assessment of a revised *DSM–5* trait model that included bipolar traits. Simms et al. (2011/this issue), in fact, are currently developing a CAT-based instrument of a trait model of personality and personality pathology that seems potentially quite useful. It is unclear whether this instrument will include bipolar traits and how closely its structure will resemble the ultimate *DSM–5* trait model.

Importantly, maladaptivity or pathology would not be synonymous with trait extremity, as clinicians would also assess the degree to which the individual evidences impairments secondary to his or her extreme standing on the traits (e.g., Widiger et al., 2002). Thus, an elevated trait standing would not be sufficient for a diagnosis of personality pathology. Instead, general diagnostic criteria, such as the set offered by the *DSM–5* Work Group, would be consulted to determine if PD is present. This is precisely the system that is used for the diagnosis of mental retardation, whereby an IQ less than 70 is necessary, but not sufficient. To qualify for the diagnosis, an individual must also demonstrate clinically significant impairment in functioning. Although the cutscore is arbitrary in the sense that it does not identify a discrete break in the distribution, it is a well-reasoned and defensible selection that was informed by the impairments in functioning commonly associated with an IQ of 70 or lower (Zachar, 2000). Similar work is needed to identify the levels of individual personality traits that are commonly associated with impairment. Additionally, it is also possible that certain organizations or combinations of traits are particularly problematic or maladaptive. Indeed, Lynam and Widiger (2001) suggested that the long-standing interest in studying antisocial PD and psychopathy results from the fact that the specific combination of impulsiveness, antagonism, anger, and thrill seeking is so particularly insidious within organized society.

Areas for Further Study

A relevant question for any dimensional model, whether bipolar or unipolar, is how to assess it within clinical practice. Implementing an adaptive assessment of personality will likely be most efficient if it were developed as a questionnaire and completed by the patient (i.e., self-report). Indeed, the research supporting the validity of trait models relies heavily, but not exclusively, on self-report data. However, a self-report questionnaire is not the only possible solution. A clinician can also complete a questionnaire based on his or her experiences with the individual or the patient's responses to standardized stimuli. There have only been a few studies that have examined clinicians' descriptions of their patients using dimensional trait models (e.g., Blais, 1997) and this research has indicated that clinicians' ratings often are quite divergent from those provided by self-report or even semistructured interview (Samuel & Widiger, 2010). Another alternative is to develop a standardized, semistructured interview that can be administered by a clinician or another trained professional. Such an interview could also be adaptive in that responses to given stimuli would determine which additional items are administered. Again, this type of approach could be modeled after intellectual functioning assessments, such as the Wechsler Adult Intelligence Scale (Wechsler, 2008), which clearly specifies discontinuation rules that depend on the performance of the individual being assessed. Future research that continues to clarify the feasibility, reliability, and validity of these alternative assessment approaches, particularly clinician descriptions, is highly warranted.

Although existing nomothetic research suggests that opposite poles of trait spectra, such as compulsivity and disinhibition, are inversely related to one another, this is not always true idiographically (e.g., Villemarette-Pittman, Stanford, Greve, Houston, & Mathias, 2004). When this occurs, it is likely due to different elevations on different facets within the same domain. It would appear nonintuitive that a person could be described as both rigid and spontaneous, but it is theoretically possible that an individual could score highly on both traits if they were assessed separately (in fact, the Millon Index of Personality Styles includes unipolar scales to assess bipolar traits precisely for this purpose; Millon, Weiss, & Millon, 2004). Research that investigates this possibility is necessary. If such situations were discovered to be common, then clinicians and researchers might also want to consider intraindividual variability for each trait (Tellegen, 1998).

Finally, additional research is needed to specify whether the traits relevant for describing personality pathology can be accommodated within a bipolar framework. Specifically, this would entail investigating whether both ends of the traits can, in fact, be maladaptive in some contexts. Consider, for example, the domain of negative emotionality, which is clearly maladaptive at the highest end. Although extremely low scores on this domain could lead to problematic functioning in concept (i.e., the absence of negative emotions such as anger, sadness, or fear might lead to impairment), it is not clear how prevalent such low scores are in the population. However, even here it is suggested that some of these low scores can involve the maladaptively low anxiousness, glib charm, and fearlessness seen in psychopathic persons (Lynam & Widiger, 2007).

CONCLUSIONS AND RECOMMENDATIONS

The *DSM–5* Personality and Personality Disorders Work Group stands poised to revolutionize the assessment and diagnosis of personality pathology by including a dimensional trait model. They have an additional opportunity to take the historic step of integrating general personality traits into the clinical nomenclature. It is also possible for the committee to use a large body of empirical research on categorical and dimensional personality models to inform its deliberation. The current *DSM–5* trait proposal risks failure on both points, but this can be remedied by the inclusion of bipolar traits that recognize the sizable research literature suggesting that personality pathology can be understood as maladaptive variants of the same traits that define general personality. Such an integrated model would hold numerous advantages in terms of efficiency. A unipolar model would ostensibly require separate assessments of both maladaptive extremes of a given trait (e.g., disinhibition and compulsivity) as well as the normative or adaptive aspects of the trait (e.g., conscientiousness). In contrast, a system that acknowledges these traits as different levels of a bipolar continuum needs only to assess those levels that are relevant to a given individual. The result is an assessment that is twice as efficient for assessing pathology and potentially three times more efficient if one also assesses normal traits separately. A bipolar system that integrates adaptive personality would also be considerably more useful to clinicians, as it would provide clinically relevant information about all individuals. For example, the current unipolar *DSM–5* proposal would provide virtually no information about an individual within the adaptive range of extraversion, other than that he or she was not introverted. In contrast, a bipolar system might recognize the individual as sociable, outgoing, and assertive and suggest meaningful ways to utilize these attributes therapeutically.

In summary, reconfiguring the current *DSM–5* proposal to reflect bipolarity would not only overcome potential limitations of the model (e.g., factor structure incongruous with previous research and incomplete coverage of personality pathology), but it would also hold numerous advantages. Perhaps most notable of these would be the formal integration of general personality assessment into the clinical context.

ACKNOWLEDGMENTS

Writing of this article was supported by the Office of Academic Affiliations, Advanced Fellowship Program in Mental Illness Research and Treatment, Department of Veterans Affairs. This article is adapted from a presentation at the 2010 Midwinter Meeting of the Society for Personality Assessment.

REFERENCES

American Psychiatric Association. (1952). *Diagnostic and statistical manual of mental disorders*. Washington, DC: Author.

American Psychiatric Association. (1994). *Diagnostic and statistical manual of mental disorders* (4th ed.). Washington, DC: Author.

Allik, J. (2005). Personality dimensions across cultures. *Journal of Personality Disorders, 19*, 212–232.

Ashton, M. C., & Lee, K. (2007). Empirical, theoretical, and practical advantages of the HEXACO model of personality structure. *Personality and Social Psychology Review, 11*, 150–166.

Blais, M. A. (1997). Clinician ratings of the five-factor model of personality and the *DSM–IV* personality disorders. *Journal of Nervous and Mental Disease, 185*, 388–393.

Blashfield, R. K., & Intoccia, V. (2000). Growth of the literature on the topic of personality disorders. *American Journal of Psychiatry, 157*, 472–473.

Carver, C. S., Scheier, M. F., & Segerstrom, S. C. (2010). Optimism. *Clinical Psychology Review, 30*, 879–889. doi:10.1016/j.cpr.2010.01.006

Caspi, A., Roberts, B. W., & Shiner, R. L. (2005). Personality development: Stability and change. *Annual Review of Psychology, 56*, 453–484.

Clark, L. A. (1993). *Schedule for Nonadaptive and Adaptive Personality (SNAP)*. Minneapolis: University of Minnesota Press.

Clark, L. A. (2005). Temperament as a unifying basis for personality and psychopathology. *Journal of Abnormal Psychology, 114*, 505–521.

Clark, L. A. (2007). Assessment and diagnosis of personality disorder: Perennial issues and an emerging reconceptualization. *Annual Review of Psychology, 58*, 227–257.

Clark, L. A., & Krueger, R. F. (2010). *Rationale for a six-domain trait dimensional diagnostic system for personality disorder*. Retrieved from http://www.dsm5.0rg/ProposedRevisions/Pages/RationaleforaSix-DomainTraitDimensionalDiagnosticSystemforPersonalityDisorder.aspx

Clark, L. A., Livesley, W. J., Schroeder, M. L., & Irish, S. L. (1996). Convergence of two systems for assessing specific traits of personality disorder. *Psychological Assessment, 8*, 294–303.

Cloninger, C. R. (2008). The psychobiological theory of temperament and character: Comment on Farmer and Goldberg (2008). *Psychological Assessment, 20*, 292–299.

Costa, P. T., Jr. (2008). Just do it: Replace Axis II with a diagnostic system based on the five-factor model of personality. In T. A. Widiger, E. Simonsen, P. J. Sirovatka, & D. A. Regier (Eds.), *Dimensional models of personality disorders: Refining the research agenda for DSM–V* (pp. 195–198). Washington, DC: American Psychiatric Association.

Costa, P. T., Jr., & McCrae, R. R. (1992). *Revised NEO Personality Inventory (NEO PI–R) and NEO Five-Factor Inventory (NEO–FFI) professional manual*. Odessa, FL: Psychological Assessment Resources.

Dillard, A. J., Midboe, A. M., & Klein, W. M. P. (2009). The dark side of optimism: Unrealistic optimism about problems with alcohol predicts subsequent negative event experiences. *Personality and Social Psychology Bulletin, 35*, 1540–1550.

DSM–5 Personality and Personality Disorders Work Group. (2010). *Personality and personality disorders*. Retrieved from http://www.dsm5.0rg/ProposedRevisions/pages/proposedrevision.aspx?rid=470

First, M. B. (2010). Commentary on: Krueger and Eaton's "Personality traits and the classification of mental disorders: Toward a more complete integration in *DSM–V* and an empirical model of psychopathology": Real-world considerations in implementing an empirically-based dimensional model of personality in *DSM–5*. *Personality Disorders: Theory, Research, and Treatment, 1*, 123–126.

Flegal, J. N., Carroll, M. D., Ogden, C. L., & Johnson, C. L. (2002). Prevalence and trends in obesity among US adults, 1999–2000. *Journal of the American Medical Association, 288*, 1723–1727.

Frances, A. J. (1993). Dimensional diagnosis of personality—Not whether, but when and which. *Psychological Inquiry, 4*, 110–111.

Golden, N. H., Jacobson, M. S., Sterling, W. M., & Hertz, S. (2008). Treatment goal weight in adolescents with anorexia nervosa: Use of BMI percentiles. *International Journal of Eating Disorders, 41*, 301–306.

Haigler, E. D., & Widiger, T. A. (2001). Experimental manipulation of NEO PI–R items. *Journal of Personality Assessment, 77*, 339–358.

Hopwood, C. J., Morey, L. C., Ansell, E. B., Grilo, C. M., Sanislow, C. A., McGlashan, T. H., . . . Skodol, A. E. (2009). The convergent and discriminant validity of five-factor traits: Current and prospective social, work, and recreational dysfunction. *Journal of Personality Disorders, 23*, 466–476.

John, O. P., Naumann, L. P., & Soto, C. J. (2008). Paradigm shift to the integrative big five trait taxonomy: History, measurement, and conceptual issues. In O. P. John, R. W. Robins, & L. A. Pervin (Eds.), *Handbook of personality* (3rd ed., pp. 1114–1158). New York, NY: Guilford.

Krueger, R. F., & Johnson, W. (2008). Behavioral genetics and personality: A new look at the integration of nature and nurture. In O. P. John, R. W. Robins, & L. A. Pervin (Eds.), *Handbook of personality* (3rd ed., pp. 287–310). New York, NY: Guilford.

Kwapil, T. R., Barrantes-Vidal, N., & Silvia, P. J. (2008). The dimensional structure of the Wisconsin Schizotypy Scales: Factor identification and construct validity. *Schizophrenia Bulletin, 34*, 444–457.

Lahey, B. B. (2009). Public health significance of neuroticism. *American Psychologist, 64*, 241–256.

Lavie, C. J., Milani, R. V., & Ventura, H. O. (2009). Obesity and cardiovascular disease. *Journal of the American College of Cardiology, 21*, 1925–1932.

Livesley, W. J. (2001). Conceptual and taxonomic issues. In W. J. Livesley (Ed.), *Handbook of personality disorders: Theory, research, and treatment* (pp. 3–38). New York, NY: Guilford.

Livesley, W. J., & Jackson, D. (2009). *Manual for the Dimensional Assessment of Personality Pathology–Basic Questionnaire*. Port Huron, MI: Sigma Press.

Lynam, D. R., & Widiger, T. A. (2001). Using the five factor model to represent the *DSM–IV* personality disorders: An expert consensus approach. *Journal of Abnormal Psychology, 110*, 401–412.

Lynam, D. R., & Widiger, T. A. (2007). Using a general model of personality to identify basic elements of psychopathy. *Journal of Personality Disorders, 21*, 160–178.

Markon, K. E., Krueger, R. F., & Watson, D. (2005). Delineating the structure of normal and abnormal personality: An integrative hierarchical approach. *Personality and Individual Differences, 88*, 139–157.

McCrae, R. R., & Costa, P. T. (2008). The five factor theory of personality. In O. P. John, R. W. Robins, & L. A. Pervin (Eds.), *Handbook of personality* (3rd ed., pp. 159–181). New York, NY: Guilford.

McCrae, R. R., Terracciano, A., & 78 members of the Personality Profiles of Cultures Project. (2005). Universal features of personality traits from the observer's perspective: Data from 50 cultures. *Journal of Personality and Social Psychology, 88*, 547–561.

Millon, T. (1981). *Disorders of personality: DSM–III: Axis II*. New York, NY: Guilford.

Millon, T., Weiss, L., & Millon, C. (2004). *Millon Index of Personality Styles revised manual*. Minneapolis, MN: NCS Pearson.

O'Connor, B. P. (2005). A search for consensus on the dimensional structure of personality disorders. *Journal of Clinical Psychology, 61*, 323–645.

Ozer, D. J., & Benet-Martinez, V. (2006). Personality and the prediction of consequential outcomes. *Annual Review of Psychology, 57*, 401–421.

Piedmont, R. L., Sherman, M. F., Sherman, N. C., Dy-Liacco, G., & Williams, J. E. G. (2009). Using the five-factor model to identify a new personality disorder domain: The case for experiential permeability. *Journal of Personality and Social Psychology, 96*, 1245–1258.

Pincus, A. L. (2002). Constellations of dependency within the five-factor model of personality. In P. T. Costa, Jr., & T. A. Widiger (Eds.), *Personality disorders and the Five-factor model of personality* (2nd ed., pp. 203–214). Washington, DC: American Psychological Association.

Pryor, L. R., Miller, J. D., & Gaughan, E. T. (2009). Testing two alternative pathological personality measures in the assessment of psychopathy: An examination of the SNAP and DAPP–BQ. *Journal of Personality Disorders, 23*(1), 85–100.

Roberts, B. W., & DelVecchio, W. F. (2000). The rank-order consistency of personality traits from childhood to old age: A quantitative review of longitudinal studies. *Psychological Bulletin, 126*, 3–25.

Roberts, B. W., Wood, D., & Caspi, A. (2008). The development of personality traits in adulthood. In O. P. John, R. W. Robins, & L. A. Pervin (Eds.), *Handbook of personality* (3rd ed., pp. 375–398). New York, NY: Guilford.

Ross, S. R., Lutz, C. J., & Bailey, S. E. (2002). Positive and negative symptoms of schizotypy and the five-factor model: A domain and facet level analysis. *Journal of Personality Assessment, 79*, 53–72.

Samuel, D. B., Simms, L. J., Clark, L. A., Livesley, W. J., & Widiger, T. A. (2010). An item response theory integration of normal and abnormal personality scales. *Personality Disorders: Theory, Research, and Treatment, 1*, 5–21.

Samuel, D. B., & Widiger, T. A. (2004). Clinicians' descriptions of prototypic personality disorders. *Journal of Personality Disorders, 18*, 286–308.

Samuel, D. B., & Widiger, T. A. (2008). A meta-analytic review of the relationships between the five-factor model and *DSM–IV–TR* personality disorders: A facet level analysis. *Clinical Psychology Review, 28*, 1326–1342.

Samuel, D. B., & Widiger, T. A. (2010). Comparing personality disorder models: Cross-method assessment of the FFM and *DSM–IV–TR*. *Journal of Personality Disorders, 24*, 721–745.

Samuel, D. B., & Widiger, T. A. (in press). Conscientiousness and obsessive–compulsive personality disorder. *Personality Disorders: Theory, Research, and Treatment*.

Sanderson, C. J., & Clarkin, J. F. (2002). Further use of the NEO PI–R personality dimensions in differential treatment planning. In P. T. Costa & T. A. Widiger (Eds.), *Personality disorders and the five-factor model of personality* (2nd ed., pp. 351–375). Washington, DC: American Psychological Association.

Saulsman, L. M., & Page, A. C. (2004). The five-factor model and personality disorder empirical literature: A meta-analytic review. *Clinical Psychology Review, 23*, 1055–1085.

Simms, L. J., Goldberg, L. R., Roberts, J. E., Watson, D., Weste, J., & Rotterman, J. H. (2011/this issue). Computerized adaptive assessment of personality disorder: Introducing the CAT–PD Project. *Journal of Personality Assessment, 93*, 380–389.

Simms, L. J., & Clark, L. A. (2005). Validation of a computerized adaptive version of the Schedule for Nonadaptive and Adaptive Personality (SNAP). *Psychological Assessment, 17*, 28–43.

Skodol, A. E (2009). *Report of the DSM–5 Personality and Personality Disorders Work Group (April, 2009)*. Retrieved from http://www.dsm5.0rg/progressreports/pages/0904reportofthedsm-vpersonalityandpersonalitydisordersworkgroup.aspx

Tackett, J. L., Silberschmidt, A. L., Krueger, R. F., & Sponheim, S. R. (2008). A dimensional model of personality disorder: Incorporating *DSM* cluster A characteristics. *Journal of Abnormal Psychology, 117*, 454–459.

Tellegen, A. (1988). The analysis of consistency in personality assessment. *Journal of Personality, 56*, 621–663.

Tesfaye, F., Nawi, N. G., Van Minh, H., Byass, P., Berhane, Y., Bonita, R., & Wall, S. (2007). Association between body mass index and blood pressure across three populations in Africa and Asia. *Journal of Human Hypertension, 21*, 28–37.

Trull, T. J., & Durrett, C. A. (2005). Categorical and dimensional models of personality disorder. *Annual Review of Clinical Psychology, 1*, 355–380.

Villemarette-Pittman, N. R., Stanford, M. S., Greve, K. W., Houston, R. L., & Mathias, C. W. (2004). Obsessive–compulsive personality disorder and behavioral disinhibition. *The Journal of Psychology, 138*, 5–22.

Watson, D., Clark, L. A., & Chmielewski, M. (2008). Structures of personality and their relevance to psychopathology: II. Further articulation of a comprehensive unified trait structure. *Journal of Personality, 76*, 1485–1522.

Wechsler, D. (2008). *WAIS–IV administration and scoring manual*. San Antonio, TX: Pearson.

Widiger, T. A., Costa, P. T., Jr., & McCrae, R. R. (2002). A proposal for Axis II: Diagnosing personality disorders using the five-factor model. In P. T. Costa, Jr., & T. A. Widiger (Eds.), *Personality disorders and the Five-factor model of personality* (2nd ed., pp. 431–456). Washington, DC: American Psychological Association.

Widiger, T. A., De Clercq, B., & De Fruyt, F. (2009). Childhood antecedents of personality disorder: An alternative perspective. *Development and Psychopathology, 21*, 771–791.

Widiger, T. A., Livesley, W. J., & Clark, L. A. (2009). An integrative dimensional classification of personality disorder. *Psychological Assessment, 21*, 243–255.

Widiger, T. A., & Samuel, D. B. (2005). Diagnostic categories or dimensions: A question for *DSM–V*. *Journal of Abnormal Psychology, 114*, 494–504.

Widiger, T. A., & Simonsen, E. (2005). Alternative dimensional models of personality disorder: Finding a common ground. *Journal of Personality Disorders, 19*, 110–130.

Widiger, T. A., & Trull, T. J. (2007). Plate tectonics in the classification of personality disorder: Shifting to a dimensional model. *American Psychologist, 62*, 71–83.

Wiggins, J. S., & Pincus, A. L. (1989). Conceptions of personality disorders and dimensions of personality. *Psychological Assessment: A Journal of Consulting and Clinical Psychology, 1*, 305–316.

Yamagata, S., Suzuki, A., Ando, J., One, Y., Kijima, N., Yoshimura, K., ... Jang, K. L. (2006). Is the genetic structure of human personality universal? A cross-cultural twin study from North America, Europe, and Asia. *Journal of Personality and Social Psychology, 90*, 987–998.

Zachar, P. (2000). Psychiatric disorders are not natural kinds. *Philosophy, Psychiatry, Psychology, 7*, 167–182.

Personality Traits in the *DSM–5*

CHRISTOPHER J. HOPWOOD

Department of Psychology, Michigan State University

Recent advances in personality research coupled with a broad acknowledgment of the limitations of the representation of personality pathology in the third and fourth editions of the *Diagnostic and Statistical Manual of Mental Disorders* (*DSM–III* and *DSM–IV*) have positioned personality science to influence the shape of personality assessment in the fifth edition (*DSM–5*). Representing normative personality with well-validated traits that are broad, normally distributed, theoretically integrative, and distinct from personality disorder constructs would take optimal advantage of this opportunity. The assessment of normative traits would also link a large body of personality research with the practice of clinical diagnosis and would encourage clinicians to consider every patient's personality regardless of his or her diagnosis. Furthermore, conceptualizing personality traits and disorders separately would promote more careful clinical consideration of the functional severity and specific symptom constellations among personality disorders. Based on these considerations I argue that Five-factor model personality traits should be assessed separately from personality disorders in the *DSM–5*.

In a report about progress toward the *Diagnostic and Statistical Manual of Mental Disorders* (3rd ed. [*DSM–III*]; American Psychiatric Association, 1987), the manual's editor, R. L. Spitzer wrote, "As part of the discussion of the multi-axial approach, the Task Force will consider requiring a personality disorder diagnosis for all patients so that personality disorders, when accompanied by more acute disorders, are not ignored, as is commonly done" (Spitzer, 1976, as quoted in Williams, 1985). It is clear from this statement that Spitzer was motivated to incorporate personality assessment into the *DSM* because of his concerns that clinicians routinely ignore personality. However, by using the term *personality disorder* (PD) rather than *personality,* Spitzer implied that the personality of any person who does not meet criteria for a PD is not clinically important.

Yet most personality assessors view normative personality traits and dynamics as an essential context within which to view psychopathology and behavior. The failure of the *DSM–III* and *Diagnostic and Statistical Manual of Mental Disorders* (4th ed. [*DSM–IV*]; American Psychiatric Association, 1994) to provide a means for assessing such characteristics, combined with multiple empirical shortcomings of the *DSM–III/DSM–IV* PD model (Clark, 2007; Krueger, Skodol, Livesley, Shrout, & Huang, 2007; Widiger & Trull, 2007) may explain the limited use of personality assessment in clinical practice both before and after *DSM–III*. Because of both the shortcomings of the *DSM–III/DSM–IV* PDs and advances in personality science, personality psychology finds itself in a potent position to influence *Diagnostic and Statistical Manual of Mental Disorder* (5th ed. [*DSM–5*]) personality assessment. However, personality psychology currently risks contributing further to the problematic conflation of personality traits and disorders by replacing disorders with traits.

In this article I describe this risk and argue for the decoupling of normative personality trait assessment and PD diagnosis in the *DSM–5*. I first review research on normative personality and its relation to personality pathology. I next critique the *DSM–5* proposal in the context of this review. I conclude with a proposal that capitalizes on the gains made in personality science toward a more valid and clinically useful conception of personality traits and disorders.

NORMATIVE PERSONALITY

Research on personality traits has progressed exponentially over the past few decades. Many in the field now recognize the Five-factor model (FFM; neuroticism, extraversion, openness, agreeableness, and conscientiousness) or one of its close cousins (e.g., models with two to seven broad dimensions) as reflecting the natural ordering of a higher order level of personality traits (Goldberg, 1993). This structure appears to generalize across cultures (McCrae & Costa, 1997) and to include traits that can be mapped onto brain regions (De Young et al., 2010) and pathways (Depue & Lenzenweger, 2004). The course of FFM traits has been studied extensively and evidence for their absolute and differential stability in adulthood is substantial (Caspi, Roberts, & Shiner, 2005). Research has also documented the heritability of traits (Loehlin, 2001), the influences of genetic factors on personality stability (Bleidorn, Kandler, Riemann, Angleitner, & Spinath, 2009; Hopwood, Donnellan, et al., 2011), and the relations of traits to childhood temperament (Caspi & Silva, 1995; Rothbart, 2007). Finally, evidence supports the predictive validity of personality constructs for a host of important life outcomes (Grucza & Goldberg, 2007; Ozer & Benet-Martinez, 2006).

Moreover, there is substantial evidence regarding the importance of normative traits for clinical assessment. FFM traits relate to most psychiatric disorders including the PDs (Samuel & Widiger, 2008) and many Axis I disorders (e.g., substance abuse: Ruiz, Pincus, & Schinka, 2008; Attention Deficit Hyperactivity Disorder: Nigg et al., 2002; mood disorders: Bagby et al., 1996; see also Kotov, Gamez, Schmidt, & Watson, 2010). Traits also increment Axis I and II diagnoses in predicting clinical dysfunction (Morey et al., 2007; Trull, Widiger, Lynam, & Costa, 2003). Personality traits, and particularly those related to affective functioning (i.e., internalizing) and behavioral constraint (i.e., externalizing), can help explain comorbidity between disorders (Krueger, 1999). Thus assessing these personality traits has the potential to refine searches for the etiology of psychopathology. Conversely, pathoplastic personality traits such as those related to interpersonal behavior can capture heterogeneity among people with similar psychopathology (Pincus, Lukowitsky, & Wright, in press). These elements of personality have the potential to depict diagnostic subtypes and thereby guide differential treatment strategy selection for individuals with the same diagnosis but varying personality characteristics.

PERSONALITY TRAITS AND DISORDERS

Emboldened by the large body of evidence on the validity and clinical utility of normative personality traits, some personality psychologists appear to view *DSM–5* as an opportunity to replace the PDs of *DSM*s past with a personality assessment system based exclusively on normative traits (e.g., Widiger & Trull, 2007). The risk in this movement is the same one that faced the authors of the *DSM–III* and *DSM–IV:* the conflation of normative and pathological personality. One argument for replacing PDs with normative traits is that doing so would integrate various trait models (Widiger & Simonsen, 2005) as well as psychological and psychiatric perspectives on personality assessment (Clark, 2007). Indeed it is well documented that personality traits and disorders systematically relate to one another (Samuel & Widiger, 2008). If traits and disorders can be integrated without losing information, why not simply eliminate PDs in the *DSM–5* and replace them with traits?

However, if personality traits and disorders are meaningfully different, efforts should be made to understand and exploit those differences. Indeed, regardless of one's theoretical orientation, personality is an incredibly complex concept that houses a variety of features and elements that can be distinguished in numerous ways. To the extent that normative personality traits and pathological personality symptoms are conceptually and empirically distinct and mutually informative in clinical assessment, it would be more clinically useful to assess routinely both traits and disorders than to limit assessment to one domain or the other. Here I offer four reasons why personality traits and disorders are distinct and why it would be important to assess normative traits and PD constructs separately in the *DSM–5*.

Normative Traits Relate to Most Forms of Psychopathology

Normative personality traits correlate with nearly every individual difference variable in psychology, including most forms of psychopathology (Kotov et al., 2010). Often these correlations are stronger for disorders other than PDs. For instance, Ruiz et al. (2008) conducted a meta-analysis of the relations between FFM traits and antisocial PD and substance abuse. Both of these diagnoses were systematically related to traits, but the magnitude was stronger for substance abuse than antisocial PD (in clinical samples, the average absolute correlation between neuroticism, extraversion, agreeableness, and conscientiousness with antisocial PD was .17, whereas the same correlation for substance use disorders was .32; their Table 5). As such, there is nothing necessarily unique about the relations between FFM traits and PDs. Demonstrating these relations is not sufficient for arguing that personality traits and disorders overlap completely.

Furthermore, some evidence suggests that FFM traits are mostly related to overall severity and are more limited in depicting stylistic differences in pathological expression. Specifically, most PDs involve relatively high neuroticism and low agreeableness, extraversion, and conscientiousness (Morey et al., 2002; Saulsman & Page, 2004). In Samuel and Widiger's (2008) meta-analysis of PD–FFM relations, all PDs had positive correlations with neuroticism; all had negative correlations with extraversion except antisocial, histrionic, and narcissistic; all had negative correlations with agreeableness except dependent; and all had negative correlations with conscientiousness except obsessive–compulsive. In a recent study (Hopwood, Malone, et al., in press), the four FFM traits just listed related strongly to the sum of all PD symptoms but showed limited relations to specific PDs with this general symptom severity component covaried. This finding suggests that differences among PD constructs would be better explained by considering features external to the influences of normative personality than by FFM traits.

Empirical Evidence Supports Distinctions Between Personality Traits and Disorders

There are several areas of empirical nonoverlap between personality traits and disorders that suggest that important information would be lost should the PDs be reconceptualized as trait constellations. Some of these findings are potentially equivocal. For instance, normative traits are unlike PDs in that they have normal distributions. However, this could be due to the fact that the PDs reflect constellations of the tail ends of normal distributions (Widiger & Simonsen, 2005). Another example is that some research suggests that PDs are less stable, in the differential (rank-order) sense, than normative traits (Durbin & Klein, 2006; Morey et al., 2007). This is the case despite the fact that PD measures often insist that respondents or raters consider stable aspects of personality functioning. Indeed, the differential stability of PDs could be overestimated when such measures are used relative to systems in which PD symptoms are rated without the presumption of stability. Alternatively, differential stability differences between PDs and normative traits observed empirically could be due to the fact that PDs are usually assessed by interviews and traits by self-report, and that self-report methods tend to demonstrate greater stability than interviews (Ferguson, 2010; Samuel et al., in press). The relative distributions and differential stabilities of normative and pathological personality constructs, assessed with the same methods, are important questions for future research.

Other differences are less equivocal. For instance, longitudinal studies in clinical (Warner et al., 2004) and nonclinical (Lenzenweger & Willett, 2007) samples have found that previous levels of normative traits influence PD symptom changes, whereas previous PD levels do not influence normative trait changes. These results suggest that traits are somewhat more basic, whereas PDs reflect symptoms that wax and wane in part as a function of underlying personality dynamics, perhaps as well as changes in environmental contexts. Related to this point, instability in normative traits appears to be diagnostic of some forms of personality pathology, and particularly borderline symptoms (Hopwood et al., 2009; Hopwood & Zanarini, in press). The fact that features of normative traits other than their levels are influential on PDs highlights that the interaction of normative and pathological personality features is more complex than can be accommodated by a single, integrated system.

Traits and PDs also increment one another in clinical predictions (Hopwood & Zanarini, 2010; Morey et al., 2007; Trull et al., 2003). For instance, Morey et al. (2007) showed that the Revised NEO Personality Inventory (NEO PI–R; Costa & McCrae, 1992) domains and *DSM–IV* PD symptom counts incremented one another in predicting baseline, 2-year, and 4-year functioning scores (assessed by both interview and self-report) as well as the total number of concurrent and prospective Axis I disorders in a sample of patients followed naturalistically. If traits and disorders were redundant or if one set of variables was more valid than the other, they would be unlikely to increment one another. In fact, traits predict concurrent and prospective patient functioning whether or not patients have a PD (Hopwood et al., 2007). This finding illustrates that traits are not just useful for conceptualizing people with PDs; they are useful for conceptualizing people.

Lower Order Facets Do Not Bridge Normative and Pathological Personality

Trait researchers often argue that a more refined picture of personality pathology can be obtained through considering lower level facets of higher order trait dimensions (Clark, 2007; Samuel & Widiger, 2008). However, lower order facets are not a viable bridge between normative and pathological personality for the following reasons.

First, studies that have used cross-validation techniques to test the incremental validity of lower order facets over higher order traits have found that they do not tend to meaningfully increment higher order trait predictions in nonclinical (Grucza & Goldberg, 2007) and clinical (Morey et al., 2007) samples. This is important because equations in the general linear model with more predictors tend to overfit data and inflate estimates of explained variance (Stevens, 2002). Thus, any time the 30 facets of the NEO PI–R are entered in a hierarchical regression model testing their increment over the five domains, the 30 facets will produce a higher R^2. However, cross-validation removes this artifact, so that more confidence should be placed in studies that have cross-validated such equations than those that have not. Overall, the results of such studies suggest that nuance in personality pathology is not likely to be found in the lower order levels of normative traits.

Second, PD symptoms vary from traits in more ways than their breadth. PD symptoms are also more pathological and narrower than traits. They might also be less stable, depending on the kind of stability being considered (e.g., results are equivocal with respect to differential stability as described earlier but less so with regard to absolute stability as described later). Because lower order traits vary in their associations to pathology, one approach to dealing with differences in pathology has involved conceptualizing only the pathological facets of traits (e.g., Clark, 2007; Krueger et al., 2007), as in the current *DSM–5* proposal. However, this necessarily leads to a limited conceptualization of the full range of personality by omitting normative or adaptive facets. Thus far, promoters of lower order facet representations of personality pathology have not effectively dealt with breadth or stability differences between traits and PD symptoms.

Third, unlike the structure of the higher levels of traits, the field has not approached consensus on the structure of lower

order facets of personality. Thus even if it were possible in the future to fully integrate the lower levels of personality hierarchies with the symptoms of personality pathology, at this point evidence in this regard is not sufficient to justify replacing PDs with lower order traits in the *DSM–5*.

It Is More Useful Clinically to Assess Personality Traits and Disorders Separately

Separating traits and disorders would be more useful clinically than collapsing them for several reasons. First, doing so would emphasize to clinicians the importance of assessing every patient's personality, regardless of his or her diagnosis. Second, the separation of personality traits and disorders would allow for a focus on those PD symptoms that are most bothersome to patients and that are most likely to be targets of intervention. The absolute (mean) levels of traits are fairly stable in adults (Caspi et al., 2005), so clinicians are unlikely to target traits for intervention. Longitudinal research has shown that group levels of PD symptoms, in contrast, can change at higher rates than was previously thought (Grilo et al., 2004; Morey et al., 2007; Zanarini et al., 2007), and therapeutic interventions have shown the ability to decrease PD symptoms (e.g., Matusiewicz, Hopwood, Banducci, & Lejuez, 2010). Thus, distinguishing stable personality characteristics from the malleable elements of PDs would facilitate the assessment of treatment effects to a greater degree than conflating personality traits and disorders. Conceptualizing these malleable elements more distinctly might also promote research on those dynamic aspects of the environment that could impact PD expression, such as life stresses, relationship dynamics, treatment, or other potential influences.

Third, conflating traits and disorders could limit the potential impact of findings from personality science on clinical diagnosis. Trait assessment would be useful to surgeons who wish to predict patient response (Swami, Chamorro-Premuzic, Bridges, & Furnham, 2009), nurses seeking to understand how to care for those they discharge or how to screen for illness (Iwasa et al., 2009), occupational therapists or social workers endeavoring to help the mentally ill find employment (De Fruyt & Mervielde, 1999), marriage counselors trying to help individuals adapt to living with one another (Humbad, Donnellan, Iacono, & Burt, 2010), and many other applications. Regarding personality traits as primarily relevant for PD limits the likelihood that clinicians will recognize the broad utility of personality for their practice. If the authors of the *DSM–5* make the same mistake as the framers of the *DSM–III* and *DSM–IV* in conflating personality traits and disorders, the full potential for the science of personality to influence clinical practice will not have been fulfilled.

Finally, traits have broad integrative potential for clinicians operating from varying perspectives. Most trait researchers recognize that many trait models can be integrated with the FFM (e.g., Widiger & Simonsen, 2005). However, some personality assessors might be concerned that assessing stable, normative traits and dynamic, pathological PD symptoms would still miss the assessment of normative but dynamic personality processes. The FFM was not designed to assess dynamic processes, which might be better represented by the interpersonal model (Pincus, Lukowitsky, & Wright, 2010) that conceptualizes personality in the dynamic social environment, the attachment model that understands personality in the context of internalized representations affected by early relationships with caregivers (Hazan

TABLE 1.—Associations of dynamic personality model dimensions with Five-factor model traits.

Theory	Neuroticism	Extraversion	Openness	Agreeableness	Conscientiousness
Interpersonal		Agency		Communion	
Attachment	Anxiety			Avoidance	
Mood	Negative affects	Positive affects			Constraint
Motivation	Behavioral inhibition	Behavioral activation			
Temperament	Negative affectivity	Surgency			Effortful control

& Shaver, 1994), mood models that capture emotional fluctuations over time (Watson & Tellegen, 1985), motivational models that correspond to dynamic behavioral and neurobiological processes (Gray, 1987), or temperament models that emphasize developmental features of personality (Rothbart, 2007).

As shown in Table 1, each of these more dynamic models can be described by dimensions that relate systematically to FFM traits (interpersonal: McCrae & Costa, 1989; attachment: Noftle & Shaver, 2006; mood: Watson & Clark, 1992; motivation: Smits & Boeck, 2006; temperament: Rothbart, 2007). As such, clinicians or researchers who work from these perspectives can make inferences that fit into their preferred theories with ratings of FFM traits, while also recognizing that dynamic features of these models are like PD symptoms in that they are not fully captured by such trait ratings. This potential suggests not only that an FFM assessment in the *DSM–5* would augment the manual's clinical utility, but also that it would pave the way for future research on the interaction among psychopathology, functioning, and important dynamic processes in personality and social behavior.

THE *DSM–5* PROPOSAL

The *DSM–5* Personality and Personality Disorder Work Group proposal as of February 2010 conceptualizes three levels of personality assessment (Skodol et al., 2011). The first is an overall severity composite that would be similar to *DSM–IV* Global Assessment of Functioning (GAF) but specific to self and interpersonal dysfunction thought to be characteristic of personality pathology. The second involves five PD prototypes that are rated according to the patient's match to the prototype description. The third involves a list of six higher order but pathological and unipolar traits, as well as facets for each of these traits.

This system is an improvement over the *DSM–III/DSM–IV* model in several respects that are not discussed here. However, there are also significant limitations of the proposed system. To be consistent with the purpose of this article, I focus my critique on the *DSM–5* proposal for assessing traits.

It is implicit in the architecture of the *DSM–5* that traits should be rated for their relevance to personality pathology, rather than for their ability to describe people more generally. This constrains what can be done with the traits. For instance, if the purpose of traits is to assess personality pathology, it is difficult to justify including general traits because specific and pathological traits are more strongly related to PDs than general and normative ones (Clark, 2007). However, it makes little sense from a predictive standpoint to rate disorders as well as pathological traits that were selected because of their ability to connote PD. The point should not be to identify trait and disorder constructs that are redundant, but instead to provide data about constructs that are relatively distinct (i.e., discriminant valid) and mutu-

ally informative. Broad normative traits have the potential to provide a greater increment of PD constructs than pathological traits because they overlap less. As one example, the ability to predict adaptive life outcomes might be limited by an exclusive focus on pathological traits.

A related problem that is likely in part a consequence of the structure of the *DSM–5* is that the traits are unipolar rather than bipolar, even though normative traits such as those in the FFM are bipolar in nature (see Samuel, 2011/this issue). The *DSM–5*'s departure from the current state of understanding about trait concepts limits the degree to which the system can be described as supported by available evidence. This also creates problems related to clinical utility. For example, in some instances the tail of a trait dimension that is usually healthy can lead to dysfunction (e.g., pathological agreeableness can connote dependency; Lowe, Edmundson, & Widiger, 2009). Another problem is that, to the extent that only the pathological tails of normally distributed traits are represented in the *DSM–5*, clinicians will not be able to use the healthier tails to indicate personality strengths or predict adaptations.

At a broader level, the proposed traits amount to a new structure for conceptualizing personality. Several decades of research has led to a point where personality psychologists can begin to agree on an integrative structure for traits. In this context, offering a new structure with limited theoretical and empirical support would appear to be a step backward. In the end, the mandate to consider those traits that are the most strongly related to personality pathology appears to have constrained the ability of the Personality and Personality Disorder Work Group to represent traits in a clinically useful, scientifically viable, and theoretically coherent way.

AN ALTERNATIVE: NORMATIVE PERSONALITY TRAIT ASSESSMENT IN THE *DSM–5*

So how could *DSM–5* personality trait assessment be clinically useful, evidence-based, and theoretically coherent? I next offer a system that could achieve these goals.

What: FFM Traits

As described earlier, the FFM has more empirical support and demonstrated clinical utility than any other model of normative personality traits. Significant advances have also occurred in developing theoretical models for the FFM (McCrae & Costa, 2003; Wiggins, 1996). The assessment of normative personality in the *DSM–5* would therefore be on the most solid empirical, clinical, and theoretical footing if it assessed FFM traits.

When: Always

FFM traits should be rated for every person who is diagnosed with the *DSM–5*, whether or not personality pathology is significant, because every person has a personality. However, it is not only the case that all people should be assessed; all trait aspects of all people should be assessed as well. To limit the possibility that important aspects of personality might be missed, the traits should be bipolar—meaning that both high and low scores on each trait should be regarded as meaningful (see Samuel, 2011/this issue). The assessment of bipolar trait dimensions would be more consistent with common personality trait models (including but not limited to the FFM) than unipolar traits. Bipolar traits would also provide greater clinical utility than unipolar traits, for example, in cases in which adaptive tails of some dimensions could be used to predict positive patient outcomes.

Where: Separate From PDs

To ensure that personality traits are treated as relevant for all people rather than as markers of specific forms of PD, all clinicians should rate all patients on FFM traits regardless of their diagnosis. This will be most likely if traits and PDs are assessed in separate sections of the manual. Using the *DSM–III* and *DSM–IV* multiaxial lingo, traits should be listed on Axis II, whereas disorders, including PDs, should be listed on Axis I (see Ruocco, 2005).

How: Clinician Ratings Potentially Supplemented by Formal Assessment Data

Rating forms have been developed for the FFM that could be adopted readily by the *DSM–5* (e.g., Mullins-Sweatt, Jamerson, Samuel, Olson, & Widiger, 2006). There are also several longer assessment methods for the FFM that could supplement or inform clinician ratings. These methods vary in format (e.g., self, other, or interview), length (e.g., long questionnaires with facet scales, brief questionnaires, or rating sheets with one item per trait), and cost (proprietary or public domain). The availability of these methods permits flexibility among clinicians, who could choose optimal assessment methods according to the clinical situation, psychometric evidence, and their preferences.

Issues and Limitations of This Proposal

Assessing FFM traits in the *DSM–5* in the manner I have proposed represents a straightforward strategy for increasing the likelihood of routine personality assessment in clinical practice and linking psychiatric diagnosis and personality science more closely. However, several issues would need to be addressed before this system could be implemented.

One issue is that openness to experience has demonstrated relatively less validity in clinical predictions than the other four FFM traits. It is also unlike the other traits in that it has not been effectively linked to biological structures or pathways (De Young et al., 2010) and is not represented consistently in either stable (Widiger & Simonsen, 2005) or dynamic models of personality (Table 1). Finally, there is the risk that, because the concept of openness is compelling, clinicians could overinterpret this dimension by making clinical inferences that are not supported by research evidence. Thus, good arguments could be made in favor of dropping this dimension. However, there are two reasons to prefer including openness to experience. First, it (or a variant often labeled intellect/imagination; cf. Goldberg, 1993) has been an important part of the FFM since the model was developed, and eliminating it would make trait assessment less comprehensive. Second, the validity of openness to experience

for clinical assessment remains an open question. From a prediction standpoint those traits that are least related to psychopathology have the most potential for incremental validity because their partial coefficients are least constrained by predictive utility of covariates. This fact of prediction suggests some potential for openness to experience in predicting outcomes that are mostly unrelated to psychopathology, such as treatment preferences, optimal work environments, or preferred recreational outlets.

A second issue involves whether or not to incorporate lower order facets of the FFM. It is intuitive that describing a person at the level of the 30 facets of the NEO PI–R provides a more nuanced portrait than a five-domain description, and many clinicians would regard facet assessment as an opportunity to add nuance to descriptions of patient personalities. It is also possible that facet-level description could have specific diagnostic or predictive purposes. For instance, it might be helpful to know if an individual's social behavior is driven primarily by affects or interpersonal motives, as might be indicated by his or her constellation of scores on extraversion facets. Facet descriptions might furthermore be useful for representing psychological traitedness, or the degree to which a given trait is relevant for a particular person (Tellegen, 1988). For instance, some patients are both neurotic (e.g., prone to self-doubt and depression) and emotionally stable (e.g., acquiescent and nonaggressive). Such a person might be described as very high in vulnerability but very low in hostility, suggesting that knowing this person's neuroticism score would not provide as fully accurate a picture of his or her behavior as would knowing the person's score on the neuroticism facets.

However, the structure of facets is not well-established and facets have not shown an ability to increment the domains in clinical predictions in cross-validated prediction models, as discussed earlier. There are also concerns related to the need to limit the complexity of the *DSM–5* system, because greater complexity increases the burden for training clinicians on how to use the manual and for the amount of time and resources required for diagnosis. With these considerations in mind, one potential compromise would be to mandate all clinicians to provide ratings on the FFM trait domains for all patients, and to give clinicians the additional option to rate facets for those cases in which the broad domains do not appear to adequately capture the personality traits of a particular patient.

A third issue involves whether this, or any other system, would increase the likelihood that clinicians would routinely assess personality. Indeed, just because a revised system would offer clinicians a better reason than in the *DSM–III* or *DSM–IV* to assess personality does not mean that clinicians will do so. Overall, personality and PD researchers need to demonstrate more effectively the utility of personality assessment to clinicians and train clinicians in how to adequately assess personality than they have in the past. One way to begin this process is to render personality assessment in the diagnostic manual as straightforward, economical, and evidence-based as possible. Listing carefully selected traits and disorders with the most robust empirical support and least overlap might thus contribute to an increased focus among clinicians on personality assessment.

COMPARISON OF THIS PROPOSAL WITH OTHER PROPOSALS FOR PERSONALITY/PD ASSESSMENT

To summarize, in this proposal FFM trait domains would be listed in a section that is completely separate from the PD

TABLE 2.—Four models proposed for *DSM–5* personality/personality disorder assessment.

Model	Normative Personality	Personality Disorder
DSM–5 Work Group	Absent	37 pathological traits 2 general severity dimensions 5 PD prototypes
FFM of PD	5 FFM traits 30 FFM facets	Absent
Bornstein (1998)	Adaptive aspects of 10 PDs	1 general severity dimension 10 PD dimensions (with separate ratings for impairment and severity)
Current proposal	5 FFM traits	1 general severity dimension 5–10 PD dimensions

Note. DSM = Diagnostic and Statistical Manual of Mental Disorders; FFM = Five-factor model; PD = personality disorder.

section. Clinicians would be required to make ratings on each of the FFM traits for all patients, with the option of also rating facets. There is not sufficient space in this article to outline in detail a model for how to assess the PDs as separate from these traits. In a previous article (Hopwood, Malone, et al., in press) my colleagues and I described a model that is based somewhat on Bornstein's (1998, 2011/this issue) proposal to assess three levels of personality functioning: overall severity, impairment and severity related to specific PDs, and adaptive features of specific PDs. The main difference involves whether or not the normative and adaptive features of personality are best assessed by normative traits or by rating the potentially adaptive features of PDs.

Thus, as shown in Table 2, the PD model in this proposal would include two of Bornstein's three levels: generalized PD severity and stylistic PD dimensions. However unlike Bornstein's proposal, clinicians would rate five normative personality dimensions in a section separate from the PDs. They would rate a global severity dimensions as well as the symptoms of between 5 (e.g., *DSM–5* proposal; Hopwood, Malone, et al., in press) and 10 (e.g., *DSM–IV*) stylistic PD dimensions in another section. A general severity dimension, analogous to the *g* factor in intelligence or the *DSM–IV* GAF score for more general functional difficulties, has been an important part of some theories of personality pathology (e.g., Kernberg's [1984] personality organization), and researchers have developed methods to assess it (e.g., Bornstein, 2011/this issue). In terms of stylistic PD dimensions, initial decisions about which constructs to retain could be based first on accumulated validity evidence. However, achieving consensus about which PDs are supported by available evidence is unlikely. As described in Hopwood, Malone, et al. (in press), a second and perhaps more influential consideration would involve identifying PD constructs that are maximally distinct from one another and from normative traits. The purpose of focusing on the discriminant validity of various elements of personality assessment would be to provide clinical information that is minimally overlapping and incrementally useful.

Table 2 shows similarities and differences between this proposal and the *DSM–5* proposal as well. There are two major differences. First, whereas in the *DSM–5* proposal traits and disorders (types) are intermingled, I would separate them to focus more on their potential discriminant validity. Not only

would traits and disorders be rated in separate sections, but they would also be constructed to differ in terms of their distributions (normal/bipolar vs. positively skewed/unipolar), stability (stable vs. dynamic), and breadth (broad vs. narrow). We (Hopwood, Malone, et al., in press) showed that orthogonal PD dimensions can be derived that correlate only modestly with normative traits but are nevertheless valid predictors of specific kinds of functioning. This finding indicates that it is possible to derive discriminantly valid and mutually informative normative and pathological personality dimensions. Second, the PDs would be diagnosed according to symptoms rather than prototype descriptions. The reasons for this are practical. Symptoms permit a more nuanced description of pathology, provide a more precise indication of treatment targets than global ratings, and allow for a more specific assessment of change. Rating PD dimensions with symptoms also encourages clinicians to think about PDs the way they think about any other Axis I diagnoses—as pathological, changeable, and meaningfully separate from the personality context in which they occur.

Finally, Table 2 shows how the proposed model is different from the FFM of PD (Widiger & Trull, 2007). Rather than presuming that the pathological elements of personality can be adequately conceptualized with normative traits, the current model explicitly separates normative and pathological personality features.

FUTURE DIRECTIONS

Whatever happens in the *DSM–5*, future research should focus on developing a better understanding of how traits predispose symptoms and what dynamic processes interact with traits to produce PD symptoms and other forms of psychopathology. Such processes are most likely to be identified if researchers balance the current focus on individual differences with an increased focus on intraindividual change (e.g., see Russell, Moskowitz, Zuroff, Sookman, & Paris, 2007, for an example of this sort of research with borderline personality) and if they balance the current overreliance on interview and self-report data with an increased use of other methods (e.g., see Klonsky & Oltmanns, 2002, for a discussion of other-report data and Huprich & Bornstein, 2007, for a discussion of performance-based personality assessment methods). That such future research will be more fruitful if it capitalizes on the accumulated knowledge of personality science represents another reason that the *DSM–5* should avoid departing from evidence-based models of personality.

CONCLUSION

It is possible that personality traits and disorders might in the end fit into an integrative framework that achieves scientific and clinical consensus and is continuous in terms of individual difference variables, but also in terms of normality–pathology, stability–change, and breadth–depth, and that can account coherently for different systems, such as affects, interpersonal behaviors, cognitions, functional outcomes, and motives. Such a system would have numerous and obvious advantages over any current or proposed diagnostic framework. It is also possible that, in the end, there is something important about the difference between enduring, normative traits and narrower, more dynamic, personality pathology symptoms, and that it is most sensible to conceptualize these as interpenetrating but meaningfully independent domains. Current evidence is insufficient to determine which of these models will end up being more viable, or if some other model will best explain future data.

What is known now is that traits are important, PDs are important, personality traits relate to but are not redundant with PDs, and traits and disorders increment one another for clinical predictions. Based on what is known, it would not be prudent to integrate personality traits and disorders in a manner that would risk missing important assessment information. Conversely, distinguishing traits, the severity of personality pathology, and the stylistic expression of PD symptoms would allow each element of personality assessment to be useful for different kinds of questions (Hopwood, Malone, et al., in press). Traits could be consulted for questions regarding the enduring and pervasive personality context of a person's difficulties and thus the likelihood of quick remittance (e.g., To what degree is this patient's depression predisposed by neuroticism vs. more contextual factors?), general severity would be relevant for making predictions about optimal levels of care (e.g., Should this patient be hospitalized?), and PD symptom constellations would be important for determining treatment strategies (e.g., Would transference-focused psychotherapy be appropriate for this patient?).

What has been presented here offers a balance between accounting for personality traits and disorders broadly and inclusively, and in such a way that most of the assessment data would be incremental rather than redundant. This model would achieve the original promise of the multiaxial format of the *DSM–III* and *DSM–IV* to explicitly separate personality from pathology by regarding PDs as more disorder than personality and liberating personality to occupy its own, unencumbered section of the manual. Given that Spitzer's goal that all clinicians would diagnose personality has not been achieved in the most recent editions of the *DSM* and in light of the significant advances in personality science over the past few decades, it is time for the official diagnostic manual to give clinicians a reason to diagnose personality in all people.

ACKNOWLEDGMENTS

I thank M. Brent Donnellan, Steven K. Huprich, Leslie C. Morey, Aaron L. Pincus, Andrew E. Skodol, Katherine M. Thomas, and Aidan G. C. Wright for their helpful feedback on earlier drafts of this article.

REFERENCES

American Psychiatric Association. (1987). *Diagnostic and statistical manual of mental disorders* (3rd ed.). Washington, DC: Author.

American Psychiatric Association. (1994). *Diagnostic and statistical manual of mental disorders* (4th ed.). Washington, DC: Author.

Bagby, R. M., Young, L. T., Schuller, D. R., Bindseil, K. D., Cooke, R. G., Dickens, S. E., . . . Joffe, R. T. (1996). Bipolar disorder, unipolar depression, and the Five-Factor Model of personality. *Journal of Affective Disorders, 41*, 25–32.

Bleidorn, W., Kandler, C., Riemann, R., Angleitner, A., & Spinath, F. M. (2009). Patterns and sources of adult personality development: Growth curve analyses of the NEO PI–R scales in a longitudinal twin study. *Journal of Personality and Social Psychology, 97*, 142–155.

Bornstein, R. F. (1998). Reconceptualizing personality disorder diagnosis in the *DSM–V*: The discriminant validity challenge. *Clinical Psychology: Science and Practice, 5*, 333–343.

Bornstein, R. F. (2011/this issue). Toward a multidimensional model of personality disorder diagnosis: Implications for *DSM–5*. *Journal of Personality Assessment, 93*, 362–369.

Caspi, A., Roberts, B. W., & Shiner, R. L. (2005). Personality development: Stability and change. *Annual Review of Psychology, 56*, 453–484.

Caspi, A., & Silva, P. A. (1995). Temperamental qualities at age three predict personality traits in young adulthood: Longitudinal evidence from a birth cohort. *Child Development, 66*, 486–498.

Clark, L. A. (2007). Assessment and diagnosis of personality disorder: Perennial issues and emerging conceptualization. *Annual Review of Psychology, 58*, 227–258.

Costa, P. T. Jr., & McCrae, R. R. (1992). *Revised NEO Personality Inventory professional manual.* Odessa, FL: Psychological Assessment Resources.

De Fruyt, F., & Mervielde, I. (1999). RIASEC types and big five traits as predictors of employment status and nature of employment. *Personnel Psychology, 52*, 701–727.

Depue, R. A., & Lenzenweger, M. F. (2004). A neurobehavioral dimensional model of personality disturbance. In M. F. Lenzenweger & J. F. Clarkin (Eds.), *Major theories of personality disorder* (2nd ed., pp. 391–454). New York, NY: Guilford.

De Young, C. G., Hirsch, J. B., Shane, M. S., Papademetris, X., Rajeevan, N., & Gray, J. R. (2010). Testing predictions from personality neuroscience: Brain structure and the big five. *Psychological Science, 21*, 820–828.

Durbin, C. E., & Klein, D. N. (2006). Ten-year stability of personality disorders among outpatients with mood disorders. *Journal of Abnormal Psychology, 115*, 75–84.

Ferguson, C. J. (2010). A meta-analysis of normative and disordered personality across the life span. *Journal of Personality and Social Psychology, 98*, 659–667.

Goldberg, L. R. (1993). The structure of phenotypic personality traits. *American Psychologist, 48*, 26–34.

Gray, J. A. (1987). *The psychology of fear and stress* (2nd ed.). New York, NY: Cambridge University Press.

Grilo, C. M., Sanislow, C. A., Gunderson, J. G., Pagano, M. E., Yen, S., Zanarini, M. C., . . . McGlashan, T. H. (2004). Two-year stability and change of schizotypal, borderline, avoidant, and obsessive-compulsive personality disorders. *Journal of Consulting and Clinical Psychology, 72*, 767–775.

Grucza, R. A., & Goldberg, L. R. (2007). The comparative validity of 11 modern personality inventories: Predictions based on behavioral acts, informant reports, and clinical indicators. *Journal of Personality Assessment, 89*, 167–187.

Hazan, C., & Shaver, P. R. (1994). Attachment as an organizational framework for research on close relationships. *Psychological Inquiry, 5*, 1–22.

Hopwood, C. J., Donnellan, M. B., Blonigen, D. M., Krueger, R. F., McGue, M., Iacono, W. G., & Burt, S. A. (2011). Genetic and environmental influences on personality trait stability and growth during the transition to adulthood: A three wave longitudinal study. *Journal of Personality and Social Psychology, 100*, 545–556.

Hopwood, C. J., Malone, J. C., Ansell, E. B., Sanislow, C. A., Grilo, C. M., McGlashan, T. H., . . . Morey, L. C. (in press). Personality assessment in *DSM–V*: Empirical support for rating severity, style, and traits. *Journal of Personality Disorders.*

Hopwood, C. J., Morey, L. C., Shea, M. T., McGlashan, T. H., Sanislow, C. A., Grilo, C.M., . . . Skodol, A. E. (2007). Personality traits predict current and future functioning comparably for individuals with major depressive and personality disorders. *Journal of Nervous and Mental Disease, 195*, 266–269.

Hopwood, C. J., Newman, D. A., Donnellan, M. B., Markowitz, J. C., Grilo, C. M., Sanislow, C. A., . . . Morey, L. C. (2009). The stability of personality traits in individuals with borderline personality disorder. *Journal of Abnormal Psychology, 118*, 806–815.

Hopwood, C. J., & Zanarini, M. C. (2010). Borderline personality traits and disorder: Predicting prospective patient functioning. *Journal of Consulting and Clinical Psychology, 78*, 585–589.

Hopwood, C. J., & Zanarini, M. C. (in press). Five factor trait instability in borderline relative to other personality disorders. *Personality Disorders: Theory, Research, and Treatment.*

Humbad, M. N., Donnellan, M. B., Iacono, W. G., & Burt, S. A. (2010). Externalizing psychopathology and marital adjustment in long-term marriages: Results from a large combined sample of married couples. *Journal of Abnormal Psychology, 119*, 151–162.

Huprich, S. K., & Bornstein, R. F. (2007). Categorical and dimensional assessment of personality disorders: A consideration of the issues. *Journal of Personality Assessment, 89*, 3–15.

Iwasa, H., Masui, Y., Gondo, Y., Yoshida, Y., Inagaki, H., Kawaai, C., ... Suzuki, T. (2009). Personality and participation in mass health checkups among Japanese community-dwelling elderly. *Journal of Psychosomatic Research, 66*, 155–159.

Kernberg, O. F. (1984). *Severe personality disorders: Psychotherapeutic strategies*. New Haven, CT: Yale University Press.

Klonsky, E. D., & Oltmanns, T. F. (2002). Informant reports of personality disorder: Relation to self-reports and future research directions. *Clinical Psychology: Science and Practice, 9*, 300–311.

Kotov, R., Gamez, W., Schmidt, F., & Watson, D. (2010). Linking "big" personality traits to anxiety, depressive, and substance use disorders: A meta-analysis. *Psychological Bulletin, 136*, 768–821.

Krueger, R. F. (1999). The structure of common mental disorders. *Archives of General Psychiatry, 56*, 921–926.

Krueger, R. F., Skodol, A. E., Livesley, W. J., Shrout, P. E., & Huang, Y. (2007). Synthesizing dimensional and categorical approaches to personality disorders: Refining the research agenda for *DSM–V* Axis II. *International Journal of Methods in Psychiatric Research, 16*, S65–S73.

Lenzenweger, M. F., & Willett, J. B. (2007). Predicting individual change in personality disorder features by simultaneous individual change in personality dimensions linked to neurobehavioral systems: The longitudinal study of personality disorders. *Journal of Abnormal Psychology, 116*, 684–700.

Loehlin, J. C. (2001). Behavior genetics and parenting theory. *American Psychologist, 56*, 169–170.

Lowe, J. R., Edmundson, M., & Widiger, T. A. (2009). Assessment of dependency, agreeableness, and their relationship. *Psychological Assessment, 21*, 543–553.

Matusiewicz, A. K., Hopwood, C. J., Banducci, A. N., & Lejuez, C. W. (2010). The effectiveness of cognitive behavioral therapy for personality disorders. *Psychiatric Clinics of North America, 33*, 657–686.

McCrae, R. R., & Costa, P. T. (1989). The structure of interpersonal traits: Wiggins's circumplex and the five-factor model. *Journal of Personality and Social Psychology, 56*, 586–595.

McCrae, R. R., & Costa, P. T. (1997). Personality trait structure as a human universal. *American Psychologist, 52*, 509–516.

McCrae, R. R., & Costa, P. T. (2003). *Personality in adulthood: A five-factor theory perspective* (2nd ed.). New York, NY: Guilford.

Morey, L. C., Gunderson, J. G., Quigley, B. D., Shea, M. T., Skodol, A. E., McGlashan, T. H., ... Zanarini, M. C. (2002). The representation of borderline, avoidant, obsessive–compulsive, and schizotypal personality disorders by the five-factor model. *Journal of Personality Disorders, 16*, 215–234.

Morey L. C., Hopwood C. J., Gunderson J. G., Skodol A. E., Shea M. T., Yen, S., ... McGlashan, T. H. (2007). Comparison of alternative models for personality disorders. *Psychological Medicine, 37*, 983–994.

Mullins-Sweatt, S. N., Jamerson, J. E., Samuel, D. B., Olson, D. R., & Widiger, T. A. (2006). Psychometric properties of an abbreviated instrument of the five-factor model. *Assessment, 13*, 119–137.

Nigg, J. T., John, O. P., Blaskey, L. G., Huang-Pollock, C. L., Willcutt, E. G., Hinshaw, S. P., & Pennington, B. (2002). Big five dimensions and ADHD symptoms: Links between personality traits and clinical symptoms. *Journal of Personality and Social Psychology, 83*, 451–469.

Noftle, E. E., & Shaver, P. R. (2006). Attachment dimensions and the big five personality traits: Associations and comparative validity to predict relationship quality. *Journal of Research in Personality, 40*, 179–208.

Ozer, D. J., & Benet-Martinez, V. (2006). Personality and the prediction of consequential life outcomes. *Annual Review of Psychology, 57*, 401–421.

Pincus, A. L., Lukowitsky, M. R., & Wright, A. G. C. (2010). The interpersonal nexus of personality and psychopathology. In T. Millon, R. F. Krueger, & E. Simonsen (Eds.), *Contemporary directions in psychopathology: Scientific foundations of the DSM–V and ICD–11* (pp. 523–552). New York, NY: Guilford.

Rothbart, M. K. (2007). Temperament, development, and personality. *Current Directions in Psychological Science, 16*, 207–212.

Ruiz, M. A., Pincus, A. L., & Schinka, J. A. (2008). Externalizing pathology and the five-factor model: A meta-analysis of personality traits associated with antisocial personality disorder, substance use disorder, and their co-occurrence. *Journal of Personality Disorders, 22*, 365–388.

Ruocco, A. C. (2005). Reevaluating the distinction between Axis I and Axis II disorders: The case of borderline personality disorder. *Journal of Clinical Psychology, 61*, 1509–1523.

Russell, J. J., Moskowitz, D. S., Zuroff, D. C., Sookman, D., & Paris, J. (2007). Stability and variability of affective experience and interpersonal behavior in borderline personality disorder. *Journal of Abnormal Psychology, 116*, 578–588.

Samuel, D. B. (2011/this issue). Assessing personality in the *DSM–5*: The utility of bipolar constructs. *Journal of Personality Assessment, 93*, 390–397.

Samuel, D. B., Hopwood, C. J., Ansell, E. B., Morey, L. C., Sanislow, C. A., Markowitz, J. C., ... Grilo, C. M. (in press). The temporal stability of self-reported personality disorder. *Journal of Abnormal Psychology*.

Samuel, D. B., & Widiger, T. A. (2008). A meta-analytic review of the relationships between the five-factor model and *DSM–IV–TR* personality disorders: A facet-level analysis. *Clinical Psychology Review, 28*, 1326–1342.

Saulsman, L. M., & Page, A. C. (2004). The five-factor model and personality disorder empirical literature: A meta-analytic review. *Clinical Psychology Review, 23*, 1055–1085.

Skodol, A. E., Clark, L. A., Bender, D. S., Krueger, R. F., Morey, L. C., Verheul, R., ... Oldham, J. M. (2011). Proposed changes in personality and personality disorder assessment and diagnosis for *DSM–5* Part I: Description and rationale. *Personality Disorders: Theory, Research, and Treatment, 2*, 4–22.

Smits, D. J. M., & Boeck, P. D. (2006). From BIS/BAS to the big five. *European Journal of Personality, 20*, 255–270.

Spitzer, R. L. (1976). *Progress report on the preparation of DSM–III*. Unpublished manuscript. Washington, DC: American Psychiatric Association Task Force on Nomenclature and Statistics.

Stevens, J. P. (2002). *Applied multivariate statistics for the social sciences* (4th ed.) Mahwah, NJ: Erlbaum.

Swami, V., Chamorro-Premuzic, T., Bridges, S., & Furnham, A. (2009). Acceptance of cosmetic surgery: Personality and individual difference predictors. *Body Image, 6*, 7–13.

Tellegen, A. (1988). The analysis of consistency in personality assessment. *Journal of Personality, 56*, 621–663.

Trull, T. J., Widiger, T. A., Lynam, D. R., & Costa, P. T. (2003). Borderline personality disorder from the perspective of general personality functioning. *Journal of Abnormal Psychology, 112*, 193–202.

Warner, M. B., Morey, L. C., Finch, J. F., Gunderson, J. G., Skodol, A. E., Sanislow, C. A., ... Grilo, C. M. (2004). The longitudinal relationship of personality traits and disorders. *Journal of Abnormal Psychology, 113*, 217–227.

Watson, D., & Clark, L. A. (1992). On traits and temperament: General and specific factors of emotional experience and their relation to the five-factor model. *Journal of Personality, 60*, 441–476.

Watson, D., & Tellegen, A. (1985). Toward a consensual structure of mood. *Psychological Bulletin, 98*, 219–235.

Widiger, T. A., & Simonsen, E. (2005). Alternative dimensional models of personality disorder: Finding a common ground. *Journal of Personality Disorders, 19*, 110–130.

Widiger, T. A., & Trull, T. J. (2007). Plate tectonics in the classification of personality disorder: Shifting to a dimensional model. *American Psychologist, 62*, 71–83.

Wiggins, J. S. (1996). *The five-factor model of personality: Theoretical perspectives*. New York, NY: Guilford.

Williams, J. B. W. (1985). The multiaxial system of *DSM–III*: Where did it come from and where should it go? *Archives of General Psychiatry, 42*, 175–180.

Zanarini, M. C., Frankenburg, F. R., Reich, D. R., Silk, K. R., Hudson, J. I., & McSweeney, L. B. (2007). The subsyndromal phenomenology of borderline personality disorder: A 10-year follow-up study. *American Journal of Psychiatry, 164*, 929–935.

Computerized Adaptive Assessment of Personality Disorder: Introducing the CAT–PD Project

Leonard J. Simms,[1] Lewis R. Goldberg,[2] John E. Roberts,[1] David Watson,[3] John Welte,[4] and Jane H. Rotterman[1]

[1]Department of Psychology, University at Buffalo, The State University of New York
[2]Oregon Research Institute, Eugene, Oregon
[3]Department of Psychology, University of Notre Dame
[4]Research Institute on Addictions, University at Buffalo, The State University of New York

Assessment of personality disorders (PD) has been hindered by reliance on the problematic categorical model embodied in the most recent *Diagnostic and Statistical Model of Mental Disorders* (*DSM*), lack of consensus among alternative dimensional models, and inefficient measurement methods. This article describes the rationale for and early results from a multiyear study funded by the National Institute of Mental Health that was designed to develop an integrative and comprehensive model and efficient measure of PD trait dimensions. To accomplish these goals, we are in the midst of a 5-phase project to develop and validate the model and measure. The results of Phase 1 of the project—which was focused on developing the PD traits to be assessed and the initial item pool—resulted in a candidate list of 59 PD traits and an initial item pool of 2,589 items. Data collection and structural analyses in community and patient samples will inform the ultimate structure of the measure, and computerized adaptive testing will permit efficient measurement of the resultant traits. The resultant Computerized Adaptive Test of Personality Disorder (CAT–PD) will be well positioned as a measure of the proposed *DSM–5 PD* traits. Implications for both applied and basic personality research are discussed.

Personality pathology is prevalent in the community and in mental health settings. In recent epidemiological surveys of *Diagnostic and Statistical Manual of Mental Disorders* (4th ed. [*DSM–IV*]; American Psychiatric Association, 1994) and *International Classification of Diseases* (10th ed. [*ICD–10*; World Health Organization, 1992]) personality disorders (PDs), prevalence rates have ranged between 9% and 14% in community samples (e.g., Ekselius, Tillfors, Furmark, & Fredrikson, 2001; Samuels et al., 2002; Torgersen, Kringlen, & Cramer, 2001) and as high as 45% in patient samples (e.g., Zimmerman, Rothschild, & Chelminski, 2005). Moreover, personality pathology is highly comorbid with Axis I disorders (Grant et al., 2005; Zimmerman et al., 2005), and such comorbidity changes or complicates the treatment course of such syndromes. Studies have indicated that personality pathology negatively affects the course and outcome of both psychotherapeutic and pharmacological treatments for Axis I disorders (e.g., Cyranowski et al., 2004; Feske et al., 2004; Reich, 2003) and is associated with higher health-care service utilization and functional impairment in a variety of important life domains (e.g., Bender et al., 2001; Skodol et al., 2005; Smith & Benjamin, 2002).

Thus, personality pathology is an important mental health concern that should be routinely assessed and treated in mental health settings. However, the length and administration time associated with most PD measures, the problems associated with the current categorical classification of PD, and the wide variety of alternative PD models and measures have interfered with the routine assessment of personality pathology in both research

and clinical settings. Both interview and questionnaire methods can be costly in terms of the time and resources required to administer, score, and interpret them properly. Unfortunately, these time and staff requirements are difficult to accommodate in most settings (e.g., Piotrowski, 1999; Piotrowski, Belter, & Keller, 1998; Yates & Taub, 2003), especially in the context of current ambiguities about how best to classify and assess personality problems. To remedy these concerns and improve the assessment of PD, new classification models are needed that bridge and improve on existing models. Moreover, measurement methods are needed that increase the efficiency of PD assessment. The development of comprehensive and efficient measures of personality pathology would be an important addition to the toolbox of mental health clinicians and researchers.

CATEGORICAL VS. DIMENSIONAL CLASSIFICATION OF PERSONALITY PATHOLOGY

Traditional nosological systems of personality pathology, such as *DSM–IV* and *ICD–10*, describe PD using a medical model within which pathological syndromes are viewed as being either present or absent. However, although the inclusion of PDs on Axis II as an independent domain in *DSM–III* (3rd ed.; American Psychiatric Association, 1980) was an important advance, the categorical model used by that and subsequent editions of the *DSM* suffers from a number of problems that limit its usefulness, including high rates of diagnostic comorbidity among purportedly distinct PDs (e.g., Clark, Watson, & Reynolds, 1995; Dolan, Evans, & Norton, 1995; Fossati et al., 2000; Oldham et al., 1995), within-disorder heterogeneity (e.g., Clark et al., 1995; Widiger, 1993), an arbitrary boundary between normal and abnormal personality traits (e.g., Clark et al., 1995; Livesley, Jang, & Vernon, 1998; Widiger & Clark, 2000), poor reliability (Dreessen & Arntz, 1998; Pilkonis et al., 1995;

Zanarini et al., 2000), and low convergent validity (see Clark, Livesley, & Morey, 1997, for a review). Moreover, categorical systems appear to result in substantial information loss, especially for individuals who manifest clinically significant signs and symptoms that do not quite reach the arbitrary thresholds specified by the *DSM*.

As a result, many have called for a dimensional approach to describing and assessing personality pathology (e.g., Clark, 2007; Livesley & Jackson, 2009; Widiger & Clark, 2000; Widiger & Simonsen, 2005). Two basic approaches have been proposed to dimensionalize Axis II. The first is to maintain the current PD category labels and simply measure them along continua, either by summing the *DSM* criteria, creating measures to tap the relevant aspects of each PD construct, or by developing rational or empirical PD prototypes that can be rated dimensionally in terms of prototype similarity (e.g., Oldham & Skodol, 2000; Shedler & Westen, 2004; Westen, Shedler, & Bradley, 2006). Such methods generally lead to increased stability of measurement (e.g., Zanarini et al., 2000); however, diagnostic overlap and within-class heterogencity are still problems (Clark, 2007). The second method involves (a) discarding the a priori assumption that personality pathology is adequately defined by the current set of *DSM–IV* PD categories, and (b) identifying and measuring the trait dimensions that underlie phenotypic manifestations of personality pathology.

A number of measures and models have been proposed along these lines. Most notably, the Five-factor model (FFM) has gathered support in recent years as a viable model for personality pathology in general and as a potential basis for describing PD in the next revision of the *DSM* (e.g., Miller et al., 2010; Widiger & Simonsen, 2005; Widiger & Trull, 2007). In addition, the interpersonal circumplex has been proposed as a dimensional framework for understanding personality pathology (e.g., Pincus & Gurtman, 2006). Both of these models represent attempts to explain personality pathology in terms of existing structural models of *normal-range* personality. In contrast, several bottom-up, PD-specific models have been offered (e.g., the Schedule for Nonadaptive and Adaptive Personality–2nd Edition [SNAP–2; Clark, Simms, Wu, & Casillas, in press] and the Dimensional Assessment of Personality Pathology–Basic Questionnaire [DAPP–BQ; Livesley & Jackson, 2009]) that first identify lower order traits relevant to PD and then let the covariance among those traits drive the ultimate structure of the domain.

In either case, the primary descriptive units in dimensional models of this second broad type are the basic personality traits that underlie the domain of personality pathology. Patients are rated on a number of distinct traits relevant to personality dysfunction, rather than being placed in one or more diagnostic categories. The distinction between normal and abnormal functioning then can be determined on the basis of empirical criteria. Statistical infrequency is a common criterion of abnormality in dimensional models, with individuals scoring, say, 1.5 or 2 *SD* above or below the norm considered to be in the "abnormal" or "pathological" range. Of course, the use and location of cut points along dimensions can be arbitrary and generally results in the loss of statistical power, leading some to eschew the use of cutoffs and interpret dimensional scores quantitatively, either relative to norms or to other dimensions within the same clinical profile. Moreover, some have argued that statistical infrequency alone is an inadequate criterion to signal the presence of personality disorder unless it is coupled with concomitant dysfunction or impairment in important areas of functioning (e.g., Livesley

& Jang, 2000; Tyrer, 2005). In any case, comprehensive dimensional systems can be used as the foundation for empirically based classification systems (e.g., based on latent class and latent profile analyses) in which diagnostic entities are formed by identifying individuals with similar profiles of personality traits (e.g., Eaton, Krueger, South, Simms, & Clark, in press). Thus, although the primary strength of trait-based systems is their ability to yield relatively homogeneous and distinctive dimensional interpretations, such systems also are flexible enough to yield empirically based categorical information.

DIMENSIONAL MODELS OF PD

A variety of dimensional models have been proposed as alternatives to the current categorical PD system (e.g., Clark, 1993; Clark et al., in press; Livesley & Jackson, 2009; Widiger & Simonsen, 2005, 2006; Widiger & Trull, 2007). Widiger and Simonsen (2005, 2006) summarized 18 dimensional PD models and organized the traits included in these models into a pathology-slanted version of the FFM: (a) extraversion versus introversion, (b) antagonism versus compliance, (c) constraint versus impulsivity, (d) emotional dysregulation versus emotional stability, and (e) unconventionality versus closedness to experience. Within this integrative framework, each broad domain is made up of a number of narrower, lower order dimensions that, when factored, should give rise to the five higher order dimensions. Table 1 includes a summary of Widiger and Simonsen's (2005, 2006) assignment of lower order dimensions to each broad domain. Several themes are apparent from this collection of dimensions. First, within each broad domain, there is substantial overlap across similarly named traits (e.g., sociability and social closeness vs. aloofness, detachment, and social avoidance all appear to tap quite similar aspects of interpersonal behavior in the extraversion–introversion domain). Second, some lower order traits are listed across multiple domains (e.g., alienation, entitlement, social closeness, dependency), which likely is due to different conceptualizations of these traits across models.

For these reasons, the lower order dimensions identified by Widiger and Simonsen are too numerous and overlapping in their current form to be of real practical value. Moreover, each of the 18 models that contributed to Table 1 (including such prominent models as the FFM, Livesley's DAPP–BQ, and Clark's SNAP–2) is incomplete in its representation of relevant dimensions of personality pathology. Widiger and Simonsen (2006) summarized their review by noting that "none of the models lacks any limitations that could not at times be well compensated through an integration with another model" (p. 3). Thus, although previous models exist to describe the lower order structure of personality pathology, no single model proposed to date encompasses the full range and breadth of dimensions relevant to personality pathology. Based on these models, Widiger and Simonsen (2006) concluded "that an important goal of future research will be the identification of a common ground among alternative dimensional models of personality disorder" (p. 15). As such, additional work is needed to refine this set of dimensions (i.e., identify the core, nonoverlapping constructs that are relevant to personality pathology) and to generate a measure that efficiently and practically assesses each of them.

WORKING TOWARD *DSM–5*

The American Psychiatric Association began the planning process for *DSM–5* in 1999. The proposed revisions were

TABLE 1.—Summary of personality-disorder dimensions identified by Widiger and Simonsen (2005, 2006), organized by the Five-factor model.

Broad Domain	Relevant Lower Order Trait Facets Identified in the Literature
Extraversion vs. introversion	Activity, aloofness, assertiveness, detachment, entitlement, excitement seeking, exhibitionism, exploratory excitability, extravagance, gregariousness, histrionic sexualization, intimacy problems, optimism, positive emotionality, restricted expression, schizoid orientation, shyness, sociability, social avoidance, social closeness, social potency, stimulus seeking, warmth, well-being
Antagonism vs. compliance	Aggression, agreeableness, alienation, altruism, attachment, callousness, compassion, compliance, conduct problems, dependency, diffidence, empathy, entitlement, helpfulness, insecure attachment, interpersonal disesteem, manipulativeness, mistrust, modesty, narcissism, passive oppositionality, psychopathy, pure-hearted, rejection, sentimentality, social acceptance, social closeness, straightforwardness, submissiveness, suspiciousness, tender-mindedness, trust
Constraint vs. impulsivity	Achievement-striving, childishness, competence, compulsivity, conscientiousness, deliberation, disorderliness, dutifulness, eagerness of effort, harm avoidance, impulsivity, irresponsibility, obsessionality, order, perfectionism, propriety, resourcefulness, responsibility, risk taking, self-discipline, traditionalism, workaholism
Emotional dysregulation vs. stability	Affective lability, alienation, angry hostility, anticipatory worry, anxiousness, dependency, depressiveness, dysphoria, emotional dysregulation, fear of uncertainty, hostility, hypochondriasis, identify problems, inferiority, introspection, irritability, negative affect, pessimism, self-acceptance, self-consciousness, self-harm, sensitivity, stress reaction, unhappiness, vulnerability, worthlessness
Unconventionality vs. closedness to experience	Absorption, dissociation, eccentric perceptions, eccentricity, openness to experience, perceptual cognitive distortion, rigidity, spiritual acceptance, thought disorder, transpersonal identification

released to the public on the DSM5.org Web site early in 2010. Based on the issues raised earlier regarding categorical PD models, the Personality and Personality Disorders (PPD) Work Group, which includes a diverse group of psychologists and psychiatrists with PD expertise, has proposed a fairly radical reformulation of the PD domain that includes, in part, a dimensional trait system. Ongoing field trials might lead to changes from what has been proposed, but the current proposal includes four primary components for PD classification: (a) a new general definition of PD focused on deficits in personality functioning and elevated pathological traits, (b) a five-tier dimensional scheme for describing personality-related functioning and impairment, (c) five PD prototypes that are based on DSM–IV disorders deemed worthy of retention by the work group, and (d) a trait system characterized by six broad, higher order personality trait domains (Negative Emotionality, Introversion, Antagonism, Disinhibition, Compulsivity, and Schizotypy), into which 37 specific trait facets are organized.

Although the proposed list of traits seems to be reasonably representative of the PD domain, the origins of this particular set of trait facets have not been described in much detail. The rationale for the selected lower order traits, as posted on the DSM5.org Web site, is limited to the following: "The pro-

posed specific trait facets were selected as representative based on existing measures of normal and abnormal personality, as well as recommendations by experts in personality assessment. Nonetheless, the proposed trait set is provisional, and currently is being tested for its structural validity before finalizing the DSM–V proposal" (Clark & Krueger, 2010). However, the nature of the experts used to guide this process, as well as how these particular traits relate to the broad PD domain, are not elaborated by Clark and Krueger. Thus, although the field trials likely will result in refinement of the initial trait set, traits not included in the initial set will have no opportunity to enter the model at this later stage. Any omissions from the initial model almost certainly will be maintained in the final scheme.

THE CAT–PD PROJECT

To summarize, accumulating evidence has revealed significant problems with the current categorical framework underlying PD description in DSM–IV, and adopting a dimensional model of the traits underlying personality pathology can ameliorate most of these problems. Moreover, the proposed DSM–5 criteria for PD include an explicitly dimensional system that, although not fully validated as yet, reflects a fundamental shift away from a purely categorical model. However, although reasonable consensus has emerged regarding the higher order trait structure of the personality/PD domains (e.g., Markon, Krueger, & Watson, 2005), no such consensus exists regarding the nature and number of the lower order traits to be included in a comprehensive PD trait system. In addition, most common measures of PD are quite inefficient and must be administered and scored by professional staff. To that end, we designed the Computerized Adaptive Test of Personality Disorder (CAT–PD) project to accomplish two related goals: (a) identify a comprehensive and integrative set of higher and lower order personality traits relevant to personality pathology, and (b) develop a computerized system, based on the principles of adaptive testing to measure the resultant traits efficiently. In addition to these primary goals, it is likely that the resultant CAT–PD model and measure has the potential to improve PD research and clinical work in a number of interesting ways, such as (a) providing a basis for richer etiological and treatment models of PD, (b) improving our understanding of the higher and lower order structure of PD-relevant personality traits, and (c) providing a flexible and comprehensive basis for clinical personality profile analyses.

We currently are in Phase 2 of a five-phase CAT–PD process:

1. Identification of all possible candidate traits to be assessed and development of the initial item pool.
2. Community and patient data collection, followed by scale development and refinement.
3. Calibration of the final item sets using item response theory (IRT) and computerized adaptive testing (CAT) simulation studies to optimize the organization and administration of the CAT–PD.
4. Development of the CAT–PD software.
5. Construct validation of the final CAT–PD test and software.

In the remainder of this article, we provide details from Phase 1 of the project, highlight the major aims of the remaining steps, and describe briefly the potential benefits of IRT and CAT for the CAT–PD project and for personality assessment more generally.

Identification of CAT–PD Candidate Traits

Given the inclusiveness and comprehensiveness of Widiger and Simonsen's (2005, 2006) summary of 18 dimensional models of PD-relevant traits, we based our construct development efforts on tapping each of the lower order dimensions listed in Table 1. To do this, we followed several steps. First, we sorted and combined these traits based on obvious redundancies in the list. Second, we reviewed the literature related to each candidate trait dimension, and each existing model and PD measure, so as to hone the list further and develop operational definitions for each trait. In general, we strived to develop operational definitions that tapped all central features of each trait (i.e., building content validity into the definitions). This process resulted in an initial list of 53 candidate traits, organized into five broad domains similar to those proposed by Widiger and Simonsen: (a) negative emotionality, (b) positive emotionality, (c) antagonism, (d) (dis)constraint, and (e) oddity.

Although the research team had considerable expertise to inform the selection and conceptualization of the traits to this point, we next opened the process up to external expert review to ensure that the candidate trait dimensions were broadly representative of the PD domain and that the results were not unduly influenced by the particular biases of the research team. To that end, we solicited feedback from a diverse sample of 28 personality and PD experts, who were selected on the basis of their published contributions to either the personality or PD literatures. Experts were drawn from academic psychology (79%) and psychiatry (21%) settings, and all held either PhD (93%) or MD (7%) degrees. They were drawn primarily from the United States (92%) and described themselves as mostly White (93%) and male (89%). Experts reported a mean of 18 years since their terminal degree ($SD = 14$), which suggests that they had ample experience to inform their work on this task. The experts expressed a range of opinions regarding the way PDs should be described in the next *DSM,* with 75% arguing for a trait dimensional system of some kind and 18% arguing for a system resembling the current *DSM–IV* model. Experts were recruited via telephone, e-mail, or both; visited a password-protected Web site that guided them through the task; and were paid $100 as compensation. Specifically, experts were asked to (a) rate the *relevance* and *representativeness* (i.e., content validity; Haynes, Richard, & Kubany, 1995) of each candidate trait with respect to personality pathology, (b) identify deficiencies in the set of candidate traits, and (c) evaluate the accuracy of the operational definitions that we developed for each trait.

The numerical ratings and open-ended feedback provided by the experts were then considered and integrated by the research team, a process that resulted in a modified set of 59 candidate dimensions and operational definitions. This revised set of candidate traits appears in Table 2, along with a rational mapping of our candidate CAT–PD traits onto the 37 traits proposed by the PPD Work Group. Interestingly, our set of candidate traits appears to cover all of the dimensions in the proposed *DSM–5* scheme. Notably, the CAT–PD set includes multiple traits relevant to 13 *DSM–5* traits, as well as six candidate traits not modeled in the *DSM–5* list. Thus, the CAT–PD candidate traits appear to be more differentiated and somewhat broader in scope than those proposed by the PPD Work Group. Of course, structural analyses following data collection in Phase 2 of the project will ultimately determine the exact nature and number of traits,

TABLE 2.—Summary of 59 CAT–PD candidate traits and conceptually relevant *DSM–5* personality traits.

Domain	CAT–PD Candidate Traits	Relevant *DSM–5* Traits
Negative emotionality	Anxious apprehension	Anxiousness
	Fearfulness	Anxiousness
	Depressive dysphoria	Depressivity
	Affective lability	Emotional lability
	Stress reactivity	Emotional lability
	Shame/guilt	Guilt/shame
	Low self-esteem	Low self-esteem
	Self-harm	Self-harm
	Suicidality	Self-harm
	Rejection sensitivity	Separation insecurity
	Submissiveness	Submissiveness
	Exploitability	Submissiveness
	Hypochondriasis	—
	Jealousy	—
Positive emotionality	Anhedonia	Anhedonia
	Exhibitionism	Histrionism
	Seductiveness	Histrionism
	Dramaticism	Histrionism
	Entitlement	Narcissism
	Arrogance	Narcissism
	Optimism/pessimism	Pessimism
	Emotional detachment	Restricted affectivity
	Social aloofness	Social detachment
	Social avoidance	Social withdrawal
	Romantic disinterest	Intimacy avoidance
	Lack of activity/energy	—
Antagonism	Aggression	Aggression
	Anger/irritability	Aggression
	Hostility	Hostility
	Callousness	Callousness
	Depravity	Callousness
	Social insensitivity	Callousness
	Deceitfulness	Deceitfulness
	Manipulativeness	Manipulativeness
	Conduct problems	Irresponsibility
	Oppositionality	Oppositionality
	Selfishness	Narcissism
	Blame externalization	—
	Domineering	—
(Dis)constraint	Urgency	Impulsivity
	Lack of premeditation	Impulsivity
	Undependability	Irresponsibility
	Rebellious nonconformity	Oppositionality
	Orderliness	Orderliness
	Perfectionism	Perfectionism
	Excessive achievement striving	Perfectionism
	Lack of perseverance	Perseveration
	Risk-taking/recklessness	Recklessness, risk aversion
	Rigid propriety	(–)
	Lack of concern for consequences	Rigidity
		Risk aversion (–)
	Excitement seeking	—
Oddity	Cognitive dysregulation	Cognitive dysregulation
	Absorption	Dissociation proneness
	Obliviousness	Distractibility
	Peculiarity/oddity	Eccentricity
	Suspiciousness	Suspiciousness
	Cynicism	Suspiciousness
	Magical thinking	Unusual beliefs
	Perceptual aberrations	Unusual perceptions

Note. CAT–PD = Computerized Adaptive Test of Personality Disorder; *DSM–5* = *Diagnostic and Statistical Manual of Mental Disorders* (5th ed.).

as well as the overall structure of the higher and lower order dimensions.

Development of the Initial Item Pool

Item-pool development was guided by the principles of *substantive validity* as elaborated by Loevinger (1957) and rearticulated by others (e.g., Clark & Watson, 1995; Simms & Watson, 2007). Most notably, the initial pool was developed to be overinclusive and representative of the operational definitions written for each candidate trait. We began with the International Personality Item Pool (IPIP; Goldberg, 1999; Goldberg et al., 2006)—a broad, public-domain collection of 2,413 personality items—as the foundation on which to base the CAT–PD item pool. IPIP items tap a wide variety of constructs, and scales have been developed to serve as proxies for a number of well-known structural models (e.g., Big Three, Big Five, and Big Seven) and for a wide assortment of measures of personality traits, PDs, and other forms of psychopathology. Its large size and public-domain status made the IPIP an ideal starting point for our pool. Although not developed explicitly to measure abnormal-range personality features, the IPIP includes numerous scales tapping traits with high or low ends that are relevant to PD. However, because most IPIP items were written to tap normal-range variation in personality, we knew a priori that we would need to develop additional items for our pool to tap PD-relevant traits that are underrepresented in the IPIP, as well as to extend the measurement range to include items reflective of the pathological extremes of each candidate trait.

We implemented an iterative rational strategy to place IPIP items into the 59 CAT–PD candidate trait "bins." Eleven trained graduate and undergraduate research assistants (RAs) completed each stage of the sorting process. In the first stage, the 2,413 IPIP items were sorted into the five broad CAT–PD domains. RAs were trained on the definitions for each domain and used a computer spreadsheet to sort each item into one or more domains. Items that were sorted into a domain by at least five RAs were provisionally assigned to that domain. At this stage, items could be assigned to multiple domains. In the second sorting stage, similar procedures were used to sort items within each domain into the lower order trait bins relevant to that domain, as listed in Table 2. This stage was completed over a series of 5 weeks, each of which was devoted to a single domain. For each domain, RAs were trained on the definitions for the traits and were given 7 days to sort the assigned items into the relevant lower order trait bins. Additional sorting stages were implemented to identify additional relevant items from established IPIP scales, review all unsorted (i.e., "leftover") IPIP items for potentially useful additions, and eliminate item overlap across trait bins and domains. This iterative process resulted in 1,570 IPIP items being selected for the CAT–PD initial item pool.

The research team also developed new items for each trait bin to tap underrepresented content in the IPIP and to broaden the measurement range of each dimension to include the extreme poles reflective of personality pathology. For this task, the IPIP items within each trait bin were carefully studied for gaps in coverage, and members of the research team generated new items to fill those gaps. This process resulted in more than 2,000 new items being written. The first author (L. J. Simms) then edited the team-created items to improve their readability, eliminate redundancy, and select the final set of new items to be included in the

CAT-PD pool. At the end of this process, 1,019 team-created items were added to the CAT–PD initial item pool.

Taken together, the CAT–PD initial item pool includes 2,589 items to be used in the first round of data collection and scale development. To maintain reasonable consistency with previous studies using the IPIP, we adopted a modified 5-point response format for the CAT–PD ranging from *very untrue of me* to *very true of me*. A preliminary study indicated that the CAT–PD modified response format is psychometrically parallel to the original IPIP format (i.e., yields equivalent descriptive statistics, reliability, and validity). Given the large size of the item pool, a balanced incomplete block design (BIBD) was developed to facilitate data collection. A BIBD is a planned-missingness design in which each participant completes only a portion of the items. These designs come in many shapes and sizes, depending on the particular needs of a given study (Cochran & Cox, 1957). Our BIBD approach was selected to optimize the pairwise sample size for conceptually similar traits and includes several important features. First, traits and items were assigned to a series of nine blocks such that conceptually similar traits appeared in the same block (i.e., to facilitate within-block structural analyses following data collection). Second, blocks were assigned to 12 "booklets" in a completely balanced manner: Each booklet included exactly three blocks, and each block was assigned to exactly four booklets. A summary of this design is presented in Table 3.

Data Collection and Scale Development Progress and Plans

We currently are in the middle of Phase 2 of the project, the focus of which is on collecting responses to the initial CAT–PD pool from more than 1,000 community-dwelling adults and 600 current or recent psychiatric patients, and later to perform struc-

TABLE 3.—Summary of the balanced incomplete block design used in the first round of data collection.

Booklet	Items	Blocks of Traits/Items								
		1	2	3	4	5	6	7	8	9
A	886	x	x	x						
B	828	x			x	x				
C	860	x					x	x		
D	831	x							x	x
E	892		x		x		x			
F	878		x			x		x		
G	899		x					x		x
H	851			x	x					x
I	866			x		x		x		
J	862			x			x		x	
K	840				x			x	x	
L	863					x	x			x

Note. 1 = Affective lability, stress reactivity, depressive dysphoria, low self-esteem, shame/guilt, self-harm, suicidality; 2 = domineering, dramaticism, exhibitionism, exploitability, jealousy, rejection sensitivity, seductiveness, submissiveness; 3 = arrogance, callousness, deceitfulness, entitlement, manipulativeness, selfishness; 4 = absorption, anxious apprehension, fearfulness, hypochondriasis, magical thinking, obliviousness, perceptual aberrations; 5 = cognitive dysregulation, conduct problems, cynicism, depravity, oppositionality, peculiarity/oddity, rebellious nonconformity, suspiciousness; 6 = aggression, anger/irritability, blame externalization, hostility, optimism vs. pessimism, social insensitivity; 7 = excessive achievement striving, orderliness, perfectionism, rigid propriety, undependability; 8 = activity/energy, anhedonia, emotional detachment, romantic disinterest, social aloofness, social avoidance; 9 = excitement seeking, lack of concern for consequences, lack of perseverance, lack of premeditation, risk-taking/recklessness, urgency.

tural analyses of these responses to guide scale development and refinement. Community participants are being recruited via random-digit dialing and computer-assisted telephone interview procedures aimed at recruiting a representative sample of participants from the Buffalo-Niagara region of New York (matched roughly on age, gender, and ethnicity to U.S. Census data). The community study is nearly finished as of this writing. Interim structural analyses—made up mostly of within-block targeted IRT and factor analyses—will be conducted following the community study to hone the item pool and develop provisional scales. The resulting reduced item pool will be used for the patient study and will serve as the basis for scale cross-validation analyses. More information about these analyses and scale development procedures will be presented in future publications. The remaining phases of the project will be focused on building cross-platform CAT–PD software, completing real-data and Monte Carlo CAT/IRT simulation studies to guide that development process, and finally conducting a construct validation study of the CAT–PD in a new sample of 300 psychiatric patients.

The exact form of the final CAT–PD model and measure will be influenced by the analyses conducted following Phase 2 of the project. In broad strokes, however, the intent of the CAT–PD development team is to develop a computerized tool that can be useful in both applied assessment and treatment settings with patients as well as research settings in which comprehensive trait coverage of the PD domain is desired. The software will be developed to work on multiple operating systems and could ultimately be delivered via the Internet via a Web browser, depending on the complexity of the IRT model selected to calibrate the items and guide the CAT. We anticipate permitting clinicians and researchers to customize the CAT–PD software for their particular needs (e.g., setting it up to administer only certain scales, etc.), and computerized interpretive reports can be included after sufficient data have been gathered to inform their development. Finally, any costs associated with use of the software will be minimal and limited to those necessary to support the software and keep administration servers running smoothly.

Computerized Adaptive Testing

Over the past three decades, computers have been used increasingly to automate the administration, scoring, and interpretation of a wide variety of psychological measures, including tests of ability and academic achievement (e.g., Mills, 1999), neuropsychological status (e.g., Russell, 2000), vocational interests (e.g., Hansen, Neuman, Haverkamp, & Lubinski, 1997), and personality traits (e.g., Simms & Clark, 2005; Vispoel, Boo, & Bleiler, 2001). Computers provide an efficient and reliable means for delivering assessment services to clients and research participants (e.g., Butcher, 1987; Gosling, Vazire, Srivastava, & John, 2004). A number of personality and measurement researchers (e.g., Reise & Henson, 2000; Simms & Clark, 2005; Waller & Reise, 1989) have discussed how a specific form of computerized assessment—CAT—might be applied to personality tests. CAT methods originally were developed in the ability testing literature and have been implemented successfully in a number of high-stakes testing programs.

In the most basic sense, CAT permits the selection and administration of items that are individually tailored to the latent trait level of a given examinee, which can lead to substantial time savings with little or no loss of reliability or validity (Sands,

Waters, & McBride, 1997; Wainer, 2000; Weiss, 1985). A typical CAT selects and administers only those items that provide the most psychometric information for each individual at a given ability or trait level, eliminating the need to present items with very low or very high endorsement probabilities given a particular examinee's trait level. For example, in a CAT version of a general arithmetic test, the computer would not administer easy items (e.g., simple addition or subtraction) once it was clear from the examinee's responses that his or her ability level exceeded that level of arithmetic skill (e.g., she or he was correctly answering trigonometry or calculus items). Applied to personality measurement, a CAT to measure, for example, trait aggression would not administer items reflecting low or normative levels of anger (e.g., "I am a person who gets angry sometimes") once the examinee endorses items reflecting higher trait aggression (e.g., "I'm the type of person who gets into lots of fistfights").

A typical CAT includes three basic elements: (a) a procedure for estimating the examinee's latent trait level, (b) a procedure for selecting items from the pool, and (c) a termination rule to determine when testing may be discontinued. In practice, CAT begins with the administration of an item representative of the median trait level. The computer then scores that item, calculates a trait level estimate, and determines whether the termination rule has been satisfied. If not, the computer administers a new item that provides maximum information at the newly calculated trait level, scores the item, reestimates the trait level, and determines whether the termination rule has been satisfied. This iterative cycle continues until the termination rule has been satisfied.

How does the computer know how much psychometric information a given item provides at different levels of a trait? The ability of a CAT application to work efficiently depends on its capacity to calibrate items properly. To do this, CATs typically are built on a foundation laid by IRT, which includes a variety of related psychometric models that characterize each test item by one or more parameters (Hambleton & Swaminathan, 1985; Lord, 1980). Although a complete treatment of IRT is well beyond the scope of this article, we present some basic details here to aid readers in understanding the method and its application to CAT. Interested readers who want more details are referred to contemporary texts on IRT that are geared toward psychologists (e.g., Embretson & Reise, 2000).

An important strength of IRT for CAT applications is that item characteristics can be combined into a single index—item information—that describes how precisely an item measures the trait at various points along the trait continuum. Item information is a function of an item's discrimination ability (i.e., the "a" parameter; akin to the item's factor loading) and its difficulty or severity (i.e., the "b" parameter), and it typically is represented graphically in an *item information curve* (IIC). On an IIC, item information is plotted as a function of trait level (theta or θ). An IIC has its peak at the difficulty or severity level of an item, and the relative height of its peak is related to the item's discrimination ability. Given these properties, CATs use information to administer only those items that provide maximum information (i.e., are most precise markers of the trait) given the currently estimated level of the trait (Weiss, 1985).

Figure 1 shows the information provided by four hypothetical test items on a particular trait dimension. Consider a CAT in which the current trait estimate is $\theta = 1.0$ (this value can be interpreted similar to a z score). In a typical *maximum-information*

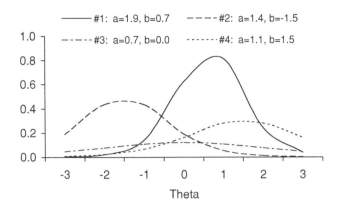

FIGURE 1.—Several prototypical item information curves. *Note.* a = discrimination; b = difficulty/severity.

item-selection strategy, assuming the trait estimate does not change markedly after each item response, the computer would present the items in the order 1, 4, 3, 2, based on the height of each IIC at the point where $\theta = 1.0$. If, however, the trait estimate was located at $\theta = -1.0$, the items would be presented in the order 2, 1, 3, 4. As mentioned earlier, another important concept in CAT is the *termination rule.* One such rule might be to stop presenting new items when reasonably informative items no longer exist in the pool. For example, Figure 1 suggests that Items 2 and 4, respectively, might not have been administered in the first and second examples earlier, because they offer negligible amounts of psychometric information at those levels of θ. Other types of termination rules are possible, but in general termination rules limit the number of items administered; marked CAT efficiency gains are possible if the item pool for a particular scale is sufficiently broad and large.

Traditional IRT models were limited to dichotomous items (e.g., true–false) from unidimensional scales. Fortunately for the CAT–PD and the field of personality assessment more generally, IRT has evolved to include (a) models for which patients are asked to rate items along a gradient of severity, frequency, or agreement (e.g., Muraki, 1990; Samejima, 1969); and (b) constructs that deviate from strict unidimensionality (e.g., Gibbons et al., 2007; Reckase, 1997).

Use of CAT for Personality and Psychopathology Assessment

Despite the widespread use of IRT and, to a lesser extent, CAT in the ability testing literature, relatively few applications of IRT-based CAT have appeared in the personality and mental health literatures, likely due to a number of factors, including (a) the greater statistical complexity of IRT/CAT compared to tests built using classical test theory, (b) the lack of user-friendly IRT/CAT software packages, and (c) the lack of consistent training in IRT/CAT methods in clinical assessment curricula. Of the limited attempts to apply IRT-based CAT in the personality literature, most of those have been based on post-hoc simulations using previously collected response data, rather than tests with live participants. For example, Waller and Reise (1989) simulated a CAT version of the Absorption scale of the Multidimensional Personality Questionnaire. Real-data CAT simulations, based on responses from 1,000 participants who previously had completed the Absorption scale in the traditional paper-

and-pencil format, yielded item savings ranging from 50% to 75%, depending on the termination rule utilized. In a similar demonstration, Kamakura and Balasubramanian (1989) found item savings ranging from 60% to 66% on the Socialization scale of the California Psychological Inventory. Reise and Henson (2000) extended the personality CAT literature to multiscale batteries, conducting real-data simulations on the 30 facet scales of the Revised NEO Personality Inventory (NEO PI–R). Using a polytomous IRT model to account for the 5-point Likert scale used to rate NEO PI–R items, they achieved average item savings of 50% per facet.

Although such simulation studies have been useful in establishing that CAT methodology can be applied effectively to personality and psychopathology constructs, live-testing studies also are important to establish the ecological validity of the technique. Simms and Clark (2005) were the first to develop a prototype CAT of personality and personality pathology that was examined in a live-testing study. Based on Clark's (1993) SNAP, Simms and Clark demonstrated that CAT methods could be effectively used for a PD assessment. In their study, the SNAP–CAT yielded significant time savings (ranging from 58%–60%) over the traditional SNAP administered using paper and pencil or computer; importantly, descriptive statistics, test–retest stability, internal factor structure, and validity patterns largely were comparable across administration modes. Moreover, participants preferred the computerized version to the paper-and-pencil version.

Unfortunately, in both the simulation studies described earlier and the SNAP–CAT study, efficiency gains were achieved at the expense of small but statistically significant losses in reliability and validity, which is an inevitable result of using an existing traditional personality measures with scales that do not include adequate information at all levels of the underlying traits. Notably, traditional scale development statistical procedures (e.g., factor analysis) favor items with moderate endorsement rates; thus, extreme items (i.e., those indicative of the pathological poles of personality traits) often are inadvertently tossed out because they tend to yield much weaker factor loadings. As such, CATs for personality pathology are needed that are built from the ground up to include much broader and larger item pools, such that all relevant levels of each dimension to be measured are represented adequately. When item pools are sufficiently broad and large, CATs can yield equivalent or better reliability and validity compared to traditional tests, with fewer items, by focusing test administration only on those items that are relevant to a given patient. Thus, the IRT-based CAT methods underlying the CAT–PD project are poised to improve the efficiency of PD measurement without any loss of reliability or validity.

Indeed, because of these features of CAT, several groups funded by the National Institutes of Health (NIH) currently are working to build CAT measures for use in various physical and mental health domains. In one such application, Gibbons et al. (2008) have been working to build a comprehensive CAT measure of depressive symptomatology. Likewise, in a large, multisite, NIH-funded effort, the PROMIS group (i.e., Patient Reported Outcomes Measurement Information System) have been developing CAT item banks for a variety of common health outcomes, such as emotional distress, chronic pain, sleep disturbance, and arthritis (Cella et al., 2010). Thus, important work is ongoing to use IRT and CAT techniques in health care settings; the CAT–PD project is an example of this growing trend.

Summary and Conclusions

PDs are prevalent in the population and associated with significant functional impairment and a complicated course of treatment in psychiatric settings. However, numerous concerns—such as psychometric problems associated with the current *DSM–IV* PDs as well as the time and resources needed to administer, score, and interpret most current measures of PD—have led to a decrease in structured personality assessment in resource-limited research and applied settings. Various trait-based dimensional models and measures have been proposed in recent decades as alternatives to the current categorical approach to PD description and assessment. Such models have been shown to have numerous advantages over category or prototype-based approaches. However, no single model encompasses all prominent PD-related traits, and there remains a lack of consensus as to the lower order structure of PD-related traits. The CAT–PD project was designed to solve these interrelated concerns by (a) developing a comprehensive and integrative model of PD-related trait dimensions, and (b) creating an efficient method for measuring those traits. We assumed that a comprehensive model of PD traits would yield too large and unwieldy an instrument to be of much practical value in applied or research settings. Thus, we have elected to adopt CAT as a measurement method, which can be expected to result in significant efficiency gains over traditional questionnaire and interview methods.

The results of Phase 1 of the project have revealed 59 candidate traits organized into five broad factors corresponding to the Big Four plus oddity. These traits and the organizational scheme are consistent with the integrative work of Widiger and Simonsen (2005, 2006) and also have been influenced by feedback solicited from a large group of personality and PD experts. Moreover, the CAT–PD candidate traits are well positioned to tap the trait system recently proposed by the *DSM–5* PPD Work Group, as the CAT–PD list includes all of the dimensions on the provisional *DSM–5* list. However, a possible limitation of the CAT–PD project is its reliance on self-report methodology in the development and implementation of the new measure. Given previous work showing blind spots for certain aspects of PD (e.g., Oltmanns & Turkheimer, 2006), it will be important to extend the initial CAT–PD project to develop an informant version once the basic CAT–PD model and measure are finished and validated.

Regardless, the use of CAT as a basis for mental and physical health measurement has shown promise as a method to efficiently measure a broad range of symptoms, features, or traits with little or no loss to measurement precision or validity. The CAT–PD will continue the trend toward sophisticated measurement systems for patient-reported problems.

Acknowledgments

We thank William Calabrese, Monica Rudick, Wern How Yam, Tom Yufik, and Kerry Zelazny for their help in coordinating the expert review study and the development of the initial item pool. In addition, we thank the experts who provided feedback on the candidate traits as well as the research assistants who sorted items into candidate trait bins. Finally, we thank Lee Anna Clark for her consultation during the early stages of the project.

The studies presented in this article were supported by a research grant to the L. J. Simms from the National Institute of Mental Health (No. R01MH080086).

References

American Psychiatric Association. (1980). *Diagnostic and statistical manual of mental disorders* (3rd ed.) Washington, DC: Author.

American Psychiatric Association. (1994). *Diagnostic and statistical manual of mental disorders* (4th ed.). Washington, DC: Author.

Bender, D. S., Dolan, R. T., Skodol, A. E., Sanislow, C. A., Dyck, I. R., McGlashan, T. H., . . . Gunderson, J. G. (2001). Treatment utilization by patients with personality disorders. *American Journal of Psychiatry, 158,* 295–302.

Butcher, J. N. (1987). The use of computers in psychological assessment: An overview of practices and issues. In J. N. Butcher (Ed.), *Computerized psychological assessment: A practitioner's guide* (pp. 292–324). New York, NY: Basic Books.

Cella, D., Riley, W., Stone, A., Rothrock, N., Reeve, B., Yount, S., . . . Hays, R. D., on behalf of the PROMIS Cooperative Group. (2010). Initial item banks and first wave testing of the Patient-Reported Outcomes Measurement Information System (PROMIS) network: 2005–2008. *Journal of Clinical Epidemiology, 63,* 1179–1194.

Clark, L. A. (1993). *Schedule for nonadaptive and adaptive personality (SNAP): Manual for administration, scoring, and interpretation.* Minneapolis: University of Minnesota Press.

Clark, L. A. (2007). Assessment and diagnosis of personality disorder: Perennial issues and an emerging reconceptualization. *Annual Review of Psychology, 58,* 227–257.

Clark, L. A., & Krueger, R. F. (2010). *Rationale for a six-domain trait dimensional diagnostic system for personality disorder.* Retrieved from http://www.dsm5.org/ProposedRevisions/Pages/RationaleforaSixDomainTraitDimensionalDiagnosticSystemforPersonalityDisorder.aspx

Clark, L. A., Livesley, W. J., & Morey, L. (1997). Personality disorder assessment: The challenge of construct validity. *Journal of Personality Disorders, 11,* 205–231.

Clark, L. A., Simms, L. J., Wu, K. D., & Casillas, A. (in press). *Schedule for nonadaptive and adaptive personality-second ed. (SNAP–2): Manual for administration, scoring, and interpretation.*

Clark, L. A., & Watson, D. (1995). Constructing validity: Basic issues in objective scale development. *Psychological Assessment, 7,* 309–319.

Clark, L. A., Watson, D., & Reynolds, S. (1995). Diagnosis and classification of psychopathology: Challenges to the current system and future directions. *Annual Review of Psychology, 46,* 121–153.

Cochran, W. G., & Cox, G. M. (1957). *Experimental designs* (2nd ed.). New York, NY: Wiley.

Cyranowski, J. M., Frank, E., Winter, E., Rucci, P., Novick, D., Pilkonis, P., . . . Kupfer, D. J. (2004). Personality pathology and outcome in recurrently depressed women over 2 years of maintenance interpersonal psychotherapy. *Psychological Medicine, 34,* 659–669.

Dolan, B., Evans, C., & Norton, K. (1995). Multiple Axis-II diagnoses of personality disorder. *British Journal of Psychiatry, 166,* 107–112.

Dreessen, L., & Arntz, A. (1998). Short-interval test–retest interrater reliability of the Structured Clinical Interview for *DSM–III–R* Personality Disorders (SCID–II) in outpatients. *Journal of Personality Disorders, 12,* 138–148.

Eaton, N. R., Krueger, R. F., South, S. C., Simms, L. J., & Clark, L. A. (in press). Contrasting prototypes and dimensions in the classification of personality pathology: Evidence that dimensions, but not prototypes, are robust. *Psychological Medicine.*

Ekselius, L., Tillfors, M., Furmark, T., & Fredrikson, M. (2001). Personality disorders in the general population: *DSM–IV* and *ICD–10* defined prevalence as related to sociodemographic profile. *Personality and Individual Differences, 30,* 311–320.

Embretson, S. E., & Reise, S. P. (2000). *Item response theory for psychologists.* Mahwah, NJ: Erlbaum.

Feske, U., Mulsant, B. H., Pilkonis, P. A., Soloff, P., Dolata, D., Sackeim, H. A., & Haskett, R. F. (2004). Clinical outcome of ECT in patients with major depression and comorbid borderline personality disorder. *American Journal of Psychiatry, 161*, 2073–2080.

Fossati, A., Maffei, C., Bagnato, M., Battaglia, M., Donati, D., Donini, M., . . . Prolo, F. (2000). Patterns of covariation of *DSM–IV* personality disorders in a mixed psychiatric sample. *Comprehensive Psychiatry, 41*, 206–215.

Gibbons, R. D., Bock, R. D., Hedeker, D., Weiss, D. J., Segawa, E., Bhaumik, D. K., . . . Stover, A. (2007). Full-information bi-factor analysis of graded response data. *Applied Psychological Measurement, 31*, 4–19.

Gibbons, R. D., Weiss, D. J., Kupfer, D. J., Frank, E., Fagiolini, A., Grochocinski, V. J., . . . Immekus, J. C. (2008). Using computerized adaptive testing to reduce the burden of mental health assessment. *Psychiatric Services, 59*, 361–368.

Goldberg, L. R. (1999). A broad-bandwidth, public-domain, personality inventory measuring the lower-level facets of several five-factor models. In I. Mervielde, I. Deary, F. De Fruyt, & F. Ostendorf (Eds.), *Personality psychology in Europe* (Vol. 7, pp. 7–28). Tilburg, The Netherlands: Tilburg University Press.

Goldberg, L. R., Johnson, J. A., Eber, H. W., Hogan, R., Ashton, M. C., Cloninger, C. R., & Gough, H. C. (2006). The International Personality Item Pool and the future of public-domain personality measures. *Journal of Research in Personality, 40*, 84–96.

Gosling, S. D., Vazire, S., Srivastava, S., & John, O. P. (2004). Should we trust web-based studies? *American Psychologist, 59*, 93–104.

Grant, B. F., Hasin, D. S., Stinson, F. S., Dawson, D. A., Chou, S. P., Ruan, W. J., & Huang, B. (2005). Co-occurrence of 12-month mood and anxiety disorders in the US: Results from the National Epidemiologic Survey on Alcohol and Related Conditions. *Journal of Psychiatric Research, 39*, 1–9.

Hambleton, R. K., & Swaminathan, H. (1985). *Item response theory: Principles and applications*. Boston, MA: Kluwer-Nijhoff.

Hansen, J. C., Neuman, J. L., Haverkamp, B. E., & Lubinski, B. R. (1997). Comparison of user reaction to two methods of Strong Interest Inventory administration and report feedback. *Measurement & Evaluation in Counseling & Development, 30*, 115–127.

Haynes, S. N., Richard, D. C. S., & Kubany, E. S. (1995). Content validity in psychological assessment: A functional approach to concepts and methods. *Psychological Assessment, 7*, 238–247.

Kamakura, W. A., & Balasubramanian, S. K. (1989). Tailored interviewing: An application of item response theory for personality measurement. *Journal of Personality Assessment, 53*, 502–519.

Livesley, W. J., & Jackson, D. N. (2009). *Dimensional assessment of personality pathology—Basic questionnaire: Technical manual*. Port Huron, MI: Sigma Assessment Systems.

Livesley, W. J., & Jang, K. L. (2000). Toward an empirically based classification of personality disorder. *Journal of Personality Disorders, 14*, 137–151.

Livesley, W. J., Jang, K. L., & Vernon, P. A. (1998). The phenotypic and genetic structure of traits delineating personality disorder. *Archives of General Psychiatry, 55*, 941–948.

Loevinger, J. (1957). Objective tests as instruments of psychological theory. *Psychological Reports, 3*, 635–694.

Lord, F. M. (1980). *Applications of item response theory to practical testing problems*. Hillsdale, NJ: Erlbaum.

Markon, K. E., Krueger, R. F., & Watson, D. (2005). Delineating the structure of normal and abnormal personality: An integrative hierarchical approach. *Journal of Personality and Social Psychology, 88*, 139–157.

Miller, J. D., Maples, J., Few, L. R., Morse, J. Q., Yaggi, K. E., & Pilkonis, P. A. (2010). Using clinician-rated five-factor model data to score the *DSM–IV* personality disorders. *Journal of Personality Assessment, 92*, 296–305.

Mills, C. N. (1999). Development and introduction of a computer adaptive Graduate Record Examinations General Test. In F. Drasgow & J. B. Olson-Buchanan (Eds.), *Innovations in computerized assessment* (pp. 117–135). Mahwah, NJ: Erlbaum.

Muraki, E. (1990). Fitting a polytomous item response model to Likert-type data. *Applied Psychological Measurement, 14*, 59–71.

Oldham, J. M., & Skodol, A. E. (2000). Charting the future of Axis II. *Journal of Personality Disorders, 14*, 17–29.

Oldham, J. M., Skodol, A. E., Kellman, H. D., Hyler, S. E., Doidge, N., Rosnick, L., & Gallaher, P. E. (1995). Comorbidity of Axis I and Axis II disorders. *American Journal of Psychiatry, 152*, 571–578.

Oltmanns, T. F., & Turkheimer, E. (2006). Perceptions of self and others regarding pathological personality traits. In R. F. Krueger & J. L. Tackett (Eds.), *Personality and psychopathology* (pp. 71–111). New York, NY: Guilford.

Pilkonis, P. A., Heape, C. L., Proietti, J. M., Clark, S. W., McDavid, J. D., & Pitts, T. E. (1995). The reliability and validity of two structured diagnostic interviews for personality disorders. *Archives of General Psychiatry, 52*, 1025–1033.

Pincus, A., & Gurtman, M. B. (2006). The interpersonal circumplex and the interpersonal theory: Perspectives of personality and its pathology. In S. Strack (Ed.), *Differentiating normal and abnormal personality* (2nd ed., pp. 83–112). New York, NY: Springer.

Piotrowski, C. (1999). Assessment practices in the era of managed care: Current status and future directions. *Journal of Clinical Psychology, 55*, 787–796.

Piotrowski, C., Belter, R. W., & Keller, J. W. (1998). The impact of "managed care" on the practice of psychological testing: Preliminary findings. *Journal of Personality Assessment, 70*, 441–447.

Reckase, M. D. (1997). The past and future of multidimensional item response theory. *Applied Psychological Measurement, 21*, 25–36.

Reich, J. (2003). The effects of Axis II disorders on the outcome of treatment of anxiety and unipolar depressive disorders: A review. *Journal of Personality Disorders, 17*, 387–405.

Reise, S. P., & Henson, J. M. (2000). Computerization and adaptive administration of the NEO-PI-R. *Assessment, 7*, 347–364.

Russell, E. W. (2000). The application of computerized scoring programs to neuropsychological assessment. In R. D. Vanderploeg (Ed.), *Clinician's guide to neuropsychological assessment* (pp. 483–515). Mahwah, NJ: Erlbaum.

Samejima, F. (1969). Estimation of latent ability using a response pattern of graded scores. *Psychometrika Monographs, 34*(4, Pt. 2, Whole No. 17).

Samuels, J., Eaton, W. W., Bienvenu, O. J., Brown, C. H., Costa, P. T., Jr., & Nestadt, G. (2002). Prevalence and correlates of personality disorders in a community sample. *British Journal of Psychiatry, 180*, 536–542.

Sands, W. A., Waters, B. K., & McBride, J. R. (1997). *Computerized adaptive testing: From inquiry to operation*. Washington, DC: American Psychological Association.

Shedler, J., & Westen, D. (2004). Refining personality disorder diagnosis: Integrating science and practice. *American Journal of Psychiatry, 161*, 1350–1365.

Simms, L. J., & Clark, L. A. (2005). Validation of a computerized adaptive version of the Schedule for Nonadaptive and Adaptive Personality. *Psychological Assessment, 17*, 28–43.

Simms, L. J., & Watson, D. (2007). The construct validation approach to personality scale construction. In R. Robins, C. Fraley, & R. Krueger (Eds.), *Handbook of research methods in personality psychology* (pp. 240–258). New York, NY: Guilford

Skodol, A. E., Oldham, J. M., Bender, D. S., Dyck, I. R., Stout, R. L., Morey, L. C., . . . Gunderson, J. G. (2005). Dimensional representations of *DSM–IV* personality disorders: Relationships to functional impairment. *American Journal of Psychiatry, 162*, 1919–1925.

Smith, T. L., & Benjamin, L. S. (2002). The functional impairment associated with personality disorders. *Current Opinion in Psychiatry, 15*, 135–141.

Torgersen, S., Kringlen, E., & Cramer, V. (2001). The prevalence of personality disorders in a community sample. *Archives of General Psychiatry, 58*, 590–596.

Tyrer, P. (2005). The problem of severity in the classification of personality disorders. *Journal of Personality Disorders, 19*, 309–314.

Vispoel, W. P., Boo, J., & Bleiler, T. (2001). Computerized and paper-and-pencil versions of the Rosenberg Self-Esteem Scale: A comparison of psychometric features and respondent preferences. *Educational and Psychological Measurement, 61*, 461–474.

Wainer, H. (2000). *Computerized adaptive testing: A primer* (2nd ed.). Mahwah, NJ: Erlbaum.

Waller, N. G., & Reise, S. P. (1989). Computerized adaptive personality assessment: An illustration with the Absorption scale. *Journal of Personality and Social Psychology, 57*, 1051–1058.

Weiss, D. J. (1985). Adaptive testing by computer. *Journal of Consulting and Clinical Psychology, 53*, 774–789.

Westen, D., Shedler, J., & Bradley, R. (2006). A prototype approach to personality disorder diagnosis. *American Journal of Psychiatry, 163*, 846–856.

Widiger, T. A. (1993). The *DSM–III–R* categorical personality disorder diagnoses: A critique and an alternative. *Psychological Inquiry, 4*, 75–90.

Widiger, T. A., & Clark, L. A. (2000). Toward *DSM–V* and the classification of psychopathology. *Psychological Bulletin, 126*, 946–963.

Widiger, T. A., & Simonsen, E. (2005). Alternative dimensional models of personality disorder: Finding a common ground. *Journal of Personality Disorders, 19*, 110–130.

Widiger, T. A., & Simonsen, E. (2006). Alternative dimensional models of personality disorder: Finding a common ground. In T. A. Widiger, E. Simonsen, P. J., Sirovatka, & D. A. Regier (Eds.), *Dimensional models of personality disorders: Refining the research agenda for DSM–V* (pp. 1–21). Washington, DC: American Psychiatric Association.

Widiger, T. A., & Trull, T. J. (2007). Plate techtonics in the classification of personality disorder: Shifting to a dimensional model. *American Psychologist, 62*, 71–83.

World Health Organization (1992). *ICD–10 Classifications of Mental and Behavioural Disorder: Clinical descriptions and diagnostic guidelines.* Geneva, Switzerland: Author.

Yates, B. T., & Taub, J. (2003). Assessing the costs, benefits, cost-effectiveness, and cost-benefit of psychological assessment: We should, we can, and here's how. *Psychological Assessment, 15*, 478–495.

Zanarini, M. C., Skodol, A. E., Bender, D., Dolan, R., Sanislow, C., Schaefer, E., . . . Gunderson, J. G. (2000). The Collaborative Longitudinal Personality Disorders Study: Reliability of Axis I and II diagnoses. *Journal of Personality Disorders, 14*, 291–299.

Zimmerman, M., Rothschild, L., & Chelminski, I. (2005). The prevalence of *DSM–IV* personality disorders in psychiatric outpatients. *American Journal of Psychiatry, 162*, 1911–1918.

Contributions From Personality- and Psychodynamically Oriented Assessment to the Development of the *DSM–5* Personality Disorders

STEVEN K. HUPRICH

Department of Psychology, Eastern Michigan University

Advances in personality assessment over the past 20 years have notably influenced the proposed assessment and classification of personality disorders in the *Diagnostic and Statistical Manual of Mental Disorders* (5th ed. [*DSM–5*]). However, a considerable body of personality assessment and psychodynamically oriented assessment research has significant relevance to the way in which personality disorders are evaluated that appears to have gone unrecognized in the current proposals for *DSM–5*. In this article, I discuss the ways in which some of these 2 bodies of literature can and should inform the *DSM–5* so that the diagnostic nomenclature can be more scientifically and comprehensively informed and consequently improve the clinical utility of a diagnostic system in need of considerable revision.

The diagnostic system is presently undergoing an evolution, and plans are underway for the fifth edition of the *Diagnostic and Statistical Manual of Mental Disorders* (*DSM–5*) to be published in 2013. Perhaps in no other area will the changes be as dramatic as they will be for the Axis II personality disorders. In this case, half of the current disorders are being removed as a valid diagnostic category—Paranoid, Schizoid, Histrionic, Narcissistic, and Dependent—and the remaining disorders are being slightly reformulated and considered to be prototypes. Here, clinicians will be asked to provide a rating for each patient to the extent to which he or she matches each of the prototypes. In addition, six trait domains are described—Negative Emotionality, Introversion, Antagonism, Disinhibition, Compulsivity, and Peculiarity—each of which will have four to eight specific traits that are associated with the broad domains. Like the prototypes, patients will be assessed on each domain and their related traits. From this system, clinicians are being asked to rate each patient's personality and to make a dichotomous decision on whether or not a person meets criteria for a personality disorder, which also is newly defined for *DSM–5*.

Such changes are not without controversy. At the time of this writing, special issues of the two leading journals on personality disorders (*Journal of Personality Disorders, Personality Disorders: Theory, Research, and Treatment*) have been published which critique the *DSM–5* proposals. A document prepared by John Gunderson, MD, and signed by many experts in the personality disorder research domain has been sent to the *DSM–5* Work Group expressing significant concerns about *DSM–5* proposal for its radical departure from the past and its exclusion of clinically useful diagnoses and constructs. A critical commentary also has appeared in the *American Journal of Psychiatry* which requests the retention of the diagnostic categories as well (Shedler et al., 2010). Similarly, this series in *JPA* will include

manuscripts that are critical of the *DSM–5* proposal. The purpose of this article is to review some of the work found in two bodies of literature—personality assessment and psychodynamically oriented assessment research—and to articulate how they can inform and expand the assessment of personality and personality pathology in the *DSM–5*. I conclude that not attending to this literature runs the risk of repeating some of the same problems found in earlier editions of the *DSM*.

PERSONALITY ASSESSMENT RESEARCH AND ITS INFLUENCE ON *DSM–5*

Obvious Influence of Personality Assessment Research on DSM–5

As noted earlier, the *DSM–5* proposal for the Axis II disorders has already incorporated many of the most significant findings from personality disorder assessment research over the past decade. First, trait domains are included as part of the assessment process, which represent the now well-established findings that there are approximately four to seven major personality trait domains that are universally identified in mainly self-reported measures of personality (Allik, 2005; Markon, Krueger, & Watson, 2005; McCrae & Costa, 2008; Widiger & Simonsen, 2005). Second, diagnostic prototypes are now included and rated, based in large part on the extensive work of Shedler and Westen (e.g., reviewed in Westen & Shedler, 2007) and of Rottman, Ahn, Sanislow, and Kim (2009), who empirically demonstrated that experienced clinicians organize their perceptions of patients to the extent to which they match well-established prototypes they have formed from their experience. Finally, *DSM–5* now asks clinicians to rate patients for their degree of functional impairment, which requires clinicians to make personality assessment ratings more clinically useful, something that has been overlooked in the personality assessment literature for some time (Bornstein, 2007; Trull, 2005).

Despite these clear advances, there are many ways in which relevant personality and psychodynamically oriented assessment research has been underincorporated into the new diagnostic framework. I articulate four major ways in which this has occurred.

The Problematic Reliance on Self-Reports to Assess Personality Pathology

In a review of the literature on personality disorder assessment, Bornstein (2003) noted that 80% of the personality disorder research conducted between 1991 and 2000 relied exclusively on self-report measures. Self-report measures are readily available, they are easy to use, and they provide a considerable amount of useful information about individuals' perceptions of what they are typically like. Because of these advantages, they will continue to remain an important medium by which to assess individuals' ideas about themselves. Despite the prominence of this mode of assessment, the problems with self-report measures of personality and personality pathology are widely documented. These concerns have been articulated in detail by Ganellen (2007), Oltmanns and Turkheimer (2006), Shedler, Mayman, and Manis (1993), and Zimmerman and Coryell (1990), but can be summarized as follows: (a) Individuals often have difficulty accurately describing themselves, due to a lack of insight into their behavior and motivations, or due to a conscious or unconscious desire to present themselves in a particularly favorable or unfavorable light. (b) Similarly, when self-reports are compared to reports of others, the degree of correspondence is usually low, with correlations ranging across studies between .10 and .60 (e.g., Oltmanns & Turkheimer, 2006; Ready & Clark, 2002). (c) Some individuals are not cognizant of what particular terms or concepts might mean on a self-report, such as knowing what it means to have highly impressionistic speech (Ganellen, 2007). Such problems could be the product of limited life or educational experiences or lack of cultural norms and expectations.

When self-reports are predominantly used to assess personality pathology, they run the risk of equating the self-report of the construct with the definition of the construct itself (Bornstein, 2010). For instance, no one would agree that a person's self-report of his or her generosity is the sine qua non way in which one's generosity is measured or recognized. Similarly, few clinicians take at face value what a person reports about his or her levels of narcissistic, paranoid, or borderline qualities; rather, it is when and how they are manifested with others and in the course of treatment that they are more clearly recognized and understood for the magnitude of their influence. Yet, the *DSM–5* Work Group appears to be relying strongly on self-report measures to develop the trait dimensions that are to be rated for each patient (e.g., Krueger & Eaton, 2010; Krueger et al., 2011/this issue). Consequently, if the field trials' research on the *DSM–5* proposals relies exclusively on self-report, and if the *DSM–5* proposal does not speak to the inherent limits of relying just on patients' self-reports and not attending to and rendering judgment on the nature and extent of the problems as they are judged by the trained professional, *DSM–5* will continue to perpetuate the limitations of the past, which likely would significantly interfere with the advancement of personality pathology assessment and diagnosis.

Mood state and personality assessment. Another way in which self-report measures are limited is that mood state notably interacts with what one reports about his or her personality. This was reported nearly three decades ago by Hirschfeld

et al. (1983), who found that scores on measures of emotional lability, hypersensitivity, passivity, resiliency, extraversion, and interpersonal dependency all moved toward the "healthy" direction in those who had recovered from depression, but not in those who remained depressed. Santor, Bagby, and Joffee (1997) found that self-reported revised NEO Personality Inventory (NEO PI–R; Costa & McCrae, 1992) personality trait scores could change by as much as 1 *SD* as an individual moved between a depressed and nondepressed state. And, in a sample of patients with depressive or anxiety disorders who were assessed for personality disorders, their personality disorder scores were found to change significantly over a 7-week interval based on the presence and severity of a mood or anxiety disorder (Ottoson, Grann, & Kullgren, 2000). Specifically, Cluster B personality disorder (PD) scores tended to decrease with decreasing depression, whereas Cluster C PD scores tended to decrease with decreasing anxiety.

Conversely, a recent study has suggested that personality trait scores could be related to how individuals' mood states are maintained. Morey et al. (2010) followed 665 patients over the course of 6 years as part of the Collaborative Longitudinal Study of Personality Disorders. They evaluated personality trait scores with the NEO PI–R and personality disorder symptoms with the Diagnostic Interview for *DSM–IV* Personality (Zanarini, Frankenburg, Sickel, & Yong, 1996) and found that NEO PI–R trait scores tended to remain as stable in patients with PDs and major depression as in patients with a PD and no depression, with the exception of Extraversion. Moreover, these trait scores tended to be higher in both PD groups compared to a major depressive disorder only group. However, at a 6-year follow-up of the patients who had major depression and a PD at baseline, those with major depression at Year 6 had a significantly higher number of self-reported PD symptoms, and significantly lower scores on Neuroticism. Thus, although the relationship of mood and personality might be more stable than previously reported, interactive effects are clearly present.

Huprich, Bornstein, and Schmitt (in press) also note how individuals' momentary affective state can influence what they report about themselves. First reported by Mayer, Gaschke, Braverman, and Evans (1992):

the mood congruency effect states that people's judgments are sensitive to the correspondence between the pleasant–unpleasant quality of their mood and the pleasant–unpleasant connotations of their ideas. An affective match between a person's moods and ideas increases the merit, broadly defined, of those ideas. For example, mood-congruent concepts will be judged richer in their associations, mood-congruent attributes will be judged as more applicable, mood-congruent examples of categories will be judged as more typical, and mood-congruent causes and outcomes will be judged more probable. (p. 129)

This could be seen in individuals with personality pathology in the following way. A patient who meets criteria for obsessive–compulsive PD might view his perfectionism as a strength when he is recognized and appreciated for his exceptional organizational skills. Such recognition might induce very positive feelings and the exclusion of any information that might contradict his opinion of himself during a clinical assessment. Yet, he might also view this quality with disdain if his partner is critical and angry with him for his frequent insistence that things be done a particular way. For instance, he might present for treatment with depression and anxiety over the frequent disruptions in his relationship and feel quite worried the relationship could end at any time.

It has also been demonstrated that different memory systems are evoked when a person is asked to describe his or her emotional experiences. For instance, Robinson and Clore (2002) found that individuals use episodic memory to describe their emotions over relatively short periods of time (e.g., within a few hours), whereas semantic memory was more likely to be used to account for emotions over longer time intervals (e.g., within a few days to weeks). They suggested that discrepancies in self-reported emotions might be due in part to the time period used as the point of reference. In the case of self-reported personality pathology, this could have considerable impact on what is reported. Using the preceding example, a patient with obsessive–compulsive PD might distort the extent of his or her emotional constriction depending on the time interval used to assess this feature. For instance, he might deny his emotional constriction altogether if having just experienced a conflict with his partner. Conversely, when considering his "typical way" of being, he might describe himself with words such as *cool-handed, reserved,* or *calm.* Hence the temporal sequence of events in his life might determine what he describes about himself on a self-report measure, or when meeting a clinician for the first time for treatment.

Clearly, emotion and self-reported information about one's personality are highly interactive. In reviewing the *DSM–5* proposal for assessing PDs and personality pathology, there is no specific articulation by the Work Group that assessment of personality pathology must consider the interactive nature of mood on self-reported personality, nor are there specific recommendations for how clinicians should consider such effects. Although mood–personality interactions might be so generally agreed on that they go without saying, the Work Group could enhance the clinical utility of personality pathology assessment by articulating ways in which mood and personality interact and call for mood–personality interaction research as part of the *DSM* field trials.

Priming affects self-report. The effects of priming are widely known. Priming occurs when material presented before a target question or stimulus has the capacity to modify what is reported or done with the target question or stimulus (e.g., Bargh, Bond, Lombardi, & Tota, 1986; DeMarree, Wheeler, & Petty, 2005; Hull, Slone, Meteyer, & Matthews, 2002; Markman & McMullen, 2003; Mussweiler, 2003; Wheeler, DeMarree, & Petty, 2005). In the case of PD assessment, Huprich et al. (in press) have described one of many possible subtle ways in which priming can affect what a person reports. The Structured Interview for *DSM–IV* Personality (SIDP–IV; Pfohl, Blum, & Zimmerman, 1997) asks the following two questions consecutively: Is the praise and admiration of others important to you? In social situations, how much do you worry about being criticized or rejected by other people? These items reflect diagnostic criteria from the *Diagnostic and Statistical Manual of Mental Disorders* (4th ed. [*DSM–IV*]; American Psychiatric Association, 1994) for narcissistic and avoidant PDs, respectively. It is possible that someone with narcissistic PD might answer "No" to the first question because he or she unconsciously feels shameful about wanting praise and admiration. However, the second question is answered "Yes" by the

same individual, because conflicts over attention and criticism are evoked, which is also a point of conflict for the individual with a narcissistic PD. In this case, the narcissistic conflict was detected in part because of the priming that occurred within the sequence of questions. Yet, the person endorsed the avoidant item when he or she really meets criteria for narcissistic PD.

To date, there has been very little studied about the effects of priming on the assessment of PDs per se, although priming effects have been documented when assessing some Axis I conditions (see Huprich et al., in press). Seasoned clinicians recognize that patients' self-reports sometimes change throughout the course of assessment and treatment, which might occur due to priming effects. Yet, without a clear consideration of priming phenomena, it remains likely that such effects could continue to occur. As discussed later, moving away from a near-exclusive reliance on self-reported methodologies in the *DSM* could help reduce this phenomenon (e.g., Bornstein, 2003, 2010).

Situational Specificity and Personality Pathology

Although evidence suggests that personality traits and dimensions of pathology tend to remain fairly stable over time (Caspi, Roberts, & Shiner, 2005; Durbin & Klein, 2006; Grilo & Mc-Glashan, 2009; Zanarini et al., 2007), it is certainly the case that categorical PD diagnoses do not. However, when the situational context is reported in which a given behavior representing a specific personality trait or quality is expressed, the temporal stability of that trait is much more stable compared to the stability of the trait across different situations. For instance, children's verbally aggressive behavior has been found to be remarkably consistent in its expression when knowing to whom it can be expressed (i.e., peer or adult) and under what social context (i.e., teasing, warning, praising, or punishing; Shoda, Mischel, & Wright, 1994). These behavioral signatures of personality (captured in "if–then" statements to detect a given behavior in a given situation) have been found to be highly consistent across a number of studies (see Mischel & Shoda, 2008), and perceivers actually consider the context and behavior to make dispositional judgments about the person. For instance, Kammrath, Mendoza-Denton, and Mischel (2005) found that individuals not only created if–then behavioral profiles for target individuals, but they also used these to infer dispositional qualities about the person. Kammrath et al. also found that if–then conditions were also created and used by perceivers to infer Big Five (Goldberg, 1992) traits.

Huprich and Bornstein (2007) suggest that Mischel and Shoda's theory could be used to help improve PD assessment. They write:

How could (PD assessment) capture situational specificity without losing the generalized behavioral predispositions that characterize different PDs? One possibility is to retain the broad-based symptom questions that currently characterize most (*DSM*-based) PD measures but follow up on positive responses (i.e., acknowledged symptoms) with more focused questions regarding situational context, antecedents, and behavioral "triggers." Such an approach has the advantage of capturing an array of PD-related behaviors with each screening question and then supplementing this information with situational detail. (p. 7)

It is not at all unreasonable to think that clinicians already use this same process to assess a patient's personality and even perhaps to arrive at a PD diagnosis. In the case of a clinician assessing a patient's personality, the disposition that he or she would be assessing is the PD construct, which is formulated from a series of situationally specific behavior exemplars of personality cognitions and emotions. This is not difficult to imagine. In an initial assessment and throughout therapy sessions, a patient describes certain behavioral patterns that occurred in response to specific situations. The clinician would listen for how the patient responded in consistent and inconsistent ways across various situations to determine the underlying disposition. He or she might also begin to consider major themes or consistencies across situations, and then use this collection of information to compare it to the criteria that represent a PD within a particular framework such as the *Diagnostic and Statistical Manual of Mental Disorders* (4th ed., text revision [*DSM–IV–TR*]; American Psychiatric Association, 2001). By doing this, the clinician is able to identify the PD construct, not to mention being able to target intervention strategies.

In fact, this appears to be what actually happens in clinical practice. In a large, national survey of more than 1,800 clinicians, Westen (1997) found that clinicians rely heavily on patients' self-reports of behaviors that are exhibited in certain contexts of patients' lives and on the behavior of the patient toward the clinician in establishing an Axis II diagnosis. These data were weighted by the clinicians as more clinically useful than data provided in a diagnostic manual. Likewise, a recent study found that personality disorder case studies written using if–then behavioral signatures of the *DSM–IV* PD symptoms were diagnosed with greater accuracy than case studies written with just NEO PI–R (Costa & McCrae, 1992) items (Rhadigan & Huprich, in press). In a review of the *DSM–5* proposals for PDs, there is little evidence to suggest that clinicians are encouraged to consider the context in which traits or prototypical qualities are expressed (outside of their cultural context). Yet, it is clear that PD assessment could move forward when considering situationally specific, behaviorally anchored markers in the assessment of personality pathology (Bornstein, 2003; Bornstein & Huprich, in press; Clarkin & Huprich, 2011).

PSYCHOANALYTIC AND PSYCHODYNAMIC MODELS' CONTRIBUTIONS TO THE ASSESSMENT OF PERSONALITY PATHOLOGY

One of the reasons the *Psychodynamic Diagnostic Manual* (PDM Task Force, 2006) was created was to describe and classify psychopathology based in large part on patients' inner subjective experiences. Indeed, understanding patients' inner subjective world and the unconscious processes associated with it as a means by which to understand their psychopathology is hardly discussed within the *DSM–IV–TR* (American Psychiatric Association, 2001). In contemporary practice, surveys of clinicians demonstrate that clinicians rely considerably on patients' subjective perceptions of their problems to conceptualize and diagnose patients (First & Westen, 2007; Westen, 1997), whereas the *DSM* plays much less of a role in their decision making. This approach to clinical assessment and diagnosis occurs in clinicians of varying years' experience and theoretical orientations (Westen & Shedler, 1999a, 1999b). Even those who strongly focus upon gene–environment interaction models of personality acknowledge that "the environment may sometimes be better conceived of as the person's psychological experience of the world, as opposed to some putatively objective aspect of the

world entirely outside the person" (Krueger & Johnson, 2008, p. 298).

At present, psychoanalytic and psychodynamic models of the mind are the most influential theories when it comes to their focus on the inner subjective world of the patient as the vehicle by which to understand and treat personality pathology. Indeed, there has been a resurgence of interest in psychoanalytic and psychodynamic theory in the domains of cognitive neuroscience, social cognition, and attachment theory (e.g., Bornstein, 2005; Huprich, 2009; Kandel, 1999; Panksepp, 1999, 2003; Schore, 2000; Westen, 1992; Westen & Gabbard, 2002a, 2002b), in which ideas and concepts about psychological functioning that once were disparate are now seen as being fully compatible with each other. Huprich et al. (in press) recently made this case:

Personality is a dynamic and complex concept, which includes an understanding of the individual's traits, self-concept, cognition, affect, behavior patterns, genetic make-up, perception, motivation, interpersonal dynamics, and resiliency (John, Robins, & Pervin, 2008). Much of what has been learned about personality over the past 50 years has focused on the dynamic interplay of two or more of these variables, and many prominent personality scholars believe it is time to "put the person back together" (John et al., 2008, p. 19) and recognize the complex dynamics and intrapersonal processes that are known to affect personality. (p. 14)

Bornstein (2010) actually suggested that "psychoanalytic theory represents the most useful overarching framework" (p. 136) for assessing personality, based on three major reasons. First, as a theory it focuses more on internal processes than any other theory (as noted earlier). Second, it assesses multiple levels of awareness, which has been and continues to be well documented in the literature (e.g., Bargh & Morsella, 2008; Panksepp, 1998, 2005; Shevrin, Bond, Brakel, Hertel, & Williams, 1996). Third, as a theory, it recognizes that individuals have limited access when introspecting and utilizes techniques to help further increase conscious access to the internal, subjective experience.

Because of these many strengths, I believe there are at least four good reasons why psychoanalytic and psychodynamic theories should be considered further for how they might be incorporated into the assessment of *DSM–5* of personality pathology.

Clinical Utility

A psychodynamic framework offers a clinically useful framework by which to assess and diagnose patients. Consider two real-life examples: Ms. Davis was a 40-year-old woman who entered treatment because of feeling depressed and self-critical after a recent divorce. At the time of treatment, she was diagnosed in the *DSM–IV* with major depressive disorder, single episode, moderate severity (296.22). Mr. Adams was a 36-year-old man who sought treatment because of increasing time he spent at work on the Internet looking at pornography. His behavior occurred in the context of being in an isolated work environment and having a sexually unavailable and critical wife. Using the *DSM–IV* standards, he was diagnosed with impulse control disorder not otherwise specified (312.30). According to the *DSM–IV* criteria, the goal of treatment for Ms. Davis would be to decrease or eliminate altogether her depressed mood, self-critical rumination, and insomnia associated with her depression. For Mr. Adams, the goal of treatment would be to decrease or eliminate the time he spent on the Internet and help him find more adaptive ways to have his sexual desires met, perhaps by including the wife as part of the treatment. Both patients would not receive a personality disorder diagnosis by *DSM–IV* or the proposed *DSM–5* standards.

However, what actually happened in treatment was the following: Ms. Davis became aware of her self-critical attitudes, based on high standards to which she held herself. These standards led her to feeling angry and guilty about not doing enough to preserve the marriage, despite the fact her then-husband was doing many things to actively leave and damage the quality of the relationship. Her problems consisted of many introjective dynamics (Blatt & Shichman, 1983), which were contained within an obsessive–compulsive personality style that operated at a neurotic level of functioning. Mr. Adams came to quickly see how the Internet was a compromise solution (Brenner, 1982) for him as a means by which to experience intimacy with another woman, who was uncritical and sexually idealized. However, his idealization involved many more core problems with tendencies to devalue and idealize himself and his significant others, including the therapist. Treatment ended prematurely because the patient stated he was angry about being charged for missed appointments, despite knowing of the policy at the beginning of his treatment. In this case, the patient's personality was not quite as high functioning as that of Ms. Davis. He had more manifestations of pathological narcissism and a narcissistic personality.

In both of these cases, the assessment and diagnosis of the patients from the *DSM–IV* was of limited clinical utility, as the diagnosis did little to inform the actual nature of each patient's problems. By contrast, a psychodynamic model, such as articulated in the *PDM,* allowed the therapist to identify more conscious level manifestations of underlying conflicts over the patients' senses of themselves. These self-representations at an unconscious level were governed by excessive superego control and pathological defense mechanisms, respectively. Furthermore, by recognizing the obsessive–compulsive and narcissistic dynamics in these two patients, other actions or behaviors that were reported could be conceptualized and explored in the course of treatment for their association to more common problems centering on their self-representations and defense style. For instance, when Mr. Adams started to protest about the fees, the therapist was able to consider his dynamic assessment of the patient, which allowed him to see that Mr. Adams had highly idealized and grandiose expectations of the therapist when it came to money—namely, that Mr. Adams's schedule and activities were so important that the framework of the treatment did not apply to him. (Of course, these were concerns addressed at a manifest level. As treatment proceeded, more latent concerns were beginning to emerge that could have led Mr. Adams to move away from treatment due to their more threatening nature. The financial issue could have been utilized defensively for this purpose.)

Looking to the future, *DSM–5* personality pathology assessment would address some of these problems in the proposed diagnostic system by emphasizing that all patients' personality should be assessed. This is an idea that is readily supported by many clinicians and researchers. However, the *DSM–5* requires personality assessment to occur on a trait profile and in a patient's match to five personality prototypes. Similarly, the *PDM* advances the idea that personality is assessed on all patients, but it relies on many more established models of personality types, which are based on more comprehensive models of personality than the *DSM–5* model. For instance, Ms. Davis would bear some degree of resemblance to the *DSM–5* obsessive–compulsive prototype, although her low-level difficulties in functioning would probably not meet the criteria for a personality disorder. Using the *DSM–5* system, the treating clinician would have to assess Ms. Davis on 37 traits, and then determine how these traits were related to the interpersonal difficulties she experienced with men in her life. If and how this would occur has yet to be determined (Clarkin & Huprich, 2011). By contrast, Mr. Adams's personality would only be represented by one trait (narcissism), which figured so prominently in his daily living. In fact, because of his otherwise good level of functioning, it is very unlikely he would even meet the *DSM–5* criteria for a PD per se, nor is it clear how his high level of the narcissistic trait would be understood and utilized given its reduced prominence in the personality pathology nomenclature. Using a psychodynamic framework, patients' personalities are seen dimensionally as representative of one of many types, from which there is a dynamic expression of self and other representations, interpersonal problems, internal conflicts, defenses, and troubling affects. Hence, having to differentiate traits from prototypes is not necessary.

From an empirical perspective, one study has found that psychodynamically informed case descriptions are preferred for their clinical utility over trait-based descriptions. Spitzer, First, Shedler, Westen, and Skodol (2008) surveyed a national sample of practicing psychologists and psychiatrists and asked them to apply five different diagnostic frameworks to patients they treated and evaluate each framework for its utility and applicability to clinical practice. They found that descriptions derived from a psychodynamically informed assessment device, the Shedler–Westen Assessment Procedure (SWAP; Westen & Shedler, 1999a, 1999b) were preferred by clinicians over those based on the Five-factor model or biologically based trait model. As in other studies with the SWAP, prototypes that incorporate psychodynamic content are well valued for their clinical utility by practicing clinicians and are empirically justified.

Every Person Assessed for Level of Personality Functioning

The *DSM–5* Work Group has indicated that patients should be assessed by their clinicians for their degree of match to PD prototypes as well as relevant personality traits. Although this requirement puts more of the focus on a patient's personality and how it can be understood in the context of an individual's psychopathology, the Work Group's model consists of a hybrid of prototype and dimensional ratings; the former is based on prior editions of the *DSM* and a compilation of theory and research from multiple theoretical perspectives, whereas the latter is based on a trait model of personality. Mixing such models is likely to be challenging to clinicians, particularly when trait models do not consider the intricate interplay of dynamics and situational specificity that often helps define what is particularly problematic in an individual's personality. By contrast, the *PDM* and dynamic models of personality and psychopathology view personality as being intertwined into understanding psychopathology in a unified model of the mind that understands the relationship of mind and behavior at multiple levels (Bornstein, 2010; Huprich, 2009; McWilliams, 1999). The *PDM* requires every patient to be evaluated for his or her level of personality functioning as being neurotic, borderline, or severe; by contrast, the Work Group's proposal asks for personality assessment, yet proposes that only a categorical, yes–no decision be made about whether an individual has a PD. Although clinicians are expected to rate the traits as part of the assessment process, it is unclear whether they will consider this in their assessment if a PD has been ruled out (Clarkin & Huprich, 2011). Considering and including this diagnostic framework as part of the *DSM–5* likely would permit greater opportunities to evaluate its validity and utility in clinical practice.

Integration With Other Models of Psychological Functioning

As noted earlier, psychoanalytic and psychodynamic theory has been integrated with many other domains of psychology, including attachment theory, social psychology, cognitive psychology, cognitive neuroscience, affective neuroscience, neuropsychology, and interpersonal theory (Bornstein, 2005, 2010; Fonagy & Target, 1997, 2006; Huprich, 2011; Panksepp, 2005; Schore, 2000; Shevrin et al., 1996; Solms, 2000a, 2000b; Westen, 1992; Westen & Gabbard, 2002a, 2002b). Many contemporary theories of personality are being described in more integrative ways, which often supports many of the major ideas inherent in the original psychodynamic model (see Fonagy & Luyten, 2009; Fonagy & Target, 1997, 2006, for good examples of how neuroscience and attachment theory are being integrated to provide more comprehensive models of attachment and problems when the attachment system is disrupted). Unlike trait theory or more biologically oriented theories, psychoanalytic theory offers a comprehensive understanding of the individual that is not present in other models. For instance, there are no traits that adequately describe the phenomenon of the erratic interpersonal and dynamics and unstable self-concept that occur with a borderline patient and significant others, although many quickly understand the concept and dynamics of splitting and projective identification.

Multiple, Psychodynamically Oriented Assessment Tools

Contrary to popular opinion, there are many psychometrically solid assessment devices available to clinicians and researchers to assess psychodynamic processes and phenomena. Huprich (2009) listed eight measures of defense mechanisms, 11 measures of object relations, and six measures of personality organization that are based in psychoanalytic theory and for which multiple studies have attested to their reliability, validity, and clinical utility. Likewise, measures such as the Rorschach Inkblot Method (Lerner, 2005; Masling, Rabie, & Blondheim, 1967) and Thematic Apperception Test (Jenkins, 2007) have been used to assess psychodynamic and psychoanalytic concepts relevant to personality, and ample evidence suggests that they provide information about personality pathology that cannot be assessed with typical self-report or *DSM*-based measures. There is no other theory on which this many measures of personality and its related constructs have been developed and tested for their empirical soundness and clinical utility. *DSM–5* would enhance its empirical credibility by developing a system of assessment that is theoretically grounded and for which there are multiple, valid assessment tools. By radically altering the current diagnostic system and framework, the *DSM–5* Work Group has created a diagnostic system that requires the creation of new

assessment tools and their empirical verification before it can be determined whether the system can be reliably applied and has validity and utility.

CONCLUDING REMARKS

The science and practice of personality assessment should be a guiding force in the development of the *DSM–5* assessment of personality and personality pathology. The Personality and Personality Disorder Work Group's proposal has made a favorable step in that direction, by considering personality prototypes and dimensional ratings of prototypes and traits in the assessment and diagnosis of PDs. Yet, their efforts have not gone far enough or have not been justified well in light of the extant literature on personality assessment, some of which I have reviewed here. Likewise, psychoanalytic and psychodynamic models of personality and psychopathology offer a logical, coherent, and integrative framework on which to organize the assessment and diagnosis of personality pathology; yet, these ideas continue to be largely unintegrated into the *DSM* system. Greater attention to these domains of research holds much promise to enhance the *DSM–5* in ways that have heretofore have gone unattended.

ACKNOWLEDGMENT

Portions of this article were presented at the 2010 Annual Midwinter Meeting of the Society for Personality Assessment, San Jose, CA.

REFERENCES

Allik, J. (2005). Personality dimensions across cultures. *Journal of Personality Disorders, 19*, 212–232.

American Psychiatric Association. (1994). *Diagnostic and statistical manual of mental disorders* (4th ed.). Washington, DC: Author.

American Psychiatric Association. (2001). *Diagnostic and statistical manual of mental disorders* (4th ed., text revision). Washington, DC: Author.

Bargh, J. A., Bond, R. N., Lombardi, W. J., & Tota, M. E. (1986). The additive nature of chronic and temporary sources of construct accessibility. *Journal of Personality and Social Psychology, 50*, 869–878.

Bargh, J. A., & Morsella, E. (2008). The unconscious mind. *Perspectives on Psychological Science, 3*, 73–79.

Blatt, S. J., & Shichman, S. (1983). Two primary configurations of psychopathology. *Psychoanalysis and Contemporary Thought, 6*, 187–254.

Bornstein, R. F. (2003). Behaviorally referenced experimentation and symptom validation: A paradigm for 21st century personality disorder research. *Journal of Personality Disorders, 17*, 1–18.

Bornstein, R. F. (2005). Reconnecting psychoanalysis to mainstream psychology: Challenges and opportunities. *Psychoanalytic Psychology, 22*, 323–340.

Bornstein, R. F. (2007). From surface to depth: Diagnosis and assessment in personality pathology. *Clinical Psychology: Science and Practice, 14*, 99–102.

Bornstein, R. F. (2010). Psychoanalytic theory as a unifying framework for 21st century personality assessment. *Psychoanalytic Psychology, 27*, 133–152.

Bornstein, R. F., & Huprich, S. K. (in press). Beyond dysfunction and threshold-based classification: A multidimensional model of PD diagnosis. *Journal of Personality Disorders.*

Brenner, C. (1982). *The mind in conflict.* New York, NY: International Universities Press.

Caspi, A., Roberts, B. W., & Shiner, R. L. (2005). Personality development: Stability and change. *Annual Review of Psychology, 56*, 453–484.

Clarkin, J. F., & Huprich, S. K. (2011). Do the *DSM–5* proposals for personality disorders meet the criteria for clinical utility? *Journal of Personality Disorders, 25*, 192–205.

Costa, P. T., Jr., & McCrae, R. R. (1992). *Revised NEO Personality Inventory (NEO PI–R) and the NEO Five-Factor Inventory (NEO–FFI) professional manual.* Odessa, FL: Psychological Assessment Resources.

Costa, P. T., Jr., & Widiger, T. A. (2002). *Personality disorders and the five-factor model of personality* (2nd ed.). Washington, DC: American Psychological Association.

DeMarree, K. G., Wheeler, S. C., & Petty, R. E. (2005). Priming a new identity: Self-monitoring moderates the effects of nonself primes on self-judgments and behavior. *Journal of Personality and Social Psychology, 89,* 657–671.

Durbin, C. E., & Klein, D. N. (2006). Ten-year stability of personality disorders among outpatients with mood disorders. *Journal of Abnormal Psychology, 115,* 75–84.

First, M. B., & Westen, D. (2007). Classification for clinical practice: How to make ICD and *DSM* better able to serve clinicians. *International Review of Psychiatry, 19,* 473–481.

Fonagy, P., & Luyten, P. (2009). A developmental, mentalization based approach to the understanding and treatment of borderline personality disorder. *Development and Psychopathology, 21,* 1355–1381.

Fonagy, P., & Target, M. (1997). Attachment and reflective function: Their role in self-organization. *Development and Psychopathology, 9,* 679–700.

Fonagy, P., & Target, M. (2006). The mentalization-focused approach to self pathology. *Journal of Personality Disorders, 20,* 544–576.

Ganellen, R. J. (2007). Assessing normal and abnormal personality functioning: Strengths and weaknesses of self-report, observer, and performance-based methods. *Journal of Personality Assessment, 89,* 30–40.

Goldberg, L. R. (1992). The development of markers for the Big-Five factor structure. *Psychological Assessment, 4,* 26–42.

Grilo, C. M., & McGlashan, T. H. (2009). Course and outcome. In J. M. Oldham, A. E. Skodol, & D. S. Bender (Eds.), *Essentials of personality disorders* (pp. 63–82). Washington, DC: American Psychiatric Publishing.

Hirschfeld, R. M. A., Klerman, G. L., Clayton, P. J., Keller, M. B., McDonald-Scott, P., & Larkin, B. H. (1983). Assessing personality: Effects of the depressive state on trait measurement. *American Journal of Psychiatry, 140,* 695–699.

Hull, J. G., Slone, L. B., Meteyer, K. B., & Matthews, A. R. (2002). The nonconsciousness of self-consciousness. *Journal of Personality and Social Psychology, 83,* 406–424.

Huprich, S. K. (2009). *Psychodynamic therapy: Conceptual and empirical foundations.* New York, NY: Routledge/Taylor & Francis.

Huprich, S. K. (2011). Reclaiming the value of assessing unconscious and subjective psychological experience. *Journal of Personality Assessment, 93,* 151–160.

Huprich, S. K., & Bornstein, R. F. (2007). Categorical and dimensional assessment of personality disorders: A consideration of the issues. *Journal of Personality Assessment, 89,* 3–15.

Huprich, S. K., Bornstein, R. F., & Schmitt, T. (in press). Self-report methodology is insufficient for improving the assessment and classification of Axis II personality disorders. *Journal of Personality Disorders.*

Jenkins, S. R. (2007). *A scoring handbook for the Thematic Apperception Test.* Mahwah, NJ: Erlbaum.

John, O. P., Robins, R. W., & Pervin, L. A. (2008). *Handbook of personality* (3rd ed.). New York, NY: Guilford.

Kammrath, L., Mendoza-Denton, R., & Mischel, W. (2005). Incorporating if … then… personality signatures in person perception: Beyond the person–situation dichotomy. *Journal of Personality and Social Psychology, 88,* 605–618.

Kandel, E. R. (1999). Biology and the future of psychoanalysis: A new intellectual framework for psychiatry revisited. *American Journal of Psychiatry, 156,* 505–524.

Krueger, R. F., & Eaton, N. R. (2010). Personality traits and the classification of mental disorders: Toward a more complete integration in *DSM–5* and an empirical model of psychopathology. *Personality Disorders: Theory, Research, and Treatment, 1,* 97–118.

Krueger, R. F., Eaton, N. R., Derringer, J., Markon, K. B., Watson, D., & Skodol, A. E. (2011/this issue). Personality in *DSM–5*: Helping delineate personality disorder content and framing the metastructure. *Journal of Personality Assessment, 93,* 325–331.

Krueger, R. F., & Johnson, W. (2008). Behavioral genetics and personality: A new look at the integration of nature and nurture. In O. P. John, R. W. Robins, & L. A. Pervin (Eds.), *Handbook of personality* (3rd ed., pp. 287–310). New York, NY: Guilford.

Lerner, P. M. (2005). Defense and its assessment: The Lerner Defense Scale. In R. F. Bornstein & J. M. Masling (Eds.), *Scoring the Rorschach: Seven validated systems* (pp. 237–269). Mahwah, NJ: Erlbaum.

Markman, K. D., & McMullen, M. N. (2003). A reflection and evaluation model of comparative thinking. *Personality and Social Psychology Review, 7,* 244–267.

Markon, K. E., Krueger, R. F., & Watson, D. (2005). Delineating the structure of normal and abnormal personality: An integrative hierarchical approach. *Journal of Personality and Social Psychology, 88,* 139–157.

Masling, J. M., Rabie, L., & Blondheim, S. H. (1967). Obesity, level of aspiration, and Rorschach and TAT measures of oral dependence. *Journal of Consulting Psychology, 31,* 233–239.

Mayer, J. D., Gaschke, Y. N., Braverman, D. L., & Evans, T. W. (1992). Mood-congruent judgment is a general effect. *Journal of Personality and Social Psychology, 63,* 119–132.

McCrae, R. R., & Costa, P. T., Jr. (2008). The five-factor theory of personality. In O. P. John, R. W. Robins, & L. A. Pervin (Eds.), *Handbook of personality* (3rd ed., pp. 159–181). New York, NY: Guilford.

McWilliams, N. (1999). *Psychoanalytic case formulation.* New York, NY: Guilford.

Mischel, W., & Shoda, Y. (2008). Toward a unified theory of personality: Integrating dispositions and processing dynamics within the cognitive-affective personality system. In O. P. John, R. W. Robins, & L. A. Pervin (Eds.), *Handbook of personality* (3rd ed., pp. 208–241). New York, NY: Guilford.

Morey, L. C., Shea, M. T., Markowitz, J. C., Stout, R. L., Hopwood, C. J., Gunderson, J. G., … Skodol, A. E. (2010). State effects of major depression on the assessment of personality and personality disorder. *American Journal of Psychiatry, 167,* 528–535.

Mussweiler, T. (2003). Comparison processes in social judgment: Mechanisms and consequences. *Psychological Review, 110,* 472–489.

Oltmanns, T. F., & Turkheimer, E. (2006). Perceptions of self and others regarding pathological personality traits. In R. F. Krueger & J. L. Tackett (Eds.), *Personality and psychopathology* (pp. 71–111). New York, NY: Guilford.

Ottoson, H., Grann, M., & Kullgren, G. (2000). Test–retest reliability of a self-report questionnaire for *DSM–IV* and ICD–10 personality disorders. *European Journal of Psychological Assessment, 16,* 53–58.

Panksepp, J. (1998). *Affective neuroscience.* New York, NY: Oxford University Press.

Panksepp, J. (1999). Emotions as viewed by psychoanalysis and neuroscience: An exercise in consilience. *Neuro-Psychoanalysis, 1,* 15–38.

Panksepp, J. (2003). At the interface of the affective, behavioral, and cognitive neurosciences: Decoding the emotional feelings of the brain. *Brain and Cognition, 52,* 4–14.

Panksepp, J. (2005). Affective consciousness: Core emotional feelings in animals and humans. *Consciousness and Cognition, 14,* 30–80.

PDM Task Force. (2006). *Psychodynamic diagnostic manual.* Silver Spring, MD: Alliance of Psychoanalytic Organizations.

Pfohl, B., Blum, N., & Zimmerman, M. (1997). *Structured Interview for DSM–IV Personality.* Washington, DC: American Psychiatric Press.

Ready, R. E., & Clark, L. A. (2002). Correspondence of psychiatric patient and informant ratings of personality traits, temperament, and interpersonal problems. *Psychological Assessment, 14,* 39–49.

Rhadigan, C., & Huprich, S. K. (in press). The utility of the cognitive-affective processing system in diagnosis personality disorders: Some preliminary evidence. *Journal of Personality Disorders.*

Robinson, M. D., & Clore, G. L. (2002). Episodic and semantic knowledge in emotional self-report: Evidence for two judgment processes. *Journal of Personality and Social Psychology, 83,* 198–215.

Rottman, B. M., Ahn, W. K., Sanislow, C. A., & Kim, N. S. (2009). Can clinicians recognize *DSM–IV* personality disorders from five-factor model descriptions of patient cases? *American Journal of Psychiatry, 166,* 427–433.

Santor, D. A., Bagby, R. M., & Joffee, R. T. (1997). Evaluating stability and change in personality and depression. *Journal of Personality and Social Psychology, 73,* 1354–1362.

Schore, A. N. (2000). Attachment and the regulation of the right brain. *Attachment & Human Development, 2*, 23–47.

Shedler, J., Beck, A. T., Fonagy, P., Gabbard, G. O., Gunderson, J. G., Kernberg, O. F., . . . Weston, D. (2010). Personality disorders in *DSM–5*. *American Journal of Psychiatry, 167*, 1026–1028.

Shedler, J., Mayman, M., & Manis, M. (1993). The illusion of mental health. *American Psychologist, 48*, 1117–1131.

Shevrin, H., Bond, J., Brakel, L., Hertel, R., & Williams, W. J. (1996). *Conscious and unconscious processes: Psychodynamic, cognitive, and neurophysiological convergences.* New York, NY: Guilford.

Shoda, Y., Mischel, W., & Wright, J. C. (1994). Intra-individual stability in the organization and patterning of behavior: Incorporating psychological situations into the idiographic analysis of personality. *Journal of Personality and Social Psychology, 67*, 674–687.

Solms, M. (2000a). Preliminaries for an integration of psychoanalysis and neuroscience. *Annals of Psychoanalysis, 28*, 179–200.

Solms, M. (2000b). A psychoanalytic contribution to contemporary neuroscience. In G. van de Vijver & F. Geerardyn (Eds.), *The pre-psychoanalytic writings of Sigmund Freud* (pp. 17–35). London, UK: Karnac Books.

Spitzer, R. L., First, M. B., Shedler, J., Westen, D., & Skodol, A. E. (2008). Clinical utility of five dimensional systems for personality diagnosis: A "consumer preference" study. *Journal of Nervous and Mental Disease, 195*, 356–374.

Trull, T. J. (2005). Dimensional models of personality disorder: Coverage and cutoffs. *Journal of Personality Disorders, 19*, 262–282.

Westen, D. (1992). Social cognition and social affect in psychoanalysis and cognitive science: From analysis of regression to regression analysis. In J. W. Barron, M. N. Eagle, & D. L. Wolitzky (Eds.), *The interface of psychoanalysis and psychology* (pp. 375–388). Washington, DC: American Psychological Association.

Westen, D. (1997). Divergences between clinical and research methods for assessing personality disorders: Implications for research and evolution of Axis II. *The American Journal of Psychiatry, 154*, 895–903.

Westen, D., & Gabbard, G. O. (2002a). Developments in cognitive neuroscience: I. Conflict, compromise, and connectionism. *Journal of the American Psychoanalytic Association, 50*, 53–98.

Westen, D., & Gabbard, G. O. (2002b). Developments in cognitive neuroscience: II. Implications for theories of transference. *Journal of the American Psychoanalytic Association, 50*, 99–134.

Westen, D., & Shedler, J. (1999a). Revising and assessing Axis II, Part I: Developing a clinically and empirically valid assessment method. *American Journal of Psychiatry, 156*, 258–272.

Westen, D., & Shedler, J. (1999b). Revising and assessing Axis II, Part II: Toward an empirically based and clinically useful classification of personality disorders. *American Journal of Psychiatry, 156*, 273–285.

Westen, D., & Shedler, J. (2007). Personality diagnosis with the Shedler–Westen Assessment Procedure: Integrating clinical and statistical measurement and prediction. *Journal of Abnormal Psychology, 116*, 810–822.

Wheeler, S. C., DeMarree, K. G., & Petty, R. E. (2005). The roles of the self in priming-to-behavior effects. In A. Tesser, J. V. Wood, & D. A. Stapel (Eds.), *On building, defending and regulating the self: A psychological perspective* (pp. 245–271). New York, NY: Psychology Press.

Widiger, T. A., & Simonsen, E. (2005). Introduction to the special section: The American Psychiatric Association's research agenda for the *DSM–V*. *Journal of Personality Disorders, 19*, 103–109.

Zanarini, M. C., Frankenburg, F. R., Reich, D. R., Silk, K. R., Hudson, J. I., & McSweeney, L. B. (2007). The subsyndromal phenomenology of borderline personality disorder: A 10-year follow-up study. *American Journal of Psychiatry, 164*, 929–935.

Zanarini, M. C., Frankenburg, F. R., Sickel, A. E., & Yong, L. (1996). *The Diagnostic Interview for DSM–IV Personality Disorders (DIPD–IV)*. Belmont, MA: McLean Hospital.

Zimmerman, M., & Coryell, W. (1990). Diagnosing personality disorders in the community: A comparison of self-report and interview measures. *Archives of General Psychiatry, 47*, 527–531.

Personality Dynamics: Insights From the Personality Social Cognitive Literature

Michael D. Robinson and Kathryn H. Gordon

Department of Psychology, North Dakota State University

Psychodynamic and social cognitive approaches to personality assessment converge now more so than at any time in the history of experimental psychology. This contribution seeks to make this point. First, the trait of neuroticism predisposes one to multiple adverse outcomes, a point not sufficiently captured by the current version of the *Diagnostic and Statistical Manual of Mental Disorders* (4th ed. [*DSM–IV*]; American Psychiatric Association, 1994). Second, though, self-reported levels of neuroticism are insufficient in understanding problematic outcomes for multiple reasons. Third, there are ways of experimentally modeling the many processes of interest to psychodynamic theorists such as unconscious affective biases, implicit representations of self and other, and underlying deficits in self- and emotion regulation. Implicit approaches to assessment also provide clues to interventions targeting the processes of interest, a point that will be made as well.

Bornstein (2010) points out that personality assessment in the middle 20th century was decidedly psychodynamic. This is no longer true as a general rule. Even in the clinical realm, the American Psychiatric Association's *Diagnostic and Statistical Manual of Mental Disorders* (*DSM*; American Psychiatric Association, 1980, 1994) sought to deemphasize psychodynamic concepts in favor of more manifest symptoms and behaviors (Shedler & Westen, 2007). The cognitive revolution in psychology led to the development of basic cognitive tasks (e.g., the Stroop task, in which individuals must override their automatic tendencies to respond on the basis of color words rather than font colors) that have potential importance in understanding dysregulated outcomes of multiple types (N. P. Friedman & Miyake, 2004). Nonclinical personality psychologists have converged on an assessment model in which individual differences in extraversion, agreeableness, conscientiousness, neuroticism, and openness to experience have been shown to predict a wide array of emotional and behavioral outcomes (McCrae & Costa, 1999), including in the realm of personality disorders (Costa & Widiger, 1994). Recent developments in assessment have also occurred in the social cognition literature, which also has rarely conceptualized such assessments in explicitly psychodynamic terms (Greenwald et al., 2002).

Regardless, there are important potential continuities between psychodynamic ideas and the modern take on how the mind functions. Westen (1998) suggests that the modern emphasis on the ubiquity and importance of unconscious processes is very much in keeping with psychodynamic ideas (also see Dixon, 1981). More recently, social psychologists have shown that our goals are often unconscious, direct attention without awareness, and produce effects—such as resistance to interference and perseverance—that were previously thought to characterize only conscious, goal-directed efforts (Chartrand, Dalton, & Cheng, 2008; Dijksterhuis & Aarts, 2010; Ferguson, Hassin, & Bargh, 2008). M. D. Robinson, Schmeichel, and Inzlicht (2010) suggested that ego strength can be viewed in terms of operations of the frontal lobes, which have been shown to both monitor and correct problematic automatic tendencies (E. K. Miller & Cohen, 2001).

Also, there are a number of excellent modern psychodynamic approaches to assessment. These seek to show that psychodynamic concepts such as such as oral dependence (Bornstein, 2009), attachment styles (Shaver & Mikulincer, 2005), or defense mechanisms (Cramer, 2000) can be measured and have predictable consequences for cognition, social cognition, and behavior. Our research program has essentially examined the reversed direction. That is, we have assessed personality traits, cognitive tendencies, and social cognitive tendencies rather than individual differences of a more explicitly defined psychodynamic type. From this reversed perspective, the question is whether such ostensibly nondynamic measures predict individual difference outcomes in a manner consistent with a broadly psychodynamic perspective, such as that captured by the *Psychodynamic Diagnostic Manual* (*PDM*; PDM Task Force, 2006).

There are reasons for expecting such points of convergence. Consistent in spirit with the *PDM* (PDM Task Force, 2006), social cognitive approaches to personality assessment focus on questions of process and dynamics. Consistent with the *PDM*, they treat seriously the idea that many such processes and dynamics are unconscious. Consistent with the *PDM*, they are based on a dimensional perspective of personality rather than one assuming that a person either has or does not have a problem. Consistent with the *PDM*, they view the individual as a complex entity, particularly in terms of potential interactions among different assessments and components of personality (Bornstein, 2009). Finally, social cognitive approaches to personality assessment can examine several key assumptions of psychodynamic frameworks, such as the notion that neurotic symptoms result from a less orderly mind or one characterized by intrapsychic conflict.

The purpose of our review, then, is to highlight the ways in which social cognitive approaches to personality assessment have been and can be used in a manner consistent with a broadly psychodynamic perspective on personality functioning. Although by no means exclusively so, studies from our lab will be highlighted in the body of the review because they allow for a consistent and linear narrative and because we have conducted a great deal of work on the questions of central interest. The first author is a personality psychologist, not a clinical psychologist, but we hope the clinical implications and future directions will be at least somewhat apparent. To make this case in more particular terms, the discussion broadens our lens by highlighting recent work in which cognitive and social cognitive assessments have been admirably used in three clinical realms. We begin by reviewing evidence for the idea that one personality trait—neuroticism—possesses broad importance to the clinical literature.[1]

NEUROTICISM AS A GENERAL RISK FACTOR FOR DISORDER

One of the problems of the *DSM–IV* (American Psychiatric Association, 1994) is its categorical approach to classifying disorders (Shedler & Westen, 2007). The categorical model assumes that disorders are discrete in nature—that is, qualitatively distinct from both each other and from normality (Kendell & Jablensky, 2003). They are definitely not so, as diagnoses are highly cooccurring or comorbid. For example, anxiety and depression diagnoses are highly comorbid (Mineka, Watson, & Clark, 1998), personality disorders are highly comorbid (Widiger & Trull, 2007), and indeed comorbidity characterizes the entire spectrum of *DSM–IV* diagnoses (Widiger, Verheul, & van den Brink, 1999). Moreover, there is evidence from taxometric analyses that many disorders, including most personality disorders (Arntz et al., 2009; Marcus, Ruscio, Lilienfeld, & Hughes, 2008), are not categorically distinct from normality, but fall on a continuum with normality. Finally, a dimensional approach can explain comorbid personality disorder diagnoses that would otherwise be puzzling. For example, especially high levels of neuroticism could explain why an individual meets criteria for both obsessive–compulsive and dependent personality disorders (Lynam & Widiger, 2001). All such considerations are consistent with the *PDM* (PDM Task Force, 2006), which argues forcefully for continuous predictors of dysfunction that underlie multiple supposedly discrete diagnostic categories.

Although psychodynamic theorists and assessors are ambivalent concerning self-reports of personality (Huprich & Bornstein, 2007; Westen & Shedler, 1999), we suggest that an exception should be made in the case of self-reports of neuroticism. When individuals are asked to characterize the self "in general," either in relation to adjectives or sentences, and such data are then factor analyzed, a broad neuroticism factor

is almost always found (Goldberg, 1993; McCrae & Costa, 1999). Individuals low in neuroticism view themselves as calm and not easily perturbed, and they report lower levels of anxiety and depression. Individuals high in neuroticism, on the other hand, view themselves as prone to negative emotions (Meyer & Shack, 1989). High neuroticism individuals also report that they have high levels of emotional reactivity, low self-esteem, more frequent experiences of anxious and depressive symptoms, and a greater number of health problems (Suls & Martin, 2005; Watson & Pennebaker, 1989).[2]

Additionally, self-reports of neuroticism predict many of the real-world outcomes that clinicians typically focus on such as clinical diagnoses of major depression (Kendler, Kuhn, & Prescott, 2004), self-harming behaviors (S. A. Brown, 2009), suicide attempts (Angst, Degonda, & Ernst, 1992), and early deaths due to cardiovascular disease (Suinn, 2001). Thus, quite aside from personality-processing studies of neuroticism (Bolger & Schilling, 1991; Bolger & Zuckerman, 1995; Donahue, Robins, Roberts, & John, 1993; Magnus, Diener, Fujita, & Pavot, 1993; Suls & Martin, 2005), higher levels of this self-reported trait appear truly problematic and dysfunctional, including in clinical and applied realms (Lahey, 2009; Widiger et al., 1999). Whether fortuitous or not, then, the self-reported trait of neuroticism appears to capture many of the maladaptive tendencies viewed as contributing to neuroses by Freud and subsequent psychodynamic theorists (e.g., Fenichel, 1945; Horney, 1945).

Indeed, there are further ways of reproaching psychodynamic and trait conceptions of neuroticism. Although psychodynamic theories might generally suggest the malleability of neurotic levels of personality organization, it is recognized that there is a great degree of stability to such modes of interacting with the world (Bellak, Hurvich, & Gediman, 1973). Although trait theories might generally suggest the stability of individual differences in neuroticism, it is now recognized that neuroticism levels decrease with adulthood maturation (Caspi, Roberts, & Shiner, 2005) and as a result of successful psychotherapy (Widiger et al., 1999). In short, it seems to us that psychodynamic and trait conceptions of neuroticism converge in suggesting a degree of stability as well as malleability. From either perspective, however, the processing substrates of neuroticism must be better understood.

UNDERSTANDING NEUROTICISM

Finding a robust dimensional predictor of psychopathological symptoms of multiple types is an achievement. However, unless the processing bases of neuroticism can be understood, its predictive value is not particularly explanatory or amenable to therapeutic interventions. Consistent with the goals of the *PDM* (PDM Task Force, 2006), recent research has sought to uncover the motivations, affective tendencies, and cognitive biases associated with neuroticism. Although much work of this type remains to be done, results have greatly clarified matters and in so doing enriched our understanding of the underlying

---

[1]Meyer and Kurtz (2006) called for the elimination of the word *objective* to describe self-reports of personality. We entirely agree, further noting that there are many subjective elements to completing personality questionnaires (M. D. Robinson & Clore, 2002). Meyer and Kurtz also suggested that the term *projective* should not be used as a catch-all phrase in describing assessments that are not self-reported in nature. We agree with this point as well. We generally refer to "self-reported" or "explicit" assessments on the one hand—in which individuals self-describe their personalities—versus "implicit" on the other hand—in which personality is defined in terms of performance (e.g., reaction times) rather than self-reports. The explicit–implicit terminology is in keeping with the cognitive memory (Schultheiss, 2007), implicit motivation (McClelland, 1987), and social cognition (Fazio & Olson, 2003) literatures.

[2]We have found a 10-item broad-bandwidth neuroticism scale to have a high degree of predictive validity. Participants are asked the extent to which (1 = *very inaccurate*; 5 = *very accurate*) they "get irritated easily," "often feel blue," and "worry about things," among other items. The scale is free for use and can be found at http://ipip.ori.org/. It takes less than 5 min to complete.

reasons why neuroticism is such a ubiquitous risk factor for psychological disorder.

Neuroticism represents, among other things, a theory of the self and its typical propensity toward higher (high neuroticism) or lower (low neuroticism) levels of negative emotion (M. D. Robinson & Clore, 2002). When experiences are consistent with the self-concept, the world as a whole might seem more predictable (Epstein, 1973). On the other hand, experiences that are inconsistent with the self-concept might engender some degree of confusion and uncertainty (Swann, 1992). Somewhat paradoxically, then, high neuroticism individuals might be motivated to experience negative affect and confused when they do not. Support for the latter point was reported in a set of studies by Tamir and Robinson (2004), who found that individuals high in neuroticism performed affective processing tasks better when experiencing high (relative to low) levels of negative affect. Support for the former point was reported by Tamir (2005), who found that neurotics were more likely than nonneurotics to choose a worry induction prior to a demanding social task (e.g., giving a speech). From an epistemic perspective, then, the neurotic might hold onto negative beliefs about the self because they seem subjectively compelling and perhaps even functional. As a point of clinical intervention, such beliefs might be effectively challenged, perhaps by highlighting the many cases in which negative self-beliefs create their own reality and cause unnecessary suffering (Ellis, 2002).

It is a general point that biological organisms are motivated to approach rewards and avoid punishments (Schneirla, 1959). However, the relative strength of these two motives is likely to systematically differ between individuals (Gray, 1981; Gray & McNaughton, 2000; Higgins, 1997). Neuroticism can be understood in terms of a particularly active avoidance-motivation system. This point has been substantiated by studies examining self-reported motivational tendencies (Elliot & Thrash, 2002; Zelenski & Larsen, 1999). More recently, implicit affective sources of evidence for neuroticism's link to punishment sensitivity have been reported (Moeller & Robinson, 2010). In two studies, it was found that error feedback led individuals high in neuroticism to switch their behaviors on the next trial, even when it was not functional to do so. Results from Study 2 of that paper, in terms of percentages of switches following correct and error feedback, are graphed in Figure 1. From a motivational perspective, then, many of the problems associated with high levels of neuroticism might be due to an overactive punishment sensitivity system.[3]

Neuroticism is a strong predictor of negative emotions (Meyer & Shack, 1989). On the basis of such sources of data, it has been

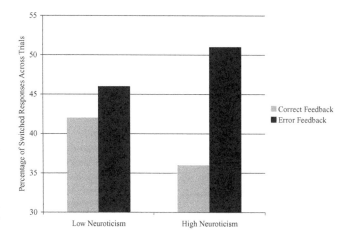

FIGURE 1.—Percentage of switched behavioral responses as a function of neuroticism and error feedback on the previous trial (Moeller & Robinson, 2010). *Note:* Partial eta squared was .07 for the neuroticism by error feedback interaction, a medium effect size.

suggested that neurotics might be accessible for, or in other words predisposed to, attribute negative meaning to affective events or stimuli. This straightforward idea has met with limited success (Matthews & Gilliland, 1999; Rusting, 1998). M. D. Robinson, Ode, Moeller, and Goetz (2007) recently revisited this search for an affective processing basis of neuroticism. Across two studies, neuroticism did not predict the speed with which negative stimuli could be evaluated. On the other hand, both studies found evidence for the idea that high neuroticism individuals possess affective networks that favor negative evaluations following negative primes on the preceding trial. In other words, neuroticism can be conceptualized in terms of an affective memory network favoring spreading activation processes from one negative thought to another. These results have implications for understanding a number of phenomena linked to higher levels of neuroticism such as stress reactivity (Suls & Martin, 2005), rumination (Trapnell & Campbell, 1999), and worry (Widiger et al., 1999).[4]

From another perspective, neuroticism is likely to have paradoxical effects on cognitive performance. On the one hand, neuroticism can be understood as a drive to performance, much as trait anxiety has been similarly characterized (Eysenck, Derakshan, Santos, & Calvo, 2007). In other words, there is an "urgency" associated with neuroticism that might often facilitate performance, especially in routine tasks. On the other hand, the doubts and worries associated with neuroticism could result in more frequent "off-task" thoughts at other times (Sarason, Sarason, & Pierce, 1990). Somewhat paradoxically, then, we

[3]Moeller and Robinson (2010) assessed punishment sensitivity in the following manner. On each trial, individuals were asked to guess whether a subsequent arrow would point upward or downward across 120 trials of a computerized task. Arrow direction was randomly manipulated by the computer, such that it was entirely unpredictable from trial to trial. Predictions would therefore be accurate approximately 50% of the time. Following each prediction, an arrow was presented and participants were told that they were "correct" or "incorrect" for the individual trial. Punishment sensitivity was implicitly assessed in terms of a higher percentage of switched predictions for the next trial (e.g., an up prediction followed by a down prediction) following incorrect relative to correct feedback on the previous trial. We view this implicit probe of punishment sensitivity as a potentially useful one in understanding clinical conditions hypothesized to reflect unduly low (e.g., psychopathy) or high (e.g., obsessive thinking) levels of punishment sensitivity. The task takes about 5 min to complete.

[4]Participants were asked to categorize words as pleasant (e.g., kiss) or unpleasant (e.g., garbage). Such word stimuli were assigned to trial at random, such that it was equally likely for a negative target (trial n) to follow a negative or positive prime (trial $n - 1$). Individual differences in negative affective priming were assessed by subtracting the individual's evaluation speed for negative–negative prime–target pairs from his or her evaluation speed for positive–negative prime–target pairs. As reported in the text, higher levels of neuroticism were associated with stronger negative affective priming effects of this type. We view this implicit probe of affective priming as a potentially useful one in understanding clinical conditions hypothesized to reflect a tendency to perseverate on negative affect, such as depression (Segal, Williams, & Teasdale, 2002). The task takes about 5 min to complete.

would expect neurotics to exhibit faster processing performance on some trials and slower processing performance on others.

Our first foray into this cognitive perspective on neuroticism combined these two perspectives by proposing that neuroticism should be associated with more variable reaction times across trials of very simple choice reaction time tasks. Indeed, across three studies, it was shown that more variable reaction times were characteristic of high neuroticism individuals relative to low neuroticism individuals (M. D. Robinson & Tamir, 2005). Similarly, more variable reaction times, independent of average speed, are reliable over time, across different cognitive tasks, and are predictive of negative emotional reactions and psychopathological symptoms in daily life (Ode, Robinson, & Hanson, in press). More recently, Bresin, Robinson, Ode, and Leth-Steenson (in press) found that high levels of anxiety and neuroticism were associated with fast typical performance but slow atypical performance, a pattern consistent with both high arousal and high distractibility. In sum, recent results reinforce the idea that neuroticism both facilitates and undermines performance, and that discrepancies between fast and slow performance appear to characterize an aspect of the intrapsychic conflict associated with high levels of neuroticism. We also suggest that reaction time variability might be useful in assessing individual differences in ego functioning, as poor ego functioning should be associated with higher levels of reaction time variability according to multiple literatures (Ode et al., in press).[5]

Freud (1926/1953) initially proposed that neurotic symptoms resulted from intrapsychic conflict, much as intrapsychic conflict has been shown to precipitate anxiety in animal models (N. E. Miller, 1944). Empirical support for this idea has been obtained. Emmons (1986) found that goal conflict was associated with anxious symptoms and indeed higher levels of neuroticism. King and Emmons (1990) found that conflict over emotional expression was predictive of higher levels of neuroticism. Donahue et al. (1993) found that conflicts among different social roles, and their requirements, were predictive of higher levels of neuroticism. More recently, M. D. Robinson and Wilkowski (2006) showed that conscious–unconscious conflicts of the social type favored by Horney (1945; getting along vs. getting ahead) predicted higher levels of neuroticism. These findings, in total, provide considerable support for the idea that neuroticism does not just predispose one to certain outcomes, but can also be viewed as an outcome itself, specifically of higher levels of intrapsychic conflict. There are many ways to be conflicted, though, and thus further demonstrations of this idea are needed.

We view neuroticism as more of a predictor of psychopathology than a target of clinical intervention. Instead, the processing correlates of neuroticism that we have identified—particularly implicit punishment sensitivity, negative affective priming, and reaction time variability—seem far more useful targets of clinical intervention and assessments of therapeutic progress. We advocate this direction of future clinical outcome research. In any case, the next section makes it clear that high levels of the trait of neuroticism are not necessarily problematic, a point that better contextualizes neuroticism as a risk factor rather than one associated with invariant problematic outcomes of a clinical type.

NEUROTICISM AS A VULNERABILITY FACTOR

Many individuals high in neuroticism never develop a psychological disorder and, perhaps equally telling, successful treatments of clinical symptoms result in relatively small decreases in self-reported neuroticism (Widiger et al., 1999). Such results necessitate that neuroticism be viewed as a vulnerability factor rather than an invariant marker of psychopathology (M. D. Robinson & Compton, 2008). If so, mechanisms and processes beyond the trait of neuroticism are necessary in understanding whether high levels of it should engender psychopathological symptoms in a particular individual. Our lab has conducted a large number of studies in examining such moderating factors and this section reviews such evidence, which we believe to be important to the clinical assessment literature.

The self-reported trait of neuroticism is a robust predictor of both self-reports of anger and aggression (Martin, Watson, & Wan, 2000) as well objective measures of behavioral aggression, particularly following provocation (Bettencourt, Talley, Benjamin, & Valentine, 2006). In addition, high levels of agreeableness are also inversely predictive of these outcomes (Bettencourt et al., 2006; Martin et al., 2000). This is likely so because agreeable individuals are motivated to self-regulate their interpersonal functioning in favor of friendly relations with others (Graziano & Eisenberg, 1997). Putting such sources of data together, agreeableness might constitute a protective factor at higher levels of neuroticism. In several studies, Ode, Robinson, and Wilkowski (2008) were able to provide support for this idea in that the highest levels of anger and aggression were particular to individuals both high in neuroticism and low in agreeableness. We should note that this very same combination might be predictive of borderline personality disorder diagnoses (Costa & Widiger, 2002; Saulsman & Page, 2004).[6]

Agreeableness is inversely predictive of anger and aggression, but typically not other psychopathological symptoms or outcomes (Watson, 2000). Thus, it is reasonable to suggest that agreeableness might moderate the problematic trait of neuroticism only in the context of anger and aggression. From another view, though, agreeableness might be linked to broader self-regulation processes than just those associated with anger and aggression (Graziano & Eisenberg, 1997). Support for this perspective has been obtained. Ode and Robinson (2007) found that that somatic symptoms interactively varied by neuroticism

---

[5]Any basic choice reaction time task can be used to assess reaction time variability. For example, Ode et al. (in press) administered a simple Stroop task in which individuals were asked to classify font colors as red or green across 252 trials. Subsequently, and for each individual separately, we quantified average speed and the standard deviation of response speed across the 252 trials. Individual differences in reaction time variability were then quantified by controlling for average speed, which often results in higher levels of reaction time variability for reasons that are psychometric rather than psychologically informative (M. D. Robinson & Tamir, 2005). We view this implicit probe of variability as a potentially useful one in understanding clinical conditions hypothesized to result from poor ego functioning. In addition, reaction time variability might prove sensitive to therapeutic progress in realms seeking to increase ego functioning (Bellak et al., 1973). The task takes about 5 min to complete.

[6]Agreeableness can be assessed by a well-validated 10-item scale asking individuals the extent to which (1 = *very inaccurate*; 5 = *very accurate*) they are "interested in people," "take time out for others" and "sympathize with others' feelings," among other items. The scale is free for use and can be found at http://ipip.ori.org/. It takes less than 5 min to complete.

and agreeableness and Ode and Robinson (2009) found similar results concerning depressive symptoms, in the latter case in terms of an implicit measure of negative affective reactivity as well. These results suggest that it might be informative to clinicians to routinely assess the trait of agreeableness as well as the trait of neuroticism, as these factors appear to interactively predict psychopathological symptoms of multiple types.

Mindfulness has been defined in terms of the extent to which the individual is aware of his or her momentary transactions with the environment (K. W. Brown & Ryan, 2004), with the idea that such enhanced awareness is crucial for effective self-regulation (M. D. Robinson, Schmeichel, & Inzlicht, 2010). Indeed, several clinical treatment literatures have shown that mindfulness meditation practices or other awareness-enhancing techniques reduce symptoms among otherwise distress-prone individuals (Baer, 2003; Grossman, Niemann, Schmidt, & Walach, 2004; Teasdale et al., 2002). Such mindfulness skills might overlap with those favored by ego psychology, which views the development of an observing ego as therapeutic to the distressed client (Bouchard et al., 2008; Fonagy & Target, 2006). Self-report scales of mindfulness have also been developed. In a set of studies assessing mindfulness in terms of the K. W. Brown and Ryan (2003) scale, Feltman, Robinson, and Ode (2009) demonstrated that higher levels of mindfulness moderated the impact of higher levels of neuroticism in two outcome realms—anger and depression. The highest such symptoms were observed among individuals both high in neuroticism and low in mindfulness. Thus, individual differences in mindfulness, like agreeableness, can possess considerable predictive validity in the clinical realm and might be worthy of wider assessment for this reason.[7]

There is a close potential relationship between cognitive control, defined in terms of being able to inhibit an unwanted thought or behavior (E. K. Miller & Cohen, 2001; van Veen & Carter, 2006), and emotion regulation processes (Zelazo & Cunningham, 2007). For example, asking individuals to reduce their negative emotional reactions to distressing stimuli (Ochsner & Gross, 2005) results in the recruitment of the same brain regions (typically the anterior cingulate cortex and the dorsolateral prefrontal cortex) also centrally implicated in cognitive control (Holroyd & Coles, 2002; Kerns et al., 2004). Accordingly, we have suggested that implicit measures sensitive to cognitive control should moderate neuroticism–outcome relations (M. D. Robinson, 2007). Support for this idea has been obtained in a number of studies assessing individual differences in cognitive control in terms of faster reaction time performance (M. D. Robinson & Clore, 2007), lesser variability in reaction time (M. D. Robinson, Wilkowski, & Meier, 2006), lesser tendencies toward habitual responding (M. D. Robinson, Goetz, Wilkowski, & Hoffman, 2006), and lesser tendencies toward response perse-

veration (M. D. Robinson, Wilkowski, Kirkeby, & Meier, 2006). Cognitive control is multifaceted, but these results leave little doubt that cognitive control is an important factor to consider in understanding whether neuroticism will result in problematic symptoms or not.[8]

The general interactive predictions emphasized in this section have recently been extended to the psychophysiology literature. Higher levels of basal heart rate variability (HRV) have been viewed as beneficial in regulating problematic emotional and social outcomes (B. H. Friedman, 2007). However, some investigators have suggested that higher levels of HRV can sometimes result in higher levels of emotional reactivity (Butler, Wilhelm, & Gross, 2006; Gyurak & Ayduk, 2008). In reconciling such perspectives on HRV, we proposed that higher levels of it might be particularly beneficial at higher levels of neuroticism. Support for this interactive framework was found in a daily protocol involving six problematic outcomes, including those related to negative affect, somatic symptoms, and impulsive behaviors (Ode, Hilmert, Zielke, & Robinson, 2010). Again, then, a purported measure of cognitive control (HRV) only appears to be beneficial to the extent that the individual is a highly neurotic one.[9]

Experience-sampling studies link neuroticism to stress reactivity (Bolger & Schilling, 1991). Stress reactivity is too general a tendency to make precise predictions concerning behavior, however, as quite a few behaviors and symptoms have been linked to it (aggression, disordered eating, heavy drinking, procrastinating, self-harming, etc.). Indeed, one might cope with stress by withdrawing from social contact or seeking it, two diametrically opposed tendencies (Taylor et al., 2000). In understanding these divergent pathways, we have turned to implicit tools capable of modeling the sort of idiographic associations posited by Mischel and Shoda's (1995) social cognitive model of personality. This model contends that (a) individuals are consistent in their behaviors within a given situation to a greater extent than across situations; (b) individuals have distinct situational signatures for many of their behaviors (e.g., aggression, talkativeness); and (c) the best prediction of behavior will take into account such individually distinctive

---

[7]K. W. Brown and Ryan's (2003) measure of mindfulness has excellent psychometric properties and is reprinted in this article. Individuals are asked to report on the frequency (1 = almost never; 6 = almost always) with which they engage in behaviors without thinking about them (e.g., "I snack without being aware that I'm eating"). Such items are reverse-scored to assess mindful attention and awareness. Mindfulness exercises are used in several validated clinical treatment protocols, including Linehan's (1993) well-known treatment for borderline personality disorder. Moreover, it has been shown that the instrument responds to multisession interventions designed to increase self-awareness and the self-regulation skills thought to result (Shapiro, Oman, Thoresen, Plante, & Flinders, 2008).

---

[8]The same or similar tasks described in footnote 4 can also be used to assess individual differences in response speed. In this case, one merely averages response speed across trials of the cognitive task. In other literatures, individuals who respond faster in choice reaction time tasks have been shown to be more intelligent (Jensen, 2006), better able to self-regulate their behaviors in health-related realms (Gottfredson & Deary, 2004), and to live for a longer period of time (Deary & Der, 2005). In all such cases, slower response speed has been shown to be problematic. Like mindfulness, M. D. Robinson and Oishi (2006) conceptualize faster response speed in terms of greater awareness of the current (stimulus) environment, which similarly should facilitate self-regulation effects (M. D. Robinson, Schmeichel, & Inzlicht, 2010). For assessments of habitual responding (M. D. Robinson, Goetz, et al., 2006) and response perseveration (M. D. Robinson, Wilkowski, Kirkeby, et al., 2006), readers are referred to the relevant publications.

[9]We omit a discussion of how to assess HRV because such assessments are costly and require considerable technical expertise. The more general point, though, is that this measure, like many others reviewed, appears protective at higher levels of neuroticism. Nonetheless, it is important to point out that HRV is a malleable entity (Garakani et al., 2009) that might reasonably be a target of therapeutic interventions among anxiety-prone individuals (B. H. Friedman, 2007).

situation-behavior profiles. For example, Harry might become aggressive in stressful situations, whereas Tom might not.

Mischel and Shoda (1995) further suggested that such individually distinctive situation-behavior profiles might be effectively understood in terms of mental associations. Reconsidering Harry and Tom, we would expect that stress-related thoughts would activate aggressive thoughts in Harry, but not Tom. Moeller, Robinson, and Bresin (2010) sought to model such intrapsychic associations and how they varied across individuals. In specific terms, we assessed the extent to which stressful primes activated aggressive thoughts (Studies 1 & 2) or eating-related thoughts (Study 3) in reaction time priming paradigms, with the idea that individuals would differ considerably in such stress-triggered thoughts due to their unique implicit associative networks involving stress. Neuroticism was also assessed. Neuroticism did not predict such stress-related priming effects. On the other hand, neuroticism interacted to predict the outcomes of interest. In Studies 1 and 2, aggression was highest among those both (a) high in neuroticism whose reaction time performance (b) indicated stronger stress–aggression associations. In Study 3, scores on a measure of disordered eating similarly varied interactively by neuroticism and stress–eating associations of an implicit type. In sum, it appears that individual differences in priming effects can be used to understand the particular problems that are likely to be exhibited among distressed individuals.[10]

UNDERSTANDING ANGER-MOTIVATED AGGRESSION

There is perhaps no interpersonal behavior as disruptive to relationships, as costly to society, and in fact as adverse to victims and perpetrators as anger-motivated aggression (Smith, Glazer, Ruiz, & Gallo, 2004; Wilkowski & Robinson, 2010a). In addition, such tendencies toward anger-motivated aggression figure prominently in a number of clinical diagnoses among both children (e.g., conduct disorder) and adults (e.g., borderline personality disorder, narcissistic personality disorder). Consistent in spirit with the *PDM* (PDM Task Force, 2006), recent studies have sought to understand the dimensional basis of anger-motivated aggression and the underlying processing dynamics involved.

This research program began with a series of studies reported by Meier and Robinson (2004). These researchers assessed the speed with which blame-implying words (e.g., malpractice, sin) could be categorized as blameworthy in nature. Such implicit tendencies were hypothesized, according to the theory of Kelly (1963), to lead to greater tendencies toward anger and aggression in everyday life and in response to a laboratory induction. Such findings were obtained, but only among low agreeable individu-

als. Because the same level of blame accessibility did not result in higher levels of anger and aggression among high agreeable individuals, Meier and Robinson proposed that agreeable individuals are capable of self-regulating their hostile thoughts in an implicit manner.[11]

To assess such purported implicit self-regulation processes more directly, Meier, Robinson, and Wilkowski (2006) administered a priming task in which primes consisted of hostile thoughts (or not) and targets consisted of words reflective of antisocial versus prosocial actions. It was found that agreeable individuals displayed a particular pattern of priming whereby hostile primes activated prosocial thoughts among agreeable individuals, but not among individuals low in agreeableness. In another cognitive paradigm, Wilkowski, Robinson, and Meier (2006) found that agreeable individuals were faster to spatially disengage from the location of a hostile prime (vs. a control prime) than were individuals low in agreeableness.

Subsequent studies have focused on the trait of anger, which is hypothesized to be more intimately linked to self-regulating hostile thoughts than is the broader construct of agreeableness (Wilkowski & Robinson, 2008a). Wilkowski and Robinson (2007) found that low anger individuals were less susceptible to hostile priming effects on judgment and also slowed down following their evaluations of hostile primes, even in a context in which targets were nonevaluative in nature. Effects of this type were recently extended by M. D. Robinson, Wilkowski, Meier, and Moeller (2010). Slowing down following problematic stimuli is likely to facilitate self-regulation efforts according to both the cognitive control (Holroyd & Coles, 2002) and anger-related (Berkowitz, 1993; Tavris, 1989) literatures.[12]

Stated in other terms, it appears that low anger individuals, but not high anger individuals, systematically recruit the cognitive control system of the brain (van Veen & Carter, 2006) to mitigate the influence of their activated hostile thoughts. More direct evidence for this idea was provided by Wilkowski and Robinson (2008b). In this set of studies, primes consisted of hostile or nonhostile words. The target tasks directly assessed cognitive control, for example in terms of flanker interference

---

[10]With reference to stress–aggression associations, the following cognitive task was used. On odd trials, individuals were asked to categorize words as stressful (e.g., *frustration*) or nonstressful (e.g., *forward*). On even trials, participants then categorized a different set of words as aggressive (e.g., *hurt*) or nonaggressive (e.g., *house*). The extent to which stressful primes activated hostile thoughts was quantified in a manner similar to footnote 3—that is, across consecutive trials of the categorization task. Here, the interest was in whether aggressive targets could be categorized more quickly following stressful primes rather than nonstressful primes. The priming procedures of Moeller et al. (2010) would seem to possess potential importance in other clinical realms as well. For example, individuals who exhibit stronger priming effects from alcohol primes to positive affective targets would likely be more vulnerable to alcoholism (Wiers & Stacy, 2006). The task takes less than 10 min to complete.

[11]Individual differences in blame accessibility were examined in a choice reaction time task. Participants were asked, as quickly and accurately as possible, whether presented words implied blame (e.g., *malpractice, sin*) or not (e.g., *baldness, earthquake*). Speed in this block was quantified. However, because individual differences in response speed, per se, are robust across different tasks (M. D. Robinson & Oishi, 2006), a control block was administered. In the control block, a neutral categorization task (distinguishing animal vs. not animal words) was used. Subsequently, residual scores for blame accessibility were created by removing the common variance to blame–not blame and animal–not animal blocks. Such procedures essentially purify the accessibility measure of interest (M. D. Robinson & Neighbors, 2006). The administration of target and control blocks took less than 5 min. Such procedures could potentially be used to assess other problematic accessible thoughts such as those associated with self-harm.

[12]Hitherto, the implicit measures reported were primarily of a reaction time type. In this context, Wilkowski and Robinson's (2007) word rating task deserves note. Participants evaluated (1 = *extremely unpleasant*; 6 = *extremely pleasant*) aggressive (e.g., *hurt, hit, punch*) and neutral (e.g., *interact, notice, talk*) words, with the words randomly intermixed. A hostility-related bias was defined in terms of more negative evaluations of neutral target (i.e., trial *n*) words that followed aggressive relative to neutral prime (i.e., trial *n*—1) words. Only angry individuals displayed such a hostility-related bias. The task takes approximately 5 min to complete and theoretically could be administered by paper and pencil rather than computer.

costs (Eriksen, 1995). It was found that low anger individuals displayed higher levels of cognitive control following the activation of hostile primes, whereas no such tendency was found among high anger individuals.[13]

To what extent can anger-motivated aggression be understood in terms of implicit processes, potentially independent of self-reported traits? Two recent investigations have sought to fill this gap in the literature. There are sources of data suggesting that hostile attribution biases, among children, are predictive of anger-motivated aggression (Orobio de Castro, Veerman, Koops, Bosch, & Monshouwer, 2002). Such hostile attribution biases involve attributing hostile intent to others when doing so is quite ambiguous or even erroneous (Crick & Dodge, 1994). Wilkowski and Robinson (2010b) used a person perception paradigm developed by Skowronski, Carlston, Mae, and Crawford (1998) and later improved by Todorov and Uleman (2002) to model erroneous tendencies to ascribe hostility to others on the basis of unconscious associative and inference processes. Individuals displaying higher levels of such hostility-related biases were angrier in their everyday lives. These results are particularly important because the only predictor of such everyday tendencies was of an implicit-unconscious type.

Wilkowski and Robinson (2008b) found that low trait anger individuals, relative to high anger individuals, displayed higher levels of cognitive control following the activation of hostile thoughts (see footnote 13 for measurement-related considerations). In a recent set of studies, Wilkowski, Robinson, and Troop-Gordon (2010) sought to determine whether such implicit tendencies could be used to understand daily functioning, independent of self-reported trait variables. Results were supportive of this implicit approach to personality assessment. In Study 1, it was found that individuals displaying greater cognitive control following hostile primes were less aggressive in a laboratory aggression paradigm and reported less vengefulness motivation. In Study 2, it was found that individuals displaying greater cognitive control following hostile primes were more forgiving of daily provocations and exhibited lower levels of anger on days subsequent to high forgiveness motivation days.

In summarizing the material presented here, important progress has been made in understanding the processes underlying individual differences in anger-motivated aggression. Such differences are facilitated by hostile attribution biases and are mitigated to the extent that the cognitive control resources of the brain are recruited in a hostile priming context. The results

reviewed here, and in other sections as well, pave the way for a psychodynamic science of emotional reactivity consistent with its purported implicit processes (PDM Task Force, 2006).

IMPLICIT SELF-REPRESENTATIONS

The Thematic Apperception Test (TAT; McClelland, Atkinson, Clark, & Lowell, 1953) literature has long suggested and supported the idea that self-reported tendencies fail to capture the implicit tendencies of the individual (McClelland, Koestner, & Weinberger, 1989). In addition, self-reports of personality are strongly influenced by social desirability factors. For example, Edwards (1953) found an $r = .9$ correlation between the social desirability of a trait and its mean level of endorsement in self-report. There are multiple potential interpretations of this strong relationship. One is that self-reports of personality are contaminated by social desirability factors; if so, controlling for individual differences in social desirability should improve trait predictions. This has not been the case (McCrae & Costa, 1983). Over time, instead, personality researchers have increasingly adopted the perspective that social desirability factors in self-report represent more substance than style—that is, evaluative factors are central to the manner in which personality is defined and potentially to its predictive core (Paulhus & John, 1998).

Nonetheless, researchers continue to pursue the premise that there are some individuals whose positive self-reported views are defensive in nature, in many cases producing informative data along such lines (Colvin, Block, & Funder, 1995; Shedler, Mayman, & Manis, 1993). The Narcissistic Personality Inventory (NPI; Raskin & Terry, 1988) was developed in the context of such psychodynamic views of the self. It is loaded with items suggestive of a grandiose view of the self, plausibly an over-grandiose one. From a defensive psychodynamic viewpoint, the most direct question is whether narcissism can be defined in terms of the discrepancy between conscious and unconscious views of the self. A series of studies by Jordan, Spencer, Zanna, and Hoshino-Browne (2003) generated great enthusiasm for this idea in that they found that narcissism could be predicted on the basis of the discrepancy between high levels of self-reported self-esteem and low levels of implicit self-esteem. Unfortunately, subsequent attempts to define NPI narcissism in this manner failed to replicate the interactive pattern (Bosson et al., 2008). At the present time, then, there is no solid evidence for the idea that narcissists of an NPI type are overcompensating for negative implicit views of the self. Rather, such individuals appear to harbor a sense of entitlement at both implicit and explicit levels of self-representation.

Bosson et al. (2008) also reviewed available measures of implicit self-esteem and concluded that two of them were reliable enough for research (and potentially clinical) purposes. The first measure quantifies implicit self-esteem in terms of a reaction time test in which individuals dually classify self-related words and unpleasant versus pleasant words. In this Implicit Association Test (IAT; Greenwald & Farnham, 2000), higher levels of implicit self-esteem are revealed to the extent that it is easier for the individual to categorize self + pleasant words when the same response is required relative to another condition in which self + unpleasant words are to be categorized by the same response key. The second implicit measure assesses

---

[13]On odd trials of the implicit task, participants categorized prime words as aggressive or nonaggressive. The primes were similar to those mentioned in footnote 12. On even trials of the task, participants completed a single trial of a flanker task by categorizing, as quickly as possible, the central letter in a five-letter array (stimuli were ppppp, qqqqq, ppqpp, and qqpqq). The flanker cost is defined in terms of difficulty (i.e., slower reaction time) with the incongruent stimuli (ppqpp and qqpqq) relative to the congruent stimuli (ppppp and qqqqq). Overcoming such flanker interference costs requires cognitive control and recruitment of regions of the frontal lobes (Kerns, 2006). Only nonangry individuals differentially recruited cognitive control following aggressive primes. The task takes approximately 5 min to complete. Tasks of this type could surely be designed to assess other processes of clinical relevance. For example, primes could consist of fatty (e.g., pizza) or healthy (e.g., celery) food words. We would expect bulimics to exhibit poorer cognitive control following fatty prime words, providing insight into their unhealthy and dysregulated eating habits.

liking for letters of one's own name (see Bosson et al., 2008, for computation considerations).[14]

It is common to suggest that implicit evaluations of the self should be more negative than self-reports of self-esteem. This perspective is incorrect on the basis of available sources of data. For example, Greenwald and Farnham (2000) reported that levels of implicit self-esteem were even more polarized in a positive evaluative direction than were levels of explicit (i.e., self-reported) self-esteem. Accordingly, implicit representations of the self seem to be especially favorable. On the other hand, implicit evaluations of the self might still possess predictive validity. In support of this idea, M. D. Robinson and Meier (2005) found that higher levels of implicit self-esteem inversely predicted negative emotional experiences and M. D. Robinson, Mitchell, Kirkeby, and Meier (2006) found an inverse relation between implicit self-esteem and somatic symptoms (e.g., headaches, nausea, etc.). Implicit self-esteem measures might also be useful for accurately tracking progress in therapy in relation to client self-views because they involve methods that are less likely to be influenced by impression management concerns.

It would be useful to develop theoretical perspectives of implicit self-representations that go beyond those of a strictly self-attitudinal type. In this connection, M. D. Robinson, Mitchell, et al. (2006) suggested that individual differences in implicit self-esteem might instead be understood in terms of an automatic form of self-protection. To score high on the self-esteem IAT (Greenwald & Farnham, 2000), one has to be particularly slow on a block in which self-responses and negative evaluations are made with the same response key. In other words, high scorers seem to "shield" negative connotations from the implicit self, thus rendering it less likely that the implicit self is "contaminated" by negative evaluative material. This interpretation of IAT self-esteem is consistent with some work on defensive processes related to the embodied self (e.g., Burris & Rempel, 2004). Accordingly, one might predict that participants scoring high in implicit self-esteem might be more easily disgusted by potential bodily contaminants (Haidt, McCauley, Dunlop, Ashmore, & Rozin, 1999). Moreover, they might exhibit higher levels of experiential avoidance (Boulanger, Hayes, & Pistorello, 2010) and might be less inclined to view aversive slides, an essentially defensive reaction (Lang, Bradley, & Cuthbert, 1997). This protective view of implicit self-esteem is plausible and—because there is yet no dominant theory of implicit self-esteem—should be systematically pursued.

M. D. Robinson, Meier, Zetocha, and McCaul (2005) demonstrated that implicit attitudes toward smoking as measured by the IAT were highly dependent on the contrast category administered. A similar conclusion has been made with respect to implicit self-esteem levels as assessed by the IAT (Karpinski, 2004). For example, Karpinski showed that implicit self-esteem scores were higher when the contrast category was Hitler relative to Santa Claus. When implicit self-esteem measures contrast "me" and "you" categories, M. D. Robinson and Wilkowski

(2006) suggested that such scores might not reflect attitudes toward the self per se, but rather tendencies to favor the self over interpersonal others more broadly (i.e., a narcissistic interpersonal tendency). Consistent with this interpretation, M. D. Robinson and Wilkowski (2006) showed that high levels of implicit self-esteem were associated with greater distress among individuals whose conscious attitudes (as assessed by the Big Five trait of agreeableness) were more egalitarian in nature, a conscious–unconscious conflict reminiscent of Horney's (1945) psychosocial theory of neurosis. If so, the IAT self-esteem test would seem to have great value in examining object relations, whether narcissistic or more egalitarian. For example, lower IAT self-esteem scores might predict greater empathy (Batson, 2010) and accommodative relationship behaviors that benefit both the self and others (Finkel & Rusbult, 2008).

Regardless, the implicit self-representation measures routinely used in the social cognition literature are of an evaluative type (Bosson et al., 2008). That is, they primarily seek to assess the extent to which implicit representations of objects are positive in attitudinal terms. Object relation theories of a psychodynamic type, on the other hand, emphasize the extent to which the individual accords greater weight to the self-object relative to the other-object in the unconscious (Klein, 1952; Kohut, 1966). To model such representations, Fetterman, Robinson, and Gilbertson (2010) developed an implicit paradigm in which the task was simply to categorize presented pronouns, one of which was self-relevant and the other of which was relevant to a potential interaction partner. To model salience processes, the font size of such pronouns varied randomly across trials, such that stimuli were sometimes larger in size (20.5 Times New Roman) and sometimes smaller in size (17.5 Times New Roman). It was found that most participants were faster to categorize the self-relevant pronoun when it was larger in size and the other-relevant pronoun when it was smaller in size. Accordingly, the paradigm appears sensitive to object representations in which the self is accorded greater salience than the other. A third study of the Fetterman et al. (2010) investigation then established that arrogant individuals displayed enhanced Pronoun × Size effects of this type. Thus, the conclusion was that arrogant individuals differentially weight the self relative to the other in object relations of an implicit type, tendencies that should have wide relevance in understanding their interpersonal behaviors.[15]

On the other hand, Pincus and colleagues have consistently suggested that there are actually two forms of narcissism—nonpathological and pathological (e.g., Cain, Pincus, & Ansell, 2008). Both forms of narcissism are marked by interpersonal coldness and a sense of entitlement, but might have very different implications for psychopathology.

---

[14]We refer the reader to Greenwald and Farnham (2000) for how to assess implicit self-esteem on the basis of the IAT. The computerized task takes approximately 5 min to complete. Implicit self-esteem can be assessed even more briefly in terms of the name-letter effect and can be done so using paper and pencil. We refer the reader to Bosson, Swann, and Pennebaker (2000) for details concerning this latter implicit measure of self-esteem.

[15]This implicit self-importance task is quite simple and takes less than 5 min to complete. Across 120 trials, the pronouns "ME" and "YOU" are presented, either in a smaller or larger font size. Reaction times in categorizing the pronouns as "me" or "you" are collected. Implicit self-importance of this dyadic object relations type is quantified in terms of the interaction between pronoun and font size. Summary scores are quantified as follows: ((ME/big reaction time + YOU/small reaction time)−(ME/small reaction time + YOU/big reaction time)), with higher scores reflecting higher levels of implicit self-importance (Fetterman et al., 2010). Arrogant individuals exhibit higher levels of implicit self-importance in this task (see text for details). The task might prove useful in assessing object relation theories of narcissism or interpersonal arrogance more generally.

Nonpathological narcissism can be assessed by the NPI (Raskin & Terry, 1988), which tends to predict greater levels of subjective well-being (Sedikides, Rudich, Gregg, Kumashiro, & Rusbult, 2004), albeit in the context of some interpersonal costs (Back, Schmukle, & Egloff, 2010; Paulhus, 1998). Pathological narcissism, on the other hand, is thought to be associated with vulnerable self-views, social withdrawal under such circumstances, and significant problems in negotiating the interpersonal world (Dickinson & Pincus, 2003). Pincus et al. (2009) created and validated a pathological narcissism scale that might have much more utility than the NPI in understanding maladaptive personality patterns. In fact, their studies showed that the two forms of narcissism were weakly correlated and that pathological narcissism levels were unique in predicting low self-esteem, suicide attempts, and aggressive behaviors among inpatients. The implications of such findings are quite clear: Pathological narcissism, relative to its nonpathological variant, is of much greater utility in understanding personality disorders and problems.

Given that the pathological narcissism inventory (Pincus et al., 2009) is a recent addition to the literature, studies linking such a form of narcissism to implicit self-representations are necessarily scarce. A study by Fetterman and Robinson (2010) is informative in this context. In this study, it was hypothesized that pathological narcissists would exhibit contingent levels of implicit self-importance, much as contingent self-views have been shown to be problematic to functioning in multiple social-personality literatures (Crocker & Knight, 2005; Donahue et al., 1993; Kernis, 2005). The dependent measure was exactly that described in footnote 15. Participants were randomly assigned to write about dominant or submissive experiences from the past, a manipulation hypothesized to strongly affect the implicit self-views of individuals high but not low in pathological narcissism. Results were in accord with predictions: The priming manipulation only influenced implicit self-importance scores at high levels of pathological narcissism. Such results need to be replicated, but they do suggest that pathological narcissism, relative to nonpathological narcissism, might be much more problematic.

DISCUSSION

Toward a Social Cognitive View of Psychodynamic Processes

More so than at any point in the history of psychology, we suggest that psychodynamic and social cognitive views of the individual can be integrated. In part, this integration potential can be attributed to a widened perspective on psychodynamic processes, one capable of meeting this integration halfway (PDM Task Force, 2006). In part, this integration potential can be attributed to work in the personality area demonstrating that implicit measures have a significant role to play in understanding individual differences in emotion and behavior (M. D. Robinson & Compton, 2008; M. D. Robinson & Neighbors, 2006). In part, this integration potential can be attributed to neurocognitive work of an individual difference type (Canli, 2004; Eisenberger, Lieberman, & Satpute, 2005). In part, finally, this integration potential can be attributed to an increased focus on individual differences in the social cognition literature (Greenwald & Farnham, 2000; Wilkowski & Robinson, 2007). Individual differences matter in all such literatures and increased cross-fertilization has occurred to some extent.

We reviewed sources of evidence for this integration potential. Consistent with Freud's (1926/1953) process-related view of neuroticism, increasing sources of evidence view it in terms of intrapsychic conflict (e.g., M. D. Robinson & Wilkowski, 2006). Consistent with ego psychology perspectives (Bellak et al., 1973), on the other hand, controlled processes can mitigate neurotic tendencies (e.g., M. D. Robinson & Clore, 2007). Anger and aggression outcomes are less instinctual in nature than sometimes proposed (Berkowitz, 1993) and more amenable to controlled processing efforts, again a set of results consistent with ego psychology perspectives. A great deal of social cognitive work has sought to understand implicit self-evaluations. There are multiple nuances to this literature (e.g., Bosson et al., 2008). However, regardless of such nuances, implicit representations of the self appear to play an important role in understanding the self's functioning in more molar terms (e.g., M. D. Robinson & Meier, 2005). New directions of research were outlined in relation to limitations of available data. Nevertheless, the review should make it clear that implicit approaches to assessment are here to stay, that psychodynamic perspectives provide useful theoretical guidance for such investigations, and that social cognitive analyses can in turn inform developments in understanding the psychodynamic self.

Revisiting the Issue of Clinical Relevance

Meyer and Kurtz (2006) highlighted the limitations of what have traditionally been referred to as "objective" tests (more recently referred to as *self-attribution tests;* Bornstein, 2007), whereby the respondent self-reports on his or her personality. Such self-reports place an onus on test respondents to understand and accurately characterize themselves on inventories using a limited set of response options, concerning which issues of memory are likely to be quite substantial (M. D. Robinson & Clore, 2002). Such responses are likely to provide useful information in some cases, but not others. For example, clients who lack insight or clients who are motivated to malinger or conceal psychopathology might provide less useful information through such methods. Although some inventories have built-in scales to detect response biases related to random responding, exaggerating psychopathology, hiding psychopathology, and defensiveness (e.g., the Minnesota Multiphasic Personality Inventory–Second Edition; Butcher, Dahlstrom, Graham, Tellegen, & Kaemmer, 1989), these scales simply tell us that caution must be taken in interpreting resulting scores. Given that invalid responding is likely somewhat prevalent, are there better or perhaps complementary assessment tools that can be administered?

As Meyer and Kurtz (2006) pointed out, some have argued that these limitations of self-attribution tests justify the use of what have traditionally been referred to as "projective" tests (e.g., the Rorschach inkblot test; Rorschach, 1921/1942), and more recently referred to as *stimulus-attribution tests* (Bornstein, 2007). Such stimulus-attribution tests address some of the aforementioned limitations of self-report assessment tools in that they provide stimuli (e.g., inkblots, pictures) and allow the respondents to provide data about themselves in a format that is more natural to them. Specifically, respondents are able to tell the assessor what they see in the stimuli by using their own words and without being forced to choose between potentially artificial response options. In addition, such tests render it substantially more difficult for clients to understand how to malinger or conceal psychopathology. Still, impression management might play a role in responding to such tests as clients are able to select which of potentially multiple responses they will share with the assessor (Bornstein, 2007). Moreover, as Meyer and Kurtz (2006) stated, issues remain in interpreting such assessments. In particular, there are difficult scoring considerations when such a wide, complex variety of test responses are obtained.

In light of the limitations of the traditional assessments made by clinicians, novel approaches to personality assessment, such as those reviewed in this article, might be desirable. Performance-based tests, in which "test scores are derived from a person's unrehearsed performance on one or more structured tasks designed to tap on-line behavior and responding" (Bornstein, 2007, p. 205), have the potential to tap implicit processes while reducing concerns related to self-attribution tests (e.g., impression management, poor insight) and stimuli attribution tests (e.g., response variability). Clinical psychologists have long used performance-based tests to measure constructs such as intelligence and cognitive functioning. However, as reviewed earlier, personality social cognitive psychologists have also used performance-based tests to measure individual differences and personality variables that are of interest to clinical psychologists (e.g., aggressiveness, narcissism). Therefore, clinical psychologists might find it useful to expand their repertoire of assessment tools by using tests of a more social cognitive type (please see the footnotes for measurement considerations). Such tests have the potential to aid in the prediction of behavior, assist in the evaluation of treatment effectiveness, and provide insight into the underlying dynamics of clients that they themselves are unaware of.

Furthermore, a number of influential psychologists have suggested that more and more diverse assessments of the individual permit insights into him or her that are simply absent when more limited assessments are used (Allport, 1937; Cattell, 1946; McClelland, 1951). This general idea has been championed by more recent personality theorists as well (Emmons, 1986; Mayer, 2005; McAdams, 1996). It has also been shown that discrepancies between implicit and self-reported personality tendencies are informative in ways that cannot be discerned on the basis of either type of data alone (Brunstein & Maier, 2005; McClelland et al., 1989; Winter, John, Stewart, Klohnen, & Duncan, 1998). Clinically, diverse sources of information surely help case conception (Bornstein, 2009). To the extent that multiple sources of data converge in identifying a pervasive issue for the client (e.g., distrust), the clinician gains valuable knowledge in setting treatment goals (Shedler & Westen, 2007). To the extent that they diverge, this divergence becomes a potentially important clue as well (Kazdin, 2008). For example, if a client receives a high intelligence score, but performs poorly in school or at work, the clinician might be well served investigating the reason(s) for this apparent discrepancy.

This said, it must be recognized that the work reviewed in the body of our article involved normal samples, focused on personality processes, and extensions to clinical assessment are needed. We recognize that there is much to do in translating the work reviewed to the clinical realm. On the other hand, we view such work in terms of opportunities rather than limitations. To better bridge this assessment–clinical interface, we close by reviewing other literatures in which such an interface has been bridged to a greater extent. In keeping with our review, we focus on cognitive and social cognitive measures of a primarily reaction time type.

Implicit Processes in Addiction

Addictions—whether to food, nicotine, or alcohol—are experienced as compelling despite their problematic nature (West, 2006). On the basis of animal models primarily, T. E. Robinson and Berridge (2001) suggested that addictions coopt an implicit neurological system responsive to rewarding cues and automatic consumptive behavior in relation to such cues. This perspective is generally known as the incentive salience model of addiction (Berridge, 2007). A variety of implicit cognitive measures have been created to assess such addictive processes and the results are strong in suggesting that such implicit probes of addiction are important to clinical realms. For example, addicted individuals exhibit higher levels of implicit attention to drug-related cues (Mogg, Bradley, Field, & De Houwer, 2003), greater difficulties in disengaging from such cues (Sayette & Hufford, 1994), and exhibit more positive implicit associations to such cues (Houben & Wiers, 2008).

Further, Stacy, Ames, and Leigh (2004) showed that an implicit measure of drug associations predicted which adolescents would later use and abuse drugs and Waters et al. (2003) showed that an implicit measure assessing attention to drug cues predicted relapse subsequent to successful treatment. Finally, Field and Eastwood (2005) showed that it was possible to train implicit tendencies to disattend from alcohol cues and doing so reduced urges to drink and alcohol consumption in a subsequent test. Data of this type are reported in an edited volume by Wiers and Stacy (2006) and they have generated considerable interest among the addiction treatment community.

Predicting Self-Harm and Suicide Attempts

There are perhaps few outcomes as problematic as self-harming behavior and suicide attempts. Such phenomena are greatly stigmatized, such that those inclined to engage in such behaviors are likely to underreport such thoughts and desires, in part to avoid involuntary hospitalization. Even more so, however, such behaviors are exhibited during particular times of emotional upset and might be disavowed at other times. Indeed, Busch, Fawcett, and Jacobs (2003) found that 78% of those who committed suicide did not communicate suicidal thoughts in their last communications before killing themselves. There is thus a great potential need for implicit measures in this context.

Nock and Banaji (2007) created a "self-injury IAT" to assess implicit self-harming associations. Associations of the self with pictures of individuals cutting themselves increased linearly from nonsuicidal adolescents to suicidal ideators to adolescents who had attempted suicide in the past. This IAT also predicted suicide ideation 6 months later, independent of a number of known risk factors. More recently, Nock et al. (2010) created a "suicide IAT" (associations of me + death relative to me + life) and found that it predicted suicide attempts in the next 6 months among 157 adults presenting to an emergency department in psychiatry. Similar results have been reported in relation to a task assessing implicit attention to suicide-related words (Cha, Najmi, Park, Finn, & Nock, 2010). As the authors noted, such implicit tendencies toward self-harm or suicide appear consequential in their prediction of future behaviors and should be taken seriously in treatment provision.

Cognitive Bias Modification as a Potential Treatment

It is now well known that clinically anxious individuals display greater attention toward threatening stimuli in implicit cognitive tasks (Mathews & MacLeod, 2005). Many theories of psychopathology, such as Beck's (e.g., Beck, Emery, & Greenberg, 2005) or that of Gray and McNaughton (2000), contend that such attentional biases might cause anxious symptoms. MacLeod (1999) reviewed evidence consistent with the idea that threat-related attentional biases predict subsequent distress reactions to stressors and thus can be considered a diathesis in understanding anxiety-proneness. Subsequently, MacLeod, Rutherford, Campbell, Ebsworthy, and Holker (2002) used an ingenious cognitive procedure to train individuals to selectively disattend to threat in a computerized task. The manipulation did not immediately reduce negative emotional states, but it did reduce negative emotional reactivity to a subsequent laboratory stressor. Such findings have been replicated and extended in several ways since then (Yiend, 2004).

This literature has grown immensely in recent years and more important has demonstrated relevance in clinical realms. See, MacLeod, and Bridle (2009) administered a home-based training program in which individuals completed a cognitive task training them to disattend to threatening stimuli in an attention paradigm. Such home-based training reduced levels of trait anxiety. Amir, Beard, Burns, and Bomyea (2009) conducted a similar eight-session treatment program that again sought to modify biases to attend to threatening stimuli. Importantly, all participants had been diagnosed with Generalized Anxiety Disorder. Training such individuals to disattend to threat, relative to a control condition in which no such training occurred, resulted in reduced levels of self-reported anxiety and also reduced levels of anxiety as exhibited in a clinical interview. Schmidt, Richey, Buckner, and Timpano (2009) trained individuals diagnosed with social anxiety disorder to disattend to disgust faces in an implicit attention task and found that (relative to a control condition) it reduced levels of social anxiety and trait anxiety. On the basis of a structural interview, it was also found that 72% of the trained individuals no longer met *DSM* criteria for social anxiety disorder, whereas only 11% of the control group no longer met such criteria, a large and clinically significant treatment effect of a purely cognitive type.

As emphasized by MacLeod, Koster, and Fox (2009), this body of work is impressive, although further work remains. A minority of the investigations, reported in a special issue of *Journal of Abnormal Psychology,* involved clinically significant problems, not all of them examined subsequent functioning in terms other than self-report, and few physiological measures were obtained across the contributions to the special issue. Regardless, the body of work suggests that implicit biases not only differentiate anxious versus nonanxious individuals, but also constitute a nexus of intervention that appears, in general, to be therapeutic.

CONCLUSIONS

The literature linking anxiety disorders to processing biases (Mathews & MacLeod, 2005) can be considered somewhat of a model for the future of the work highlighted in this re-

view. In particular, many of the processing tendencies highlighted here can also lead to interventions. For example, Meier, Wilkowski, and Robinson (2008) showed that a manipulation targeting agreeable processes of self-regulation (Meier et al., 2006), implicitly and subtly so, reduced aggression levels among all individuals, whether agreeable or disagreeable. A processing view of personality belongs to multiple subdisciplines of psychology. Accordingly, cognitive, social, personality, and clinical researchers all have a role to play. A truly integrated understanding of the person is closer at hand than ever before.

REFERENCES

Allport, G. W. (1937). *Personality: A psychological interpretation.* Oxford, UK: Holt.

American Psychiatric Association. (1980). *Diagnostic and statistical manual of mental disorders* (3rd ed.). Washington, DC: Au.

American Psychiatric Association. (1994). *Diagnostic and statistical manual of mental disorders* (4th ed.). Washington, DC: Au.

Amir, N., Beard, C., Burns, M., & Bomyea, J. (2009). Attention modification program in individuals with generalized anxiety disorder. *Journal of Abnormal Psychology, 118,* 28–33.

Angst, J., Degonda, M., & Ernst, C. (1992). The Zurich Study: XV. Suicide attempts in a cohort from age 20 to 30. *European Archives of Psychiatry and Clinical Neuroscience, 242,* 135–141.

Arntz, A., Bernstein, D., Gielen, D., van Nieuwenhuyzen, M., Penders, K., Haslam, N., & Ruscio, J. (2009). Taxometric evidence for the dimensional structure of Cluster-C, Paranoid, and Borderline personality disorders. *Journal of Personality Disorders, 23,* 606–628.

Back, M. D., Schmukle, S. C., & Egloff, B. (2010). Why are narcissists so charming at first sight? Decoding the narcissism–popularity link at zero acquaintance. *Journal of Personality and Social Psychology, 98,* 132–145.

Baer, R. A. (2003). Mindfulness training as a clinical intervention: A conceptual and empirical review. *Clinical Psychology: Science and Practice, 10,* 125–143.

Batson, C. D. (2010). Empathy-induced altruistic motivation. In M. Mikulincer & P. R. Shaver (Eds.), *Prosocial motives, emotions, and behavior: The better angels of our nature* (pp. 15–34). Washington, DC: American Psychological Association.

Beck, A. T., Emery, G., & Greenberg, R. L. (2005). *Anxiety disorders and phobias: A cognitive perspective.* New York, NY: Basic Books.

Bellak, L., Hurvich, M., & Gediman, H. K. (1973). *Ego functions in schizophrenics, neurotics, and normals.* New York, NY: Wiley.

Berkowitz, L. (1993). *Aggression: Its causes, consequences, and control.* New York, NY: McGraw-Hill.

Berridge, K. C. (2007). The debate over dopamine's role in reward: The case for incentive salience. *Psychopharmacology, 191,* 391–431.

Bettencourt, B. A., Talley, A., Benjamin, A. J., & Valentine, J. (2006). Personality and aggressive behavior under provoking and neutral conditions: A meta-analytic review. *Psychological Bulletin, 132,* 751–777.

Bolger, N., & Schilling, E. A. (1991). Personality and the problems of everyday life: The role of neuroticism in exposure and reactivity to daily stressors. *Journal of Personality, 59,* 355–386.

Bolger, N., & Zuckerman, A. (1995). A framework for studying personality in the stress process. *Journal of Personality and Social Psychology, 69,* 890–902.

Bornstein, R. F. (2007). Toward a process-based framework for classifying personality traits: Comment on Meyer and Kurtz (2006). *Journal of Personality Assessment, 89,* 202–207.

Bornstein, R. F. (2009). Heisenberg, Kandinsky, and the heteromethod convergence problem: Lessons from within and beyond psychology. *Journal of Personality Assessment, 91,* 1–8.

Bornstein, R. F. (2010). Psychoanalytic theory as a unifying framework for 21st century personality assessment. *Psychoanalytic Psychology, 27,* 133–152.

Bosson, J. K., Lakey, C. E., Campbell, W. K., Zeigler-Hill, V., Jordan, C. H., & Kernis, M. H. (2008). Untangling the links between narcissism and self-esteem: A theoretical and empirical review. *Personality and Social Psychology Compass, 2,* 1415–1439.

Bosson, J. K., Swann, W. B., & Pennebaker, J. W. (2000). Stalking the perfect measure of implicit self-esteem: The blind men and the elephant revisited? *Journal of Personality and Social Psychology, 79,* 631–643.

Bouchard, M., Target, M., Lecours, S., Fonagy, P., Tremblay, L., Schachter, A., & Stein, H. (2008). Mentalization in adult attachment narratives: Reflective functioning, mental states, and affect elaboration compared. *Psychoanalytic Psychology, 25,* 47–66.

Boulanger, J. L., Hayes, S. C., & Pistorello, J. (2010). Experiential avoidance as a functional contextual concept. In A. M. Kring & D. M. Sloan (Eds.), *Emotion regulation and psychopathology: A transdiagnostic approach to etiology and treatment* (pp. 107–136). New York, NY: Guilford.

Bresin, K., Robinson, M. D., Ode, S., & Leth-Steenson, C. (in press). Driven, distracted, or both? A performance-based ex-Gaussian analysis of individual differences in anxiety. *Journal of Personality.*

Brown, K. W., & Ryan, R. M. (2003). The benefits of being present: Mindfulness and its role in psychological well-being. *Journal of Personality and Social Psychology, 84,* 822–848.

Brown, K. W., & Ryan, R. M. (2004). Perils and promise in defining and measuring mindfulness: Observations from experience. *Clinical Psychology: Research and Practice, 11,* 242–248.

Brown, S. A. (2009). Personality and non-suicidal deliberate self-harm: Trait differences among a non-clinical population. *Psychiatry Research, 169,* 28–32.

Brunstein, J. C., & Maier, G. W. (2005). Implicit and self-attributed motives to achieve: Two separate but interacting needs. *Journal of Personality and Social Psychology, 89,* 205–222.

Burris, C. T., & Rempel, J. K. (2004). "It's the end of the world as we know it": Threat and the spatial-symbolic self. *Journal of Personality and Social Psychology, 86,* 19–42.

Busch, K. A., Fawcett, J., & Jacobs, D. G. (2003). Clinical correlates of inpatient suicide. *Journal of Clinical Psychiatry, 64,* 14–19.

Butcher, J. N., Dahlstrom, W. G., Graham, J. R., Tellegen, A., & Kaemmer, B. (1989). *MMPI–2 (Minnesota Multiphasic Personality Inventory–2): Manual for administration and scoring.* Minneapolis: University of Minnesota Press.

Butler, E. A., Wilhelm, F. H., & Gross, J. J. (2006). Respiratory sinus arrhythmia, emotion, and emotion regulation during social interaction. *Psychophysiology, 43,* 612–622.

Cain, N. M., Pincus, A. L., & Ansell, E. B. (2008). Narcissism at the crossroads: Phenotypic description of pathological narcissism across clinical theory, social/personality psychology, and psychiatric diagnosis. *Clinical Psychology Review, 28,* 638–656.

Canli, T. (2004). Functional brain mapping of extraversion and neuroticism: Learning from individual differences in emotion processing. *Journal of Personality, 72,* 1105–1132.

Caspi, A., Roberts, B. W., & Shiner, R. L. (2005). Personality development: Stability and change. *Annual Review of Psychology, 56,* 453–484.

Cattell, R. B. (1946). *Description and measurement of personality.* Oxford, UK: World Book Company.

Cha, C. B., Najmi, S., Park, J. M., Finn, C. T., & Nock, M. K. (2010). Attentional bias toward suicide-related stimuli predicts suicidal behavior. *Journal of Abnormal Psychology, 119,* 616–622.

Chartrand, T. L., Dalton, A. N., & Cheng, C. M. (2008). The antecedents and consequences of nonconscious goal pursuit. In J. Y. Shah & W. L. Gardner (Eds.), *Handbook of motivational science* (pp. 342–355). New York, NY: Guilford.

Colvin, C. R., Block, J., & Funder, D. C. (1995). Overly positive self-evaluations and personality: Negative implications for mental health. *Journal of Personality and Social Psychology, 68,* 1152–1162.

Costa, P. T., & Widiger, T. A. (1994). *Personality disorders and the five-factor model of personality.* Washington, DC: American Psychological Association.

Costa, P. T., & Widiger, T. A. (2002). *Personality disorders and the five-factor model of personality* (2nd ed.). Washington, DC: American Psychological Association.

Cramer, P. (2000). Defense mechanisms in psychology today: Further processes for adaptation. *American Psychologist, 55,* 637–646.

Crick, N. R., & Dodge, K. A. (1994). A review and reformulation of social information processing mechanisms in children's social adjustment. *Psychological Bulletin, 115,* 74–101.

Crocker, J., & Knight, K. M. (2005). Contingencies of self-worth. *Current Directions in Psychological Science, 14,* 200–203.

Deary, I. J., & Der, G. (2005). Reaction time explains IQ's association with death. *Psychological Science, 16,* 64–69.

Dickinson, K., & Pincus, A. (2003). Interpersonal analysis of grandiose and vulnerable narcissism. *Journal of Personality Disorders, 17,* 188–207.

Dijksterhuis, A., & Aarts, H. (2010). Goals, attention, and (un)consciousness. *Annual Review of Psychology, 61,* 467–490.

Dixon, N. F. (1981). *Preconscious processing.* New York, NY: Wiley.

Donahue, E. M., Robins, R. W., Roberts, B. W., & John, O. P. (1993). The divided self: Concurrent and longitudinal effects of psychological adjustment and social roles on self-concept differentiation. *Journal of Personality and Social Psychology, 64,* 834–846.

Edwards, A. L. (1953). The relationship between the judged desirability of a trait and the probability that the trait will be endorsed. *Journal of Applied Psychology, 37,* 90–93.

Eisenberger, N. I., Lieberman, M. D., & Satpute, A. B. (2005). Personality from a controlled processing perspective: An fMRI study of neuroticism, extraversion, and self-consciousness. *Cognitive, Affective & Behavioral Neuroscience, 5,* 169–181.

Elliot, A. J., & Thrash, T. M. (2002). Approach-avoidance motivation in personality: Approach and avoidance temperaments and goals. *Journal of Personality and Social Psychology, 82,* 804–818.

Ellis, A. (2002). *Overcoming resistance: A rational emotive behavior therapy integrated approach* (2nd ed.). New York, NY: Springer.

Emmons, R. A. (1986). Personality strivings: An approach to personality and subjective well-being. *Journal of Personality and Social Psychology, 51,* 1058–1068.

Epstein, S. (1973). The self-concept revisited: Or a theory of a theory. *American Psychologist, 28,* 404–416.

Eriksen, C. W. (1995). The flankers task and response competition: A useful tool for investigating a variety of cognitive problems. In C. Bundesen & H. Shibuya (Eds.), *Visual selective attention* (pp. 101–118). Hillsdale, NJ: Erlbaum.

Eysenck, M. W., Derakshan, N., Santos, R., & Calvo, M. G. (2007). Anxiety and cognitive performance: Attentional control theory. *Emotion, 7,* 336–353.

Fazio, R. H., & Olson, M. A. (2003). Implicit measures in social cognition research: Their meaning and uses. *Annual Review of Psychology, 54,* 297–327.

Feltman, R., Robinson, M. D., & Ode, S. (2009). Mindfulness as a moderator of neuroticism-outcome relations: A self-regulation perspective. *Journal of Research in Personality, 43,* 953–961.

Fenichel, O. (1945). *The psychoanalytic theory of neurosis.* New York, NY: Norton.

Ferguson, M. J., Hassin, R., & Bargh, J. A. (2008). Implicit motivation: Past, present, and future. In J. Y. Shah & W. L. Gardner (Eds.), *Handbook of motivation science* (pp. 150–166). New York, NY: Guilford.

Fetterman, A. K., & Robinson, M. D. (2010). Contingent self-importance among pathological narcissists: Evidence from an implicit task. *Journal of Research in Personality, 44,* 691–697.

Fetterman, A. K., Robinson, M. D., & Gilbertson, E. P. (2010). *Size matters: Implicit interpersonal narcissism in a pronoun categorization task.* Manuscript submitted for publication.

Field, M., & Eastwood, B. (2005). Experimental manipulation of attentional bias increases the motivation to drink alcohol. *Psychopharmacology, 183,* 350–357.

Finkel, E. J., & Rusbult, C. E. (2008). Prorelationship motivation: An interdependence theory analysis of situations with conflicting interests. In J. Y. Shah & W. L. Gardner (Eds.), *Handbook of motivation science* (pp. 547–560). New York, NY: Guilford.

Fonagy, P., & Target, M. (2006). The mentalization-focused approach to self pathology. *Journal of Personality Disorders, Journal of Personality Disorders, 20,* 544–576.

Freud, S. (1953). Symptoms, inhibitions, and anxiety. In J. Strachey (Ed. & Trans.), *The standard edition of the complete psychological works of Sigmund Freud* (pp. 77–175). London, UK: Hogarth Press. (Original work published 1926)

Friedman, B. H. (2007). An autonomic flexibility-neurovisceral integration model of anxiety and cardiac vagal tone. *Biological Psychology, 74*, 185–199.

Friedman, N. P., & Miyake, A. (2004). The relations among inhibition and interference control functions: A latent-variable analysis. *Journal of Experimental Psychology: General, 133*, 101–135.

Garakani, A., Martinez, J. M., Aaronson, C. J., Vourstianiouk, A., Kaufmann, H., & Gorman, J. M. (2009). Effects of medication and psychotherapy on heart rate variability in panic disorder. *Depression and Anxiety, 26*, 251–258.

Goldberg, L. R. (1993). The structure of phenotypic personality traits. *American Psychologist, 48*, 26–34.

Gottfredson, L. S., & Deary, I. J. (2004). Intelligence predicts health and longevity, but why? *Current Directions in Psychological Science, 13*, 1–4.

Gray, J. A. (1981). A critique of Eysenck's theory of personality. In H. J. Eysenck (Ed.), *A model for personality* (pp. 246–276). Berlin, Germany: Springer.

Gray, J. A., & McNaughton, N. (2000). *The neuropsychology of anxiety: An enquiry into the functions of the septo-hippocampal system* (2nd ed.). Oxford, UK: Oxford University Press.

Graziano, W. G., & Eisenberg, N. (1997). Agreeableness: A dimension of personality. In R. Hogan, J. A. Johnson, & S. R. Briggs (Eds.), *Handbook of personality* (pp. 795–824). San Diego, CA: Academic.

Greenwald, A. G., Banaji, M. R., Rudman, L. A., Farnham, S. D., Nosek, B. A., & Mellott, D. S. (2002). A unified theory of implicit attitudes, stereotypes, self-esteem, and self-concept. *Psychological Review, 109*, 3–25.

Greenwald, A. G., & Farnham, S. D. (2000). Using the Implicit Association Test to measure self-esteem and self-concept. *Journal of Personality and Social Psychology, 79*, 1022–1038.

Grossman, P., Niemann, L., Schmidt, S., & Walach, H. (2004). Mindfulness-based stress reduction and health benefits: A meta-analysis. *Journal of Psychosomatic Research, 57*, 35–43.

Gyurak, A., & Ayduk, Ö. (2008). Resting respiratory sinus arrhythmia buffers against rejection sensitivity via emotion control. *Emotion, 8*, 458–467.

Haidt, J., McCauley, C., Dunlop, L., Ashmore, M., & Rozin, P. (1999). Individual differences in disgust sensitivity: Comparisons and evaluations of paper-and-pencil versus behavioral measures. *Journal of Research in Personality, 33*, 330–351.

Higgins, E. T. (1997). Beyond pleasure and pain. *American Psychologist, 52*, 1280–1300.

Holroyd, C. B., & Coles, M. G. H. (2002). The neural basis of human error processing: Reinforcement learning, dopamine, and the error-related negativity. *Psychological Review, 109*, 679–709.

Horney, K. (1945). *Our inner conflicts: A constructive theory of neurosis.* New York, NY: Norton.

Houben, K., & Wiers, R. W. (2008). Implicitly positive about alcohol? Implicit positive associations predict drinking behavior. *Addictive Behaviors, 33*, 979–986.

Huprich, S. K., & Bornstein, R. F. (2007). An overview of issues related to categorical and dimensional models of personality disorder assessment. *Journal of Personality Assessment, 89*, 3–15.

Jensen, A. R. (2006). *Clocking the mind: Mental chronometer individual differences.* Amsterdam, The Netherlands: Elsevier.

Jordan, C. H., Spencer, S. J., Zanna, M. P., & Hoshino-Browne, E. (2003). Secure and defensive high self-esteem. *Journal of Personality and Social Psychology, 85*, 969–978.

Karpinski, A. (2004). Measuring self-esteem using the Implicit Association Test: The role of the other. *Personality and Social Psychology Bulletin, 30*, 22–34.

Kazdin, A. E. (2008). Evidence-based treatment and practice: New opportunities to bridge clinical research and practice, enhance the knowledge base, and improve patient care. *American Psychologist, 63*, 146–159.

Kelly, G. A. (1963). *A theory of personality: The psychology of personal constructs.* Oxford, UK: Norton.

Kendell, R., & Jablensky, A. (2003). Distinguishing between the validity and utility of psychiatric diagnoses. *The American Journal of Psychiatry, 160*, 4–12.

Kendler, K. S., Kuhn, J., & Prescott, C. A. (2004). The interrelationship of neuroticism, sex, and stressful life events in the prediction of episodes of major depression. *The American Journal of Psychiatry, 161*, 631–636.

Kernis, M. H. (2005). Measuring self-esteem in context: The importance of stability of self-esteem in psychological functioning. *Journal of Personality, 73*, 1569–1605.

Kerns, J. G. (2006). Anterior cingulate and prefrontal cortex activity in an fMRI study of trial-to-trial adjustments on the Simon task. *NeuroImage, 33*, 399–405.

Kerns, J. G., Cohen, J. D., MacDonald, A. W., Cho, R. Y., Stenger, V. A., & Carter, C. S. (2004). Anterior cingulate conflict monitoring and adjustments in control. *Science, 303*, 1023–1026.

King, L. A., & Emmons, R. A. (1990). Conflict over emotional expression: Psychological and physical correlates. *Journal of Personality and Social Psychology, 58*, 864–877.

Klein, M. (1952). The origins of transference. *The International Journal of Psychoanalysis, 33*, 433–438.

Kohut, H. (1966). Forms and transformations of narcissism. *Journal of the American Psychoanalytic Association, 14*, 243–272.

Lahey, B. B. (2009). Public health significance of neuroticism. *American Psychologist, 64*, 241–256.

Lang, P. J., Bradley, M. M., & Cuthbert, B. N. (1997). Motivated attention: Affect, activation, and action. In P. J. Lang, R. F. Simons, & M. T. Balaban (Eds.), *Attention and orienting: Sensory and motivational processes* (pp. 97–135). Mahwah, NJ: Erlbaum.

Linehan, M. M. (1993). *Cognitive-behavioral treatment of borderline personality disorder.* New York, NY: Guilford.

Lynam, D. R., & Widiger, T. A. (2001). Using the five-factor model to represent the *DSM–IV* personality disorders: An expert consensus approach. *Journal of Abnormal Psychology, 110*, 401–412.

MacLeod, C. (1999). Anxiety and anxiety disorders. In T. Dalgleish & M. J. Power (Eds.), *Handbook of cognition and emotion* (pp. 447–477). New York, NY: Wiley.

MacLeod, C., Koster, E. H. W., & Fox, E. (2009). Whither cognitive bias modification research? Commentary on the special section articles. *Journal of Abnormal Psychology, 118*, 89–99.

MacLeod, C., Rutherford, E., Campbell, L., Ebsworthy, G., & Holker, L. (2002). Selective attention and emotional vulnerability: Assessing the causal basis of their association through the experimental manipulation of attentional bias. *Journal of Abnormal Psychology, 111*, 107–123.

Magnus, K., Diener, E., Fujita, F., & Pavot, W. (1993). Extraversion and neuroticism as predictors of objective life events: A longitudinal analysis. *Journal of Personality and Social Psychology, 65*, 1046–1053.

Marcus, D. K., Ruscio, J., Lilienfeld, S. O., & Hughes, K. T. (2008). Converging evidence for the latent structure of antisocial personality disorder: Consistency of taxometric and latent class analyses. *Criminal Justice and Behavior, 35*, 284–293.

Martin, R., Watson, D., & Wan, C. K. (2000). A three-factor model of trait anger: Dimensions of affect, behavior, and cognition. *Journal of Personality, 68*, 869–897.

Mathews, A., & MacLeod, C. (2005). Cognitive vulnerability to emotional disorders. *Annual Review of Clinical Psychology, 1*, 167–195.

Matthews, G., & Gilliland, K. (1999). The personality theories of H. J. Eysenck and J. A. Gray: A comparative review. *Personality and Individual Differences, 26*, 583–626.

Mayer, J. D. (2005). A tale of two visions: Can a new view of personality help integrate psychology? *American Psychologist, 60*, 294–307.

McAdams, D. P. (1996). Alternative futures for the study of human individuality. *Journal of Research in Personality, 30*, 374–388.

McClelland, D. C. (1951). *Personality.* New York, NY: William Sloane Associates.

McClelland, D. C. (1987). *Human motivation.* New York, NY: Cambridge University Press.

McClelland, D. C., Atkinson, J. W., Clark, R. A., & Lowell, E. (1953). *The achievement motive.* East Norwalk, CT: Appleton-century-Crafts.

McClelland, D. C., Koestner, R., & Weinberger, J. (1989). How do self-attributed and implicit motives differ? *Psychological Review, 96,* 690–702.

McCrae, R. R., & Costa, P. T. (1983). Social desirability scales: More substance than style. *Journal of Consulting and Clinical Psychology, 51,* 882–888.

McCrae, R. R., & Costa, P. T. (1999). A five-factor theory of personality. In L. A. Pervin & O. P. John (Eds.), *Handbook of personality: Theory and research* (2nd ed., pp. 139–153). New York, NY: Guilford.

Meier, B. P., & Robinson, M. D. (2004). Does quick to blame mean quick to anger? The role of agreeableness in dissociating blame and anger. *Personality and Social Psychology Bulletin, 30,* 856–867.

Meier, B. P., Robinson, M. D., & Wilkowski, B. M. (2006). Turning the other cheek: Agreeableness and the regulation of aggression-related primes. *Psychological Science, 17,* 136–142.

Meier, B. P., Wilkowski, B. M., & Robinson, M. D. (2008). Bringing out the agreeableness in everyone: Using a cognitive self-regulation model to reduce aggression. *Journal of Experimental Social Psychology, 44,* 1383–1387.

Meyer, G. J., & Kurtz, J. E. (2006). Advancing personality assessment terminology: Time to retire "objective" and "projective" as personality test descriptors. *Journal of Personality Assessment, 87,* 223–225.

Meyer, G. J., & Shack, J. R. (1989). Structural convergence of mood and personality: Evidence for old and new directions. *Journal of Personality and Social Psychology, 57,* 691–706.

Miller, E. K., & Cohen, J. D. (2001). An integrative theory of prefrontal cortex function. *Annual Review of Neuroscience, 24,* 167–202.

Miller, N. E. (1944). Experimental studies of conflict. In J. M. Hunt (Ed.), *Personality and behavior disorders* (pp. 431–465). Oxford, UK: Ronald Press.

Mineka, S., Watson, D., & Clark, L. A. (1998). Comorbidity of anxiety and unipolar mood disorders. *Annual Review of Psychology, 49,* 377–412.

Mischel, W., & Shoda, Y. (1995). A cognitive affective system theory of personality: Reconceptualizing situations, dispositions, dynamics, and invariance of personality structure. *Psychological Review, 102,* 246–286.

Moeller, S. K., & Robinson, M. D. (2010). Cognitive sources of evidence for neuroticism's link to punishment reactivity processes. *Cognition and Emotion, 24,* 741–759.

Moeller, S. K., Robinson, M. D., & Bresin, K. (2010). Integrating trait and social cognitive views of personality: Neuroticism, implicit stress priming, and neuroticism-outcome relationships. *Personality and Social Psychology Bulletin, 36,* 677–689.

Mogg, K., Bradley, B. P., Field, M., & De Houwer, J. (2003). Eye movements to smoking-related pictures in smokers: Relationship between attentional biases and implicit and explicit measures of stimulus valence. *Addiction, 98,* 825–836.

Nock, M. K., & Banaji, M. R. (2007). Prediction of suicide ideation and attempts among adolescents using a brief performance-based test. *Journal of Consulting and Clinical Psychology, 75,* 707–715.

Nock, M. K., Park, J. M., Finn, C. T., Deliberto, T. L., Dour, H. J., & Banaji, M. R. (2010). Measuring the suicidal mind: Implicit cognition predicts suicidal behavior. *Psychological Science, 21,* 511–517.

Ochsner, K. N., & Gross, J. J. (2005). The cognitive control of emotion. *Trends in Cognitive Sciences, 9,* 242–249.

Ode, S., Hilmert, C. J., Zielke, D. J., & Robinson, M. D. (2010). Neuroticism's importance in understanding the daily life correlates of heart rate variability. *Emotion, 10,* 536–543.

Ode, S., & Robinson, M. D. (2007). Agreeableness and the self-regulation of negative affect: Findings involving the neuroticism/somatic distress relationship. *Personality and Individual Differences, 43,* 2137–2148.

Ode, S., & Robinson, M. D. (2009). Can agreeableness turn gray skies blue? A role for agreeableness in moderating neuroticism-linked dysphoria. *Journal of Social and Clinical Psychology, 28,* 436–462.

Ode, S., Robinson, M. D., & Hanson, D. M. (in press). Cognitive-emotional dysfunction among noisy minds: Predictions from individual differences in reaction time variability. *Cognition and Emotion.*

Ode, S., Robinson, M. D., & Wilkowski, B. M. (2008). Can one's temper be cooled? A role for agreeableness in moderating neuroticism's influence on anger and aggression. *Journal of Research in Personality, 42,* 295–311.

Orobio de Castro, B., Veerman, J. W., Koops, W., Bosch, J. D., & Monshouwer, H. J. (2002). Hostile attribution of intent and aggressive behavior: A meta-analysis. *Child Development, 73,* 916–934.

Paulhus, D. L. (1998). Interpersonal and intrapsychic adaptiveness of trait self-enhancement: A mixed blessing? *Journal of Personality and Social Psychology, 74,* 1197–1208.

Paulhus, D. L., & John, O. P. (1998). Egoistic and moralistic biases in self-perception: The interplay of self-deceptive styles with basic traits and motives. *Journal of Personality, 66,* 1025–1060.

PDM Task Force. (2006). *Psychodynamic diagnostic manual.* Silver Springs, MD: Alliance of Psychoanalytic Associations.

Pincus, A., Ansell, E., Pimentel, C., Cain, N., Wright, A., & Levy, K. (2009). Initial construction and validation of the Pathological Narcissism Inventory. *Psychological Assessment, 21,* 365–379.

Raskin, R., & Terry, H. (1988). A principal-components analysis of the Narcissistic Personality Inventory and further evidence of its construct validity. *Journal of Personality and Social Psychology, 54,* 890–902.

Robinson, M. D. (2007). Personality, affective processing, and self-regulation: Toward process-based views of extraversion, neuroticism, and agreeableness. *Social and Personality Psychology Compass, 1,* 223–235.

Robinson, M. D., & Clore, G. L. (2002). Belief and feeling: Evidence for an accessibility model of emotional self-report. *Psychological Bulletin, 128,* 934–960.

Robinson, M. D., & Clore, G. L. (2007). Traits, states, and encoding speed: Support for a top-down view of neuroticism/state relations. *Journal of Personality, 75,* 95–120.

Robinson, M. D., & Compton, R. J. (2008). The happy mind in action: The cognitive basis of subjective well-being. In M. Eid & R. J. Larsen (Eds.), *The science of subjective well-being* (pp. 220–238). New York, NY: Guilford.

Robinson, M. D., Goetz, M. C., Wilkowski, B. M., & Hoffman, S. J. (2006). Driven to tears or to joy: Response dominance and trait-based predictions. *Personality and Social Psychology Bulletin, 32,* 629–640.

Robinson, M. D., & Meier, B. P. (2005). Rotten to the core: Neuroticism and implicit evaluations of the self. *Self and Identity, 4,* 361–372.

Robinson, M. D., Meier, B. P., Zetocha, K. J., & McCaul, K. D. (2005). Smoking and the Implicit Association Test: When the contrast category determines the theoretical conclusions. *Basic and Applied Social Psychology, 27,* 201–212.

Robinson, M. D., Mitchell, K. A., Kirkeby, B. S., & Meier, B. P. (2006). The self as a container: Implications for implicit self-esteem and somatic symptoms. *Self and Identity, 21,* 147–167.

Robinson, M. D., & Neighbors, C. (2006). Catching the mind in action: Implicit methods in personality research and assessment. In M. Eid & E. Diener (Eds.), *Handbook of multimethod measurement in psychology* (pp. 115–125). Washington, DC: American Psychological Association.

Robinson, M. D., Ode, S., Moeller, S. K., & Goetz, P. W. (2007). Neuroticism and affective priming: Evidence for a neuroticism-linked negative schema. *Personality and Individual Differences, 42,* 1221–1231.

Robinson, M. D., & Oishi, S. (2006). Trait self-reports as a "fill in" belief system: Categorization speed moderates the extraversion/life satisfaction relation. *Self and Identity, 5,* 15–34.

Robinson, M. D., Schmeichel, B. J., & Inzlicht, M. (2010). A cognitive control perspective of self-control strength and its depletion. *Social and Personality Psychology Compass, 4,* 189–200.

Robinson, M. D., & Tamir, M. (2005). Neuroticism as mental noise: A relation between neuroticism and reaction time standard deviations. *Journal of Personality and Social Psychology, 89,* 107–114.

Robinson, M. D., & Wilkowski, B. M. (2006). Loving, hating, vacillating: Agreeableness, implicit self-esteem, and neurotic conflict. *Journal of Personality, 74,* 935–978.

Robinson, M. D., Wilkowski, B. M., Kirkeby, B. S., & Meier, B. P. (2006). Stuck in a rut: Perseverative response tendencies and the neuroticism/distress relationship. *Journal of Experimental Psychology: General, 135,* 78–91.

Robinson, M. D., Wilkowski, B. M., & Meier, B. P. (2006). Unstable in more ways than one: Reaction time variability and the neuroticism/distress relationship. *Journal of Personality, 74,* 311–343.

Robinson, M. D., Wilkowski, B. M., Meier, B. P., & Moeller, S. K. (2010). *Counting to ten milliseconds: Individual differences in anger and affective processing.* Manuscript submitted for publication.

Robinson, T. E., & Berridge, K. C. (2001). Incentive-sensitization and addiction. *Addiction, 96,* 103–114.

Rorschach, H. (1942). *Psychodiagnostics* (5th ed.). Berne, Switzerland: Verlag Hans Huber. (Original work published 1921)

Rusting, C. L. (1998). Personality, mood, and cognitive processing of emotional information: Three conceptual frameworks. *Psychological Bulletin, 124,* 165–196.

Sarason, I. G., Sarason, B. R., & Pierce, G. R. (1990). Anxiety, cognitive interference, and performance. *Journal of Social Behavior and Personality, 5,* 1–18.

Saulsman, L. M., & Page, A. C. (2004). The five-factor model and personality disorder empirical literature: A meta-analytic review. *Clinical Psychology Review, 23,* 1055–1085.

Sayette, M. A., & Hufford, M. R. (1994). Effects of cue exposure and deprivation on cognitive resources in smokers. *Journal of Abnormal Psychology, 103,* 812–818.

Schmidt, N. B., Richey, J. A., Buckner, J. D., & Timpano, K. R. (2009). Attention training for generalized social anxiety disorder. *Journal of Abnormal Psychology, 118,* 5–14.

Schneirla, T. C. (1959). An evolutionary and developmental theory of biphasic processes underlying approach and withdrawal. In M. R. Jones (Ed.), *Nebraska symposium on motivation* (pp. 1–42). Oxford, UK: University of Nebraska Press.

Schultheiss, O. C. (2007). A memory-systems approach to the classification of personality tests: Comment on Meyer and Kurtz (2006). *Journal of Personality Assessment, 89,* 197–201.

Sedikides, C., Rudich, E. A., Gregg, A. P., Kumashiro, M., & Rusbult, C. (2004). Are normal narcissists psychologically healthy?: Self-esteem matters. *Journal of Personality and Social Psychology, 87,* 400–416.

See, J., MacLeod, C., & Bridle, R. (2009). The reduction of anxiety vulnerability through the modification of attentional bias: A real-world study using a home-based cognitive bias modification procedure. *Journal of Abnormal Psychology, 118,* 65–75.

Segal, Z. V., Williams, J. M. G., & Teasdale, J. D. (2002). *Mindfulness-based cognitive therapy for depression: A new approach to preventing relapse.* New York, NY: Guilford.

Shapiro, S. L., Oman, D., Thoresen, C. E., Plante, T. G., & Flinders, T. (2008). Cultivating mindfulness: Effects on well-being. *Journal of Clinical Psychology, 64,* 840–862.

Shaver, P. R., & Mikulincer, M. (2005). Attachment theory and research: Resurrection of the psychodynamic approach to personality. *Journal of Research in Personality, 39,* 22–45.

Shedler, J., Mayman, M., & Manis, M. (1993). The illusion of mental health. *American Psychologist, 48,* 1117–1131.

Shedler, J., & Westen, D. (2007). The Shedler–Westen Assessment Procedures (SWAP): Making personality diagnosis clinically meaningful. *Journal of Personality Assessment, 89,* 41–55.

Skowronski, J. J., Carlston, D. E., Mae, L., & Crawford, M. T. (1998). Spontaneous trait transference: Communicators take on the qualities they describe in others. *Journal of Personality and Social Psychology, 74,* 837–848.

Smith, T. W., Glazer, K., Ruiz, J. M., & Gallo, L. C. (2004). Hostility, anger, aggressiveness, and coronary heart disease: An interpersonal perspective on personality, emotion, and health. *Journal of Personality, 72,* 1217–1270.

Stacy, A. W., Ames, S. L., & Leigh, B. C. (2004). An implicit cognition assessment approach to relapse, secondary prevention, and media effects. *Cognitive and Behavioral Practice, 11,* 139–149.

Suinn, R. M. (2001). The terrible twos—Anger and anxiety: Hazardous to your health. *American Psychologist, 56,* 27–36.

Suls, J., & Martin, R. (2005). The daily life of the garden-variety neurotic: Reactivity, stressor exposure, mood spillover, and maladaptive coping. *Journal of Personality, 73,* 1485–1510.

Swann, W. B. (1992). Seeking "truth," finding despair: Some unhappy consequences of a negative self-concept. *Current Directions in Psychological Science, 1,* 15–18.

Tamir, M. (2005). Don't worry, be happy? Neuroticism, trait-consistent affect regulation, and performance. *Journal of Personality and Social Psychology, 89,* 449–461.

Tamir, M., & Robinson, M. D. (2004). Knowing good from bad: The paradox of neuroticism, negative affect, and evaluative processing. *Journal of Personality and Social Psychology, 87,* 913–925.

Tavris, C. (1989). *Anger: The misunderstood emotion* (rev. ed.). New York, NY: Touchstone Books.

Taylor, S. E., Klein, L. C., Lewis, B. P., Gruenewald, T. L., Gurung, R. A. R., & Updegraff, J. A. (2000). Biobehavioral responses to stress in females: Tend-and-befriend, not fight-or-flight. *Psychological Review, 107,* 411–429.

Teasdale, J. D., Moore, R. G., Hayhurst, H., Pope, M., Williams, S., & Segal, Z. V. (2002). Metacognitive awareness and prevention of relapse in depression: Empirical evidence. *Journal of Consulting and Clinical Psychology, 70,* 275–287.

Todorov, A., & Uleman, J. S. (2002). Spontaneous trait inferences are bound to actors' faces: Evidence from a false recognition paradigm. *Journal of Personality and Social Psychology, 83,* 1051–1065.

Trapnell, P. D., & Campbell, J. D. (1999). Private self-consciousness and the five-factor model of personality: Distinguishing rumination from reflection. *Journal of Personality and Social Psychology, 76,* 284–304.

van Veen V., & Carter, C. S. (2006). Conflict and cognitive control in the brain. *Psychological Science, 15,* 237–240.

Waters, A. J., Shiffman, S., Sayette, M. A., Paty, J. A., Gwaltney, C. J., & Balabanis, M. H. (2003). Attentional bias predicts outcome in smoking cessation. *Health Psychology, 22,* 378–387.

Watson, D. (2000). *Mood and temperament.* New York, NY: Guilford.

Watson, D., & Pennebaker, J. W. (1989). Health complaints, stress, and distress: Exploring the central role of negative affectivity. *Psychological Review, 96,* 234–254.

West, R. (2006). *Theory of addiction.* Oxford, UK: Blackwell.

Westen, D. (1998). The scientific legacy of Sigmund Freud: Toward a psychodynamically informed psychological science. *Psychological Bulletin, 124,* 333–371.

Westen, D., & Shedler, J. (1999). Revising and assessing Axis II, part II: Toward an empirically based and clinically useful classification of personality disorders. *The American Journal of Psychiatry, 156,* 273–285.

Widiger, T. A., & Trull, T. J. (2007). Plate tectonics in the classification of personality disorder: Shifting to a dimensional model. *American Psychologist, 62,* 71–83.

Widiger, T. A., Verheul, R., & Van Den Brink, W. (1999). Personality and psychopathology. In L. A. Pervin & O. P. John (Eds.), *Handbook of personality: Theory and research* (2nd ed., pp. 347–366). New York, NY: Guilford.

Wiers, R. W., & Stacy, A. W. (2006). *Handbook of implicit cognition and addiction.* Thousand Oaks, CA: Sage.

Wilkowski, B. M., & Robinson, M. D. (2007). Keeping one's cool: Trait anger, hostile thoughts, and the recruitment of limited capacity control. *Personality and Social Psychology Bulletin, 33,* 1201–1213.

Wilkowski, B. M., & Robinson, M. D. (2008a). The cognitive basis of trait anger and reactive aggression: An integrative analysis. *Personality and Social Psychology Review, 12,* 3–21.

Wilkowski, B. M., & Robinson, M. D. (2008b). Guarding against hostile thoughts: Trait anger and the recruitment of cognitive control. *Emotion, 8,* 578–583.

Wilkowski, B. M., & Robinson, M. D. (2010a). The anatomy of anger: An integrative cognitive model of trait anger and reactive aggression. *Journal of Personality, 78,* 9–38.

Wilkowski, B. M., & Robinson, M. D. (2010b). Associative and spontaneous appraisal processes independently contribute to anger elicitation in daily life. *Emotion, 10,* 181–189.

Wilkowski, B. M., Robinson, M. D., & Meier, B. P. (2006). Agreeableness and the prolonged spatial processing of antisocial and prosocial information. *Journal of Research in Personality, 40,* 1152–1168.

Wilkowski, B. M., Robinson, M. D., & Troop-Gordon, W. (2010). How does cognitive control reduce anger and aggression? The role of conflict monitoring and forgiveness processes. *Journal of Personality and Social Psychology, 98,* 830–840.

Winter, D. G., John, O. P., Stewart, A. J., Klohnen, E. C., & Duncan, L. E. (1998). Traits and motives: Toward an integration of two traditions in personality research. *Psychological Review, 105,* 230–250.

Yiend, J. (2004). *Cognition, emotion and psychopathology: Theoretical, empirical and clinical directions.* New York, NY: Cambridge University Press.

Zelazo, P. D., & Cunningham, W. A. (2007). Executive function: Mechanisms underlying emotion regulation. In J. J. Gross (Ed.), *Handbook of emotion regulation* (pp. 135–158). New York, NY: Guilford.

Zelenski, J. M., & Larsen, R. J. (1999). Susceptibility to affect: A comparison of three personality taxonomies. *Journal of Personality, 67,* 761–791.

Toward a Multidimensional Model of Personality Disorder Diagnosis: Implications for *DSM–5*

ROBERT F. BORNSTEIN

Derner Institute of Advanced Psychological Studies, Adelphi University

This article outlines a model of personality disorder (PD) diagnosis that combines clinically useful constructs from the *Diagnostic and Statistical Manual of Mental Disorders* (*DSM*) with assessment procedures that maximize reliability and clinical utility while minimizing problems associated with threshold-based PD classification. I begin by addressing limitations in the current *DSM* conceptualization of PDs: excessive comorbidity, use of arbitrary cutoffs to distinguish normal from pathological functioning, failure to capture variations in the adaptive value of PD symptoms, and inattention to situational influences that shape PD-related behaviors. The revisions proposed by the *DSM–5* Personality and Personality Disorders Work Group help resolve some of these issues, but create new problems in other areas. A better solution would be to employ a multidimensional model of PD diagnosis in which clinicians (a) assign a single dimensional rating of overall level of personality dysfunction, (b) provide separate intensity and impairment ratings for each PD dimension, and (c) list those personality traits—including PD-related traits—that enhance adaptation and functioning. Preliminary evidence bearing on the multidimensional model is reviewed, and broader clinical and empirical implications of the model are discussed.

Regardless of whether one conceptualizes personality pathology in terms of underlying psychodynamics, acquired behavior patterns, self-defeating thoughts and dysfunctional beliefs, or neurological and neurochemical abnormalities, one truth is self-evident: Once *homo sapiens* evolved to the point that early humans had personalities, some of those personalities were bound to be disordered. As Millon (2009) noted, virtually every diagnostic system that emerged over the centuries has attempted to account for the fact that certain people behave in self-defeating ways, repeat the same dysfunctional patterns over time, and lack insight into the negative impact of their behavior on self and others.

As research on personality pathology evolved during the 20th century it became clear that whereas describing the prototypic features of different personality disorders (PDs) is comparatively straightforward, diagnosing PDs in vivo is far more challenging. Many patients show features of more than one PD (Y. R. Kim & Tyrer, 2010), and in some samples one of the most common Axis II diagnoses is mixed PD or PD not otherwise specified (PD NOS; see Madeddu, Prunas, & Hartmann, 2009; Zimmerman & Coryell, 1989). PDs show high rates of comorbidity, and in many instances PDs that co-occur at higher-than-expected rates bear little resemblance either dynamically or phenomenologically (e.g., schizoid and antisocial, dependent and paranoid; see Bornstein, 2003). Interdiagnostician reliability for PDs is generally lower than that for Axis I disorders suggesting that although clinicians can agree regarding whether a given patient has personality pathology, they cannot agree regarding how best to categorize that pathology (Blais, Benedict, & Norman, 1996).

Refining our approach to conceptualizing, diagnosing, and assessing PDs is important for several reasons. Studies show that personality pathology can lead to significant impairments in social and occupational functioning (Johnson, Rabkin, Williams, Remien, & Gorman, 2000; Sansone & Sansone, 2010), and complicate treatment for Axis I symptom disorders (Rathus, Sanderson, Miller, & Wetzler, 1995). PDs are associated with increased health care costs and decreased treatment efficacy (Soeteman, Hakkaart-van Roijen, Verheul, & Busschbach, 2008). Moreover, certain PDs (e.g., antisocial) are associated with increased risk for legal problems (Wong & Hare, 2005), and some PDs (e.g., borderline) have been linked with increased likelihood of self-harm (Paris, 2008).

This article outlines a model of PD diagnosis that combines clinically useful constructs from the most recent edition of the *Diagnostic and Statistical Manual of Mental Disorders* (4th ed., text revision [*DSM–IV–TR*]; American Psychiatric Association, 2000) with assessment procedures that maximize reliability and clinical utility while minimizing problems associated with categorical, threshold-based PD diagnosis. After addressing limitations in the current *DSM* conceptualization of PDs, and the revisions proposed by the *DSM–5* Personality and Personality Disorders (PPD) Work Group to resolve some of these issues, I outline a multidimensional model of PD diagnosis that has the potential to improve diagnostic reliability, enhance clinical utility, and reconnect PD theory and research with ideas and findings from mainstream personality psychology.

LIMITATIONS IN THE *DSM–IV* CONCEPTUALIZATION AND ASSESSMENT OF PDs

As Lenzenweger and Clarkin (2005) and Strack (2005) noted, the *DSM* conceptualization of PDs has evolved considerably since the multiaxial system was first introduced in *DSM–III* (3rd ed.; American Psychiatric Association, 1980). Among the most noteworthy shifts in this regard are (a) a trend toward increasingly atheoretical, jargon-free PD symptom descriptions (see Bornstein, 2006, for a discussion of this issue); (b) increased attention to differential diagnosis in an effort to increase interdiagnostician reliability and reduce PD overlap (Livesley, 1998;

Widiger & Trull, 2007); (c) conceptualization of personality pathology in terms of four core domains of impairment (cognition, affectivity, interpersonal functioning, and impulse control; see American Psychiatric Association, 2000); and (d) grouping of PD syndromes into three clusters (eccentric, dramatic, and anxious), based primarily on patterns of expressed behavior, a change first introduced in *DSM–III–R* (3rd ed., revised; American Psychiatric Association, 1987).

These changes have enhanced PD diagnosis in certain respects, but problems remain (see Huprich, Bornstein, & Schmitt, in press, and Y. R. Kim & Tyrer, 2010, for discussions of these issues). Four limitations in the *DSM–IV* (4th ed.; American Psychiatric Association, 1994) conceptualization and assessment of PDs are particularly noteworthy.

Arbitrary Diagnostic Thresholds

As Widiger and Clark (2000) pointed out (see also Costello, 1996), there is little evidence that patients who qualify for a PD diagnosis differ appreciably from those who have enough symptoms to be near (but not quite reach) the diagnostic threshold. Moreover, because not all PD criteria are equally severe and pathognomic, a raw symptom count is an inherently flawed method for rendering diagnoses. It is possible, for example, that one patient could qualify for a borderline PD diagnosis by meeting criteria for five *DSM–IV–TR* symptoms that reflect the milder manifestations of borderline pathology (e.g., unstable interpersonal relationships, chronic feelings of emptiness, efforts to avoid real or imagined abandonment), whereas a second patient might qualify for a smaller number of more severe symptoms (e.g., dissociative episodes, recurrent suicidal behavior) but not meet the threshold for formal diagnosis. This situation could be remedied by differentially weighting symptoms according to their associated degree of impairment or dysfunction, but such a strategy has never been employed in the *DSM*.

Excessive Overlap and Comorbidity

PDs differ considerably with respect to number of differential diagnoses on Axis II (i.e., the number of other Axis II disorders whose symptoms overlap substantially with the symptoms of that particular PD). According to *DSM–IV–TR* (American Psychiatric Association, 2000), the number of differential diagnoses per PD ranges from three (dependent, obsessive–compulsive) to seven (paranoid), with the mean number of differential diagnoses being 4.5 (median = 4, mode = 4). These figures dovetail with empirical findings regarding PD overlap and comorbidity: When Ekselius, Lindstrom, Knorring, Bodlund, and Kullgren (1994) calculated correlations among interview-derived PD symptom ratings in a heterogeneous sample of psychiatric patients and nonclinical participants, they obtained a mean interscale correlation (*r*) of .41, and statistically significant correlations in 41 of 45 comparisons (91%). More recent comorbidity investigations (e.g., Sinha & Watson, 2001) obtained similar patterns. Oldham, Skodol, Kellman, Hyler, and Rosnick (1992) found that cross-cluster *DSM–III–R* PD comorbidity rates were comparable to those for PDs within a given cluster.

Failure to Capture the Adaptive Value of PD Symptoms

Millon's (1990, 1996) biopsychosocial model of personality pathology conceptualizes PD-related responding as a dysfunctional variant of normative trait-based behavior patterns, a view

shared by several other PD models (e.g., Benjamin, 2004; Costa & Widiger, 2002; Pincus, 2005). According to this view narcissistic grandiosity can be seen as an excessive expression of normal self-confidence, and problematic obsessiveness an exaggerated form of everyday attention to detail. Studies have shown that the same dependency-related behavior—frequent help-seeking—that leads to difficulties in certain contexts (e.g., in romantic relationships) can be an asset in others (e.g., following detection of a medical symptom; see Bornstein, 2007; Bornstein, Riggs, Hill, & Calabrese, 1996). The possibility that some PD-related behaviors might enhance adaptation and functioning is not acknowledged by the *DSM–IV–TR* (American Psychiatric Association, 2000), which focuses exclusively on the harmful features of PD symptoms.

Inattention to Situational Influences on PD-Related Behavior

Studies confirm that the interpersonal behavior of narcissistic and dependent individuals varies predictably in response to changing environmental cues and contingencies (see Bornstein et al., 1996; Morf, 2006; Morf & Rhodewalt, 2001). As Huprich et al. (in press) pointed out, the implicit *DSM* assumption that personality-disordered behavior will be exhibited consistently across different contexts is not supported by empirical studies of PD-related responding, nor is it consistent with findings from mainstream personality research that demonstrate that personality-driven behavior patterns are best conceptualized in terms of trait by situation interactions (see Mischel & Shoda, 1995; Mischel, Shoda, & Mendoza-Denton, 2002). In this context both Bornstein (2005) and Morf (2006) argued that the locus of stability in personality pathology lies not in expressed behavior (which varies from situation to situation), but in core beliefs about the self, other people, and self–other interactions (which remain relatively stable over time and across context).

TOWARD *DSM–5:* PROPOSALS FROM THE PPD WORK GROUP

The *DSM–5* PPD Work Group released their draft revisions for professional and public comment in early 2010, proposing a hybrid model that combines traditional categorical diagnosis with a series of trait and impairment ratings (see Skodol, 2010, for an overview). In this model the number of PDs in *DSM–5* would be reduced by half, with five *DSM–IV* PDs retained in modified form (antisocial/psychopathic, avoidant, borderline, obsessive–compulsive, and schizotypal), and five PDs eliminated as formal diagnostic categories (paranoid, schizoid, histrionic, narcissistic, and dependent). Patients whose pathology lies in one of the five eliminated categories would be evaluated on six broad trait domains—negative emotionality, introversion, antagonism, disinhibition, compulsivity, and schizotypy—receiving a series of 4-point ratings reflecting the degree to which they display traits in each of the six domains, ranging from 0 (*very little or not at all*) to 3 (*extremely descriptive*).

Those patients who meet the criteria for a PD from one of the five retained categories in *DSM–5* would be assigned a categorical diagnosis akin to that in the *DSM–IV* (e.g., avoidant PD), along with a 5-point rating of overall level of self and interpersonal functioning ranging from 0 (*no impairment*) to 4 (*extreme impairment*). These patients would also receive 4-point ratings of the degree to which they display each of the six broad trait domains used to describe paranoid, schizoid, histrionic, narcissistic, and dependent patients (i.e., negative emotionality, disinhibition, etc.).

IMPACT OF PROPOSED PD CHANGES

The changes proposed by the *DSM–5* PPD Work Group have several potential benefits. Because the number of formal PD categories would be reduced substantially, there is a reasonable likelihood that PD comorbidity would decrease.[1] Including an overall rating of self and interpersonal functioning—a mechanism similar to that used to rate severity of personality impairment in the *Psychodynamic Diagnostic Manual* (*PDM;* Alliance of Psychoanalytic Organizations, 2006)—would have the dual advantages of calling clinicians' attention to underlying dynamic processes that appear to play an important role in various forms of personality pathology (Bornstein, 2006; Clarkin, 2006; Fowler, Brunnschweiler, Swales, & Brock, 2005; Shaver & Mikulincer, 2002) while simultaneously providing an overall index of level of inter- and intrapersonal impairment that is conceptually similar to the current Global Assessment of Functioning (GAF) scale on *DSM–IV* Axis V (see Bornstein, 2011, for a discussion of this issue).

The proposed changes have some costs as well. Most important among these is the elimination of several PDs (e.g., narcissistic, dependent, paranoid) that have demonstrable value in predicting patient functioning, response to treatment, social and occupational adjustment, and health care utilization (see Bienvenu et al., 2009; Bornstein, 2005, Ellett & Chadwick, 2007; Freeman, 2007; Ronningstam, 2005, 2009). The inclusion of separate trait domain ratings, although useful, is based primarily on factor-analytic studies of patient and clinician reports, was not validated externally using behavioral outcome criteria (Bornstein, 2003), and was not informed by research examining relevant personality dynamics (e.g., dependent, obsessive–compulsive, narcissistic) in nonclinical participants (see Bornstein, 1997; Morf & Rhodewalt, 2001; Samuel & Widiger, 2010). The proposed model does not acknowledge or account for situational variations in PD-related behavior, nor the possibility that some PD symptoms could enhance adaptation and functioning in certain contexts.

In addition to these conceptual and empirical problems, the proposed model creates an assessment dilemma that was not present in earlier *DSM* PD frameworks. Because certain syndromes (e.g., borderline) are diagnosed categorically and others (e.g., schizoid) are represented exclusively by a series of trait ratings, different syndromes are quantified using different metrics. This makes direct comparison of the antecedents, correlates, and consequences of different PDs within a given sample (or across samples) difficult. Although standardized scores and effect size

coefficients can facilitate comparison of categorical and continuous data, there are limits in the degree to which such statistical adjustments can overcome fundamental differences in how two predictors are classified and quantified (see Hunter & Schmidt, 2004; Lipsey & Wilson, 2001; Rosenthal, 1991).[2]

AN INTEGRATED MULTIDIMENSIONAL FRAMEWORK FOR PD DIAGNOSIS

To overcome the difficulties inherent in categorical, threshold-based PD diagnosis, Bornstein (1998) and Bornstein and Huprich (2011) outlined an integrated multidimensional framework. This framework not only helps correct some longstanding difficulties with *DSM* PD conceptualization and classification (see, e.g., Cooper, 2004), but utilizes a more effective PD assessment strategy than that proposed by the *DSM–5* PPD Work Group. PD diagnosis in the multidimensional model involves three steps.

Step 1: Assign Every Patient a Single Dimensional Rating of Overall Level of Personality Dysfunction

Studies suggest that the best predictor of long-term outcome for PD patients is severity (not type) of personality pathology (Peters, 1990; Tyrer & Johnson, 1996; Zikos, Gill, & Charney, 2010). Thus, PD diagnosis should begin with the assignment of a single overall rating of level of personality impairment. Structurally, the scale used to assign this rating is modeled after the *DSM–IV–TR* GAF scale, and is presented in Table 1; see Alliance for Psychoanalytic Organizations, 2006, for an alternative dimensional index of severity of personality pathology).

Because personality dysfunction is more narrowly determined than GAF-defined global psychological functioning (which is influenced by a broad array of environmental and socioeconomic variables as well as dispositional factors), use of a more truncated rating scale in the multidimensional framework seems warranted. Thus, in contrast to the GAF (where ratings are made on a 100-point continuum) the Personality Pathology Rating Scale (PPRS) uses a 50-point continuum, with lower scores reflecting greater dysfunction. As Table 1 shows, the PPRS employs anchor points (akin to those in the GAF scale) that capture the four essential features of personality pathology described in *DSM–IV–TR* (American Psychiatric Association, 2000): distorted cognition, inappropriate affectivity, impaired interpersonal functioning, and difficulties with impulse control.

The differential scaling of the PPRS and GAF warrant brief discussion in this context. Although one might argue that an optimal personality pathology index would employ the same 100-point scale as the GAF, from a psychometric standpoint use of a 50- versus 100-point PPRS scale range will have no appreciable impact on statistical analyses involving the PPRS—including those wherein PPRS and GAF scores are compared. As long as PPRS ratings are reasonably normally distributed within a

---

[1]Although reducing the total number of categories might help reduce PD comorbidity, the impact of PD syndrome reduction on comorbidity rates is in part a function of which PDs are eliminated. If those with the highest comorbidity rates are removed, overall comorbidity should indeed decrease, but if those with average or below average comorbidity rates are removed, comorbidity among the remaining syndromes might remain unchanged, or increase. In this context it is worth noting that the PDs proposed for retention in *DSM–5* include some with relatively high comorbidity rates (e.g., borderline), and those proposed for elimination have comparatively modest comorbidity with other Axis II syndromes (e.g., histrionic; see Ekselius et al., 1994; Oldham et al., 1992; Zimmerman, Rothchild, & Chelminski, 2005).

---

[2]To illustrate this dilemma, consider the researcher who hopes to compare the relative impact of early parental neglect on the subsequent development of schizoid PD and borderline PD. Using the *DSM–5* PPD Work Group model, the researcher must use indexes of early neglect to predict categorical or threshold-based borderline PD diagnoses, then use these same indexes of neglect to predict a series of dimensional trait ratings associated with schizoid PD. Even if such a comparison is statistically feasible, it is conceptually uninterpretable.

TABLE 1.—The Personality Pathology Rating Scale.

50	Perceptions of self and others are generally accurate; range and intensity of affectivity is appropriate for patient's background and culture; relationships are stable and experienced as satisfying; impulse control and affect tolerance are good.
41	
40	Perceptions of self and others are somewhat distorted; range and/or intensity of affectivity differ from what is expected based on patient's background and culture; most relationships are stable and satisfying, with significant difficulties in certain relationships; impulse control and affect tolerance are generally good.
31	
30	Perceptions of self and others are either significantly distorted or variable over time; range and/or intensity of affectivity differ significantly from what is expected based on patient's background and culture; many relationships are either unstable or unsatisfying; impulse control and affect tolerance are somewhat impaired.
21	
20	Perceptions of self and others are significantly distorted and variable over time; range and/or intensity of affectivity differ significantly from what is expected based on patient's background and culture and cause significant interpersonal conflict or distress; most or all relationships are unstable or unsatisfying; impulse control and affect tolerance are significantly impaired.
11	
10	Patient shows gross distortions in perception of self and others; inappropriate affectivity in a broad range of situations; unstable, conflicted, and/or impoverished relationships; poor impulse
1	control and an inability to tolerate or modulate affect effectively.

Note. Personality Pathology Rating Scale ratings are made on a 50-point scale, with lower scores reflecting greater impairment in personality functioning.

particular population, and show acceptable (i.e., modest) degrees of skewness and kurtosis, correlations between PPRS scores and scores on other psychometrically sound, continuous scales are minimally affected by the actual scale range (see, e.g., Markauskaite, Freebody, & Irwin, 2010; Niemi, Carmines, & McIver, 1986). If preliminary findings point to difficulties in PPRS interrater reliability or predictive validity, use of alternative scale ranges can be explored.[3]

Step 2: Assign Separate Intensity and Impairment Ratings for Each PD Dimension

In addition to an overall rating of personality pathology, patients are assigned separate intensity and impairment ratings for each PD dimension (e.g., narcissism, avoidance, dependency). These ratings not only capture *DSM–IV* PD diagnoses in dimensional form, but have the additional advantage of distinguishing PD intensity from PD impairment, which affords the clinician a more nuanced and clinically useful perspective on a patient's personality dynamics. After all, it is possible that a patient's PD symptoms are extremely intense (e.g., powerful obsessions), but that these symptoms do not lead to severe impairment or subjective discomfort (e.g., if the patient is in a profession where obsessive behavior is rewarded). Conversely, a patient's PD symptoms might be comparatively mild (e.g., moderate avoidant behavior), yet cause considerable distress and impairment (e.g., social isolation, inability to initiate and sustain romantic relationships).

Intensity and impairment ratings are made on 9-point scales, with higher scores reflecting greater symptom intensity and more severe impairment. A score of 0 would be assigned when an individual has no clinically significant symptoms in a particular PD dimension. Only those PD dimensions for which a patient received an intensity or impairment rating greater than 0 would be included in the diagnostic (chart) record, so the diagnostician need not list PD dimensions that are not salient in describing a particular patient. Note, however, that even though they are not enumerated in chart records, intensity and impairment scores of 0 can still be used for research purposes, to validate and refine the model and test predictions regarding various PD categories.

Step 3: Note Any Personality Traits—Including PD-Related Traits—That Enhance Adaptation and Functioning

As clinicians and clinical researchers have noted, many PD-related traits and behaviors actually enhance adaptation and functioning in certain circumstances. Histrionic theatricality might be a problem at work, but an asset in social settings (Apt & Hurlbert, 1994). Obsessive perfectionism is not only associated with increased risk for depression, but also with increased achievement motivation and higher probability of career success (Blatt, 1995). High levels of interpersonal dependency lead to overuse of health services, but they also predict more rapid medical help-seeking following symptom onset, with increased likelihood of early detection and successful intervention (Bornstein, 2005). Because PD diagnoses are intended to help clinicians make informed decisions regarding therapeutic strategy and accurate predictions regarding symptom and syndrome course, Axis II should include information regarding adaptation as well as dysfunction.

Thus, after rating the intensity and impairment of each PD dimension, the clinician lists those PD-related traits and behaviors that enhance adaptation (e.g., histrionic theatricality, obsessive perfectionism, dependency-related help-seeking), along with the domains of functioning enhanced by each trait (e.g., interpersonal, intrapersonal, occupational, recreational, sexual, physical or health-related). This list of adaptive traits and domains is structurally similar to the list of Psychosocial and Environmental Problems categories now used on Axis IV. Inclusion of this information not only reinforces the link between healthy and disordered personality functioning (a link that is not explicit in the current *DSM* conceptualization of PDs), but also formalizes the well-established finding that personality traits influence human behavior in situation-specific (not global) ways (Mischel et al., 2002). It is true that certain extreme variants of personality can be almost entirely maladaptive (e.g., severe borderline pathology), but it is far more common for a trait to be adaptive in certain contexts and problematic in others.[4]

---

[3]In situations wherein PPRS and GAF scores are to be contrasted directly, the scales can be rendered equivalent by (a) multiplying PPRS scores by two, or (b) converting both PPRS and GAF ratings to standardized *Z* scores (see Rosenthal, 1991).

[4]A skeptic might argue that inclusion of adaptive personality features in a diagnostic record is inappropriate because diagnoses are intended to identify areas of dysfunction and suggest possible interventions. Information regarding adaptation and healthy functioning can be useful in this regard as well. Consider, for example, a medical patient with a diagnosis of elevated blood glucose. If this patient also has normal blood pressure (an adaptive feature of physical functioning), medication options are available to treat this patient's elevated blood glucose that would not be available if the patient was hypertensive. The same is true of personality pathology: Knowing that a narcissistic person has

PROTOTYPIC PD DIAGNOSES IN THE MULTIDIMENSIONAL MODEL

Examples of PD diagnoses rendered via the multidimensional model are provided by Bornstein (1998), and Bornstein and Huprich (2011). Because the proposed model requires the diagnostician to code more information than is included in the current Axis II, diagnoses become more labor-intensive under the proposed system. This increase in effort is offset by the incremental gain in clinical utility and predictive validity that could result if the system becomes widely adopted. A relatively straightforward Axis II diagnosis might look like this:

PPRS = 41
Narcissistic: Intensity = 3, Impairment = 2
Adaptive: Self-confidence (interpersonal, sexual, occupational)
         Sense of entitlement (interpersonal, sexual)

A more complicated Axis II diagnosis would look like this:

PPRS = 24
Dependent: Intensity = 7, Impairment = 5
Borderline: Intensity = 4, Impairment = 5
Histrionic: Intensity = 3, Impairment = 2
Adaptive: Cooperativeness/compliance (occupational)
         Gregariousness (interpersonal, sexual, occupational)
         Seductiveness (interpersonal, sexual)

ADVANTAGES OF THE MULTIDIMENSIONAL PD MODEL

The multidimensional model has at least five advantages over the *DSM–IV* PD framework, and that proposed by the *DSM–5* PPD Work Group.

Fewer Comorbidity Problems

A central goal of the *DSM–5* PPD Work Group was to reduce excessive overlap among PDs (see Skodol, 2010). The multidimensional model approaches this issue from a different perspective: Because patients receive continuous ratings on all PD (syndrome-level) dimensions, the comorbidity problem as it exists in traditional threshold-based systems is rendered moot. Some patients will show features of one PD, some will show features of two or three, and others might show features of more (or none). Comorbidity per se is not an issue. An additional advantage of the multidimensional model in this regard is that it eliminates altogether the category of PD NOS: By definition, any patient with significant personality pathology will receive intensity and impairment ratings for all PD dimensions (even if many—perhaps most—of those ratings end up being 0; see Wilberg, Hummelen, Pedersen, & Karterud, 2008, for a discussion of clinical characteristics of PD NOS patients).

Greater Flexibility

Although the multidimensional model as initially outlined employed the 10 PD dimensions used in *DSM–IV* (see Bornstein, 1998), and continues to use those 10 dimensions in its current form, the model is not tied to any particular set of personality traits or PD syndromes. If an existing PD label (e.g.,

avoidant) proves to be of limited value it can be dropped without altering the fundamental structure of the multidimensional model. If additional PD dimensions (e.g., self-defeating, sadistic) prove heuristic and clinically useful, they can be added without altering the model's basic structure.

More Nuanced and Informative Diagnoses

Use of separate PD intensity and impairment ratings increases the amount of information contained in any PD diagnosis, leading to a more nuanced view of the patient, and suggesting useful starting points for treatment (e.g., those PD-related behaviors that are associated with greatest impairment). Clinical prediction and treatment planning are both enhanced. In addition, the differential impact of any given intervention on PD intensity and impairment can be evaluated using the multidimensional model. It is possible, for example, that a particular treatment will reduce the intensity of a patient's histrionic symptoms but have more modest impact on the degree of functional impairment associated with these symptoms (or vice versa). For some patients (and certain PDs), separate interventions might be required to reduce symptom intensity and lessen PD-related impairment (see Benjamin, 2004; Bornstein, 2005; Silverstein, 2007, for discussions of symptom-focused and impairment-focused interventions for various forms of personality pathology).

Use of Common Metrics for All PDs

The multidimensional model represents a potential improvement over the *DSM–5* PPD Work Group model from an assessment standpoint as well. Because overall impairment (i.e., PPRS) ratings and PD intensity and impairment ratings are made on continua, PD assessment in the multidimensional model circumvents a key difficulty inherent in the PPD model, wherein certain syndromes are diagnosed categorically whereas others are represented by trait ratings. The multidimensional model facilitates direct comparison of the antecedents, correlates, and consequences of different PDs (e.g., avoidant vs. schizoid) in ways that the PPD Work Group model cannot.

Increased Interdiagnostician Reliability

As Heumann and Morey (1990) and others (e.g., Cuthbert, 2005) noted, interdiagnostician reliability for dimensional ratings tends to be higher than that obtained when categorical diagnoses are rendered. Use of dimensional ratings rather than fixed thresholds in the multidimensional model also has the potential to enhance the methodological rigor of PD treatment outcome studies. When treatment efficacy is operationalized in terms of diagnostic remission (i.e., a reduction in symptomatology from above threshold to subthreshold), a given treatment might have a very similar impact on two patients (e.g., a significant reduction in three PD symptoms), but ostensibly appear effective for one patient (who moves from having seven symptoms to four, and is now subthreshold), but not for the other (who moves from having eight symptoms to five, and still qualifies for the diagnosis). Such problematic outcomes are not obtained when dimensional PD ratings are used.

PRELIMINARY SUPPORT FOR A MULTIDIMENSIONAL APPROACH

Hopwood et al. (in press) examined the utility of a multidimensional approach to PD assessment analogous to that pro-

---

good impulse control opens avenues for possible intervention that would not be available if that narcissistic patient showed poor impulse control.

posed by Bornstein (1998) and Bornstein and Huprich (in press). Using data from the Collaborative Longitudinal Personality Disorders Study (CLPS)—one of several large data sets used by the PPD Work Group to evaluate empirical evidence bearing on their proposed revisions—Hopwood et al. followed 605 adults prospectively for 3 years. Baseline (Time 1) assessments were made in three domains: (a) overall severity of dysfunction, (b) specific *DSM–IV* PD dimensions (referred to in this investigation as PD "style"), and (c) normative personality traits (which were quantified using the NEO Personality Inventory–Revised [NEO PI–R; Costa & McCrae, 1992] and Schedule for Nonadaptive and Adaptive Personality [SNAP; Clark, 1993]). Consistent with tenets of the multidimensional model, results revealed a strongly unitary overall severity dimension (α = .90), along with five independent PD dimensions: peculiarity (associated primarily with paranoid, schizoid, and schizotypal symptoms), withdrawal (associated with avoidance), fearfulness (which tapped both dependency and avoidance), instability (borderline), and deliberateness (obsessive–compulsive).

Hopwood et al. (in press) further found that overall personality pathology severity ratings best predicted global, social, and leisure dysfunction at 3-year (Time 2) follow-up, with peculiarity, withdrawal, and (to a lesser extent) fearfulness, instability, and deliberateness all adding unique incremental validity to the prospective prediction of dysfunction. NEO- and SNAP-derived personality trait scores were only modestly related to PD dimensional scores, leading Hopwood et al. to note that "separating severity and style ... offers a useful heuristic framework for conceptualizing and researching personality pathology" (p. 16). Hopwood et al. further noted that their findings "support assessing personality traits separately from either PD severity or style" (p. 17). They went on to conclude, "We therefore suggest a three-stage personality assessment process for *DSM–V* similar to that proposed by Bornstein (1998): a global rating of personality disorder severity, ratings of meaningful stylistic dimensions of personality pathology, and ratings of normative personality traits" (p. 18).

Although Hopwood et al.'s (in press) study examined a multidimensional PD assessment model analogous to—but not identical to—that initially proposed by Bornstein (1998), their results offer compelling support for a tripartite assessment strategy involving overall personality dysfunction, individual PD dimensions, and normative personality traits.

UNRESOLVED QUESTIONS AND FUTURE DIRECTIONS

Although use of an integrated multidimensional model for PD diagnosis in *DSM–5* and beyond has a number of advantages, and has garnered preliminary support, challenges remain. Four stand out.

Increased Clinician Effort

As Bornstein (1998) and Bornstein and Huprich (2011) noted, rendering PD diagnoses using the multidimensional model is more labor-intensive than rendering PD diagnoses using extant theoretical frameworks, and whether diagnosticians will devote the additional time and effort to employing the model appropriately remains open to question. To the degree that diagnoses derived from the multidimensional PD model provide clinicians with information regarding patient functioning that enhances their everyday clinical work, compliance is likely to increase; to the degree that the model cannot yield information that demon-

strably enhances clinical work in vivo, it will not. In this context it is worth noting that the model proposed by the *DSM–5* PPD Work Group also requires substantially greater time and effort than the current *DSM–IV–TR* PD framework.

Inclusion of Separate Global-, Syndrome-, and Symptom-Level Ratings

A central feature of the multidimensional model is its inclusion of separate global (PPRS), syndrome-level (i.e., intensity and impairment), and symptom-level ratings within every diagnosis. Although one might argue that global personality pathology ratings obscure interrelations among core elements of dysfunction (e.g., impairment in self-concept vs. interpersonal relations, difficulties in affect regulation vs. impulse control), several lines of evidence argue for the utility of such global ratings. First, as Hopwood et al. (in press) and others (e.g., Y. R. Kim & Tyrer, 2010; Peters, 1990) have shown, personality pathology can be usefully operationalized as a unitary dimension with considerable predictive value. Second, research confirms that—although conceptually and empirically distinguishable—the various elements that make up personality pathology tend to be at least moderately intercorrelated (see Hesse & Moran, 2010; Hesse, Rasmussen, & Pedersen, 2008; J. Kim, Cicchetti, Rogosch, & Manly, 2009). Finally, as Bornstein (1998) and Bornstein and Huprich (2011) noted, the intra- and interpersonal factors that underlie different forms of personality pathology are specified alongside global PPRS ratings when syndrome- and symptom-level information is included in the diagnostic record.

Capturing Adaptation and Dysfunction at the Symptom Level

As currently conceived, the multidimensional model quantifies the maladaptive elements of personality pathology via global PPRS impairment scores, and syndrome-specific intensity and impairment ratings; adaptation is captured via a listing of adaptive traits associated with each syndrome (e.g., conscientiousness, self-confidence). As evidence regarding the utility and predictive validity of the multidimensional model accumulates, it might be useful to expand the list of traits to include those that play a particularly prominent role in propagating pathology and dysfunction—a listing of the patient's most maladaptive traits (e.g., impulsivity, poor affect regulation). The decision regarding whether or not to expand this portion of the model must balance considerations regarding incremental validity with the increased time and effort it would take to enumerate additional situation-specific traits (and the potential decrease in diagnostician compliance that might occur if the procedure became too lengthy).

Revision of PD Dimensions Going Forward

Initial descriptions of the multidimensional model (Bornstein, 1998) used *DSM–IV* PD category labels so that the logic of the framework would not be confused by simultaneous introduction of novel PD categories. Because the multidimensional model is not linked to any particular set of PD dimensions, new dimensions can be introduced and eliminated as needed based on accumulating empirical findings. Refinement of the multidimensional model requires that two tasks be performed in parallel: (a) assessment of the concurrent and predictive validity of ratings derived from the model (which will yield information regarding the effectiveness of the model's *structure*), and (b) adjustment of the PD dimensions that form Step 2 in the model (to optimize the model's *content*). This latter task will likely involve a series of iterative revisions to balance parsimony with comprehensiveness, so that the multidimensional model ultimately incorporates the smallest number of PD dimensions required for maximal heuristic value and clinical utility.

Conclusion

The additional information contained in PD diagnoses using the multidimensional model will lead to a richer, more informative PD database, with stronger connections to basic research in personality than are afforded by the current *DSM–IV–TR* framework or the *DSM–5* PPD Work Group proposal. In contrast to the *DSM* and PPD frameworks, the multidimensional model incorporates findings from nonclinical as well as clinical participants, and from studies of normative personality traits as well as personality pathologies. Thus, the model has the potential to facilitate exchange between personality researchers and PD investigators, and increase the likelihood that research findings from nonclinical samples will be applied directly to questions regarding the etiology and dynamics of PDs (see Hopwood, Koonce, & Morey, 2009; Oltmanns & Turkheimer, 2009, for examples of this approach).

In addition to connecting more strongly with ideas and findings from mainstream personality research, the multidimensional model provides a useful framework for tracking therapeutic progress along multiple independent dimensions in a way that allows for focused comparison across different PDs. Because the PPD Work Group framework operationalizes some PD syndromes (e.g., borderline) as formal categories, and others (e.g., narcissistic) solely as trait constellations, comparative assessment of treatment efficacy across syndromes is more difficult within this framework (e.g., it would be difficult to ascertain whether a given intervention had a greater impact on avoidant than schizoid pathology because avoidance is diagnosed categorically in the PPD framework, whereas schizoid pathology is represented exclusively by trait ratings). Thus, the multidimensional model not only has significant assessment advantages over the PPD framework, but these assessment gains could enhance treatment efficacy and effectiveness studies.

Finally, it is important to note that despite its dimensional emphasis, the proposed model allows for both dimensional and category-based analyses (see Huprich & Bornstein, 2007): Even if intensity and impairment ratings are used to capture the essential features of PDs, cutoff points distinguishing normal from pathological functioning can still be derived for the population as a whole, or on a sample-by-sample (or syndrome-by-syndrome) basis. Just as a physician begins by quantifying a patient's blood pressure on a continuum, then uses these continuous data to classify that patient's blood pressure as being elevated or within the normal range, once clinically useful cutoff points are derived, the continuous impairment and intensity ratings that form the core of the multidimensional PD model can be used to classify patients dichotomously while retaining the myriad advantages that continuous impairment and severity ratings provide.

References

Alliance of Psychoanalytic Organizations. (2006). *Psychodynamic diagnostic manual*. Silver Spring, MD: Author.

American Psychiatric Association. (1980). *Diagnostic and statistical manual of mental disorders* (3rd ed.). Washington, DC: Author.

American Psychiatric Association. (1987). *Diagnostic and statistical manual of mental disorders* (3rd ed., revised). Washington, DC: Author.

American Psychiatric Association. (1994). *Diagnostic and statistical manual of mental disorders* (4th ed.). Washington, DC: Author.

American Psychiatric Association. (2000). *Diagnostic and statistical manual of mental disorders* (4th ed., text revision). Washington, DC: Author.

Apt, C., & Hurlbert, D. F. (1994). The sexual attitudes, behavior, and relationships of women with histrionic personality disorder. *Journal of Sex and Marital Therapy, 20*, 125–133.

Benjamin, L. S. (2004). *Personality guided interpersonal reconstructive therapy for anger, anxiety, and depression*. Washington, DC: APA Books.

Bienvenu, O. J., Stein, M. B., Samuels, J. F., Okyike, C. U., Eaton, W. W., & Nestadt, G. (2009). Personality disorder traits as predictors of subsequent first-onset panic disorder or agoraphobia. *Comprehensive Psychiatry, 50*, 209–215.

Blais, M. A., Benedict, K. B., & Norman, D. K. (1996). The perceived clarity of Axis II criteria sets. *Journal of Personality Disorders, 10*, 16–22.

Blatt, S. J. (1995). The destructiveness of perfectionism. *American Psychologist, 50*, 1003–1020.

Bornstein, R. F. (1997). Dependent personality disorder in the *DSM–IV* and beyond. *Clinical Psychology: Science and Practice, 4*, 175–187.

Bornstein, R. F. (1998). Reconceptualizing personality disorder diagnosis in the *DSM–V*: The discriminant validity challenge. *Clinical Psychology: Science and Practice, 5*, 333–343.

Bornstein, R. F. (2003). Behaviorally referenced experimentation and symptom validation: A paradigm for 21st century personality disorder research. *Journal of Personality Disorders, 17*, 1–18.

Bornstein, R. F. (2005). *The dependent patient: A practitioner's guide*. Washington, DC: APA Books.

Bornstein, R. F. (2006). A Freudian construct lost and reclaimed: The psychodynamics of personality pathology. *Psychoanalytic Psychology, 23*, 339–353.

Bornstein, R. F. (2007). Dependent personality disorder: Effective time-limited therapy. *Current Psychiatry, 6*, 37–45.

Bornstein, R. F. (2011). Reconceptualizing personality pathology in *DSM–5*: Limitations in evidence for eliminating dependent personality disorder and other *DSM–IV* syndromes. *Journal of Personality Disorders, 25*, 237–250.

Bornstein, R. F., & Huprich, S. K. (2011). Beyond dysfunction and threshold-based classification: A multidimensional model of personality disorder diagnosis. *Journal of Personality Disorders, 25*, 331–337.

Bornstein, R. F., Riggs, J. M., Hill, E. L., & Calabrese, C. (1996). Activity, passivity, self-denigration and self-promotion: Toward an interactionist model of interpersonal dependency. *Journal of Personality, 64*, 637–673.

Clark, L. A. (1993). *Manual for the Schedule for Nonadaptive and Adaptive Personality (SNAP)*. Minneapolis: University of Minnesota Press.

Clarkin, J. F. (2006). Conceptualization and treatment of personality disorders. *Psychotherapy Research, 16*, 1–11.

Cooper, R. (2004). What is wrong with the *DSM*? *History of Psychiatry, 15*, 5–25.

Costa, P. T., & McCrae, R. R. (1992). *Revised NEO Personality Inventory (NEO PI–R) and NEO Five-Factor Inventory (NEO–FFI) professional manual*. Odessa, FL: Psychological Assessment Resources.

Costa, P. T., & Widiger, T. A. (Eds.). (2002). *Personality disorders and the five-factor model of personality*. Washington, DC: APA Books.

Costello, C. G. (Ed.). (1996). *Personality characteristics of the personality disordered*. New York, NY: Wiley.

Cuthbert, B. N. (2005). Dimensional models of psychopathology: Research agenda and clinical utility. *Journal of Abnormal Psychology, 114*, 565–569.

Ekselius, L., Lindstrom, E., Knorring, L., Bodlund, O., & Kullgren, G. (1994). Comorbidity among the personality disorders in *DSM–III–R*. *Personality and Individual Differences, 17*, 155–160.

Ellett, L., & Chadwick, P. (2007). Paranoid cognitions, failure, and focus of attention in college students. *Cognition and Emotion, 21*, 558–576.

Fowler, J. C., Brunnschweiler, B., Swales, S., & Brock, J. (2005). Assessment of Rorschach dependency measures in female inpatients diagnosed with borderline personality disorder. *Journal of Personality Assessment, 85*, 146–153.

Freeman, D. (2007). Suspicious minds: The psychology of persecutory delusions. *Clinical Psychology Review, 27*, 425–457.

Hesse, M., & Moran, P. (2010). Screening for personality disorder with the Standardised Assessment of Personality: Further evidence of concurrent validity. *BMC Psychiatry, 10*, 1–6.

Hesse, M., Rasmussen, J., & Pedersen, M. K. (2008). Standardised assessment of personality—A study of validity and reliability in substance abusers. *BMC Psychiatry, 8*, 7–12.

Heumann, K. A., & Morey, L. C. (1990). Reliability of categorical and dimensional judgments of personality disorder. *American Journal of Psychiatry, 147*, 498–500.

Hopwood, C. J., Koonce, E. A., & Morey, L. C. (2009). An exploratory study of integrative personality pathology systems and the interpersonal circumplex. *Journal of Psychopathology and Behavioral Assessment, 31*, 331–339.

Hopwood, C. J., Malone, J. C., Ansell, E. B., Pinto, A., Markowitz, J. C., Shea, M. T., . . . Morey, L. C. (in press). Personality assessment in *DSM–V*: Empirical support for rating severity, style, and traits. *Journal of Personality Disorders*.

Hunter, J. E., & Schmidt. F. L. (2004). *Methods of meta-analysis: Correcting error and bias in research findings* (2nd ed.). Thousand Oaks, CA: Sage.

Huprich, S. K., & Bornstein, R. F. (2007). An overview of issues related to categorical and dimensional models of personality disorder assessment. *Journal of Personality Assessment, 89*, 3–15.

Huprich, S. K., Bornstein, R. F., & Schmitt, T. (in press). Self-report methodology is insufficient for improving the assessment and classification of Axis II personality disorders. *Journal of Personality Disorders*.

Johnson, J. G., Rabkin, J. G., Williams, J. B. W., Remien, R. H., & Gorman, J. M. (2000). Difficulties in interpersonal relationships associated with personality disorders and Axis I disorders. *Journal of Personality Disorders, 14*, 42–56.

Kim, J., Cicchetti, D., Rogosch, F. A., & Manly, J. T. (2009). Child maltreatment and trajectories of personality and behavioral functioning: Implications for the development of personality disorder. *Developmental Psychopathology, 21*, 889–912.

Kim, Y. R., & Tyrer, P. (2010). Controversies surrounding classification of personality disorder. *Psychiatry Investigations, 7*, 1–8.

Lenzenweger, M. F., & Clarkin, J. F. (Eds.). (2005). *Major theories of personality disorder*. New York, NY: Guilford.

Lipsey, M. W., & Wilson, D. B. (2001). *Practical meta-analysis*. Thousand Oaks, CA: Sage.

Livesley, W. J. (1998). Suggestions for a framework for an empirically based classification of personality disorder. *Canadian Journal of Psychiatry, 43*, 137–147.

Madeddu, F., Prunas, A., & Hartmann, D. (2009). Prevalence of Axis II disorders in a sample of clients undertaking psychiatric evaluation for sex reassignment surgery. *Psychiatric Quarterly, 80*, 261–267.

Markauskaite, L., Freebody, L., & Irwin, P. (Eds.). (2010). *Methodological choice and design*. New York, NY: Springer.

Millon, T. (1990). *Toward a new personology: An evolutionary model*. New York, NY: Wiley.

Millon, T. (1996). *Disorders of personality: DSM–IV and beyond*. New York, NY: Wiley.

Millon, T. (2009). A brief history of psychopathology. In P. H. Blaney & T. Millon (Eds.), *Oxford textbook of psychopathology* (2nd ed., pp. 3–34). New York, NY: Oxford University Press.

Mischel, W., & Shoda, Y. (1995). A cognitive-affective system theory of personality: Reconceptualizing situations, dispositions, dynamics, and invariance in personality structure. *Psychological Review, 102*, 246–268.

Mischel, W., Shoda, Y., & Mendoza-Denton, R. (2002). Situation-behavior profiles as a locus of consistency in personality. *Current Directions in Psychological Science, 11*, 50–54.

Morf, C. C. (2006). Personality reflected in a coherent idiosyncratic interplay of intra- and interpersonal self-regulatory processes. *Journal of Personality, 74*, 1527–1556.

Morf, C. C., & Rhodewalt, F. (2001). Unraveling the paradoxes of narcissism: A dynamic self-regulatory processing model. *Psychological Inquiry, 12*, 177–196.

Niemi, R. G., Carmines, E. G., & McIver, J. P. (1986). The impact of scale length on reliability and validity. *Quality and Quantity, 20*, 371–376.

Oldham, J. M., Skodol, A. E., Kellman, H. D., Hyler, S. E., & Rosnick, L. (1992). Diagnosis of *DSM–III–R* personality disorders by two structured interviews: Patterns of comorbidity. *American Journal of Psychiatry, 149*, 213–220.

Oltmanns, T. F., & Turkheimer, E. (2009). Person perception and personality pathology. *Current Directions in Psychological Science, 18*, 32–36.

Paris, J. (2008). *Treatment of borderline personality disorder: A guide to evidence-based practice*. New York, NY: Guilford.

Peters, C. P. (1990). The inpatient treatment of severe personality disorders. *New Directions for Mental Health Services, 47*, 65–85.

Pincus, A. L. (2005). A contemporary integrative interpersonal theory of personality disorders. In M. F. Lenzenweger & J. F. Clarkin (Eds.), *Major theories of personality disorder* (2nd ed., pp. 282–331). New York, NY: Guilford.

Rathus, J. H., Sanderson, W. C., Miller, A. L., & Wetzler, S. (1995). Impact of personality functioning on cognitive behavioral treatment of panic disorder: A preliminary report. *Journal of Personality Disorders, 9*, 160–168.

Ronningstam, E. (2005). *Identifying and understanding the narcissistic personality*. New York, NY: Oxford University Press.

Ronningstam, E. (2009). Narcissistic personality disorder. In P. H. Blaney & T. Millon (Eds.), *Oxford textbook of psychopathology* (2nd ed., pp. 752–771). New York, NY: Oxford University Press.

Rosenthal, R. (1991). *Meta-analytic procedures for social research* (2nd ed.). Thousand Oaks, CA: Sage.

Samuel, D. B., & Widiger, T. A. (2010). A comparison of obsessive–compulsive personality disorder scales. *Journal of Personality Assessment, 92*, 232–240.

Sansone, R. A., & Sansone, L. A. (2010). Personality dysfunction and employment dysfunction: Double, double, toil and trouble. *Psychiatry, 7*, 12–16.

Shaver, P. R., & Mikulincer, M. (2002). Attachment related psychodynamics. *Attachment and Human Development, 4*, 133–161.

Silverstein, M. L. (2007). *Disorders of the self: A personality-guided approach*. Washington, DC: APA Books.

Sinha, B. K., & Watson, D. C. (2001). Personality disorder in university students: A multitrait–multimethod matrix study. *Journal of Personality Disorders, 15*, 235–244.

Skodol, A. E. (2010). *Rationale for proposing five specific personality disorder subtypes*. Retrieved from http://www.dsm5.0rg/ProposedRevisions

Soeteman, D. I., Hakkaart-van Roijen, L., Verheul, R., & Busschbach, J. J. (2008). The economic burden of personality disorders in mental health care. *Journal of Clinical Psychiatry, 69*, 259–265.

Strack, S. (2005). Preface. In S. Strack (Ed.), *Handbook of personology and psychopathology* (pp. xi–xv). Hoboken, NJ: Wiley.

Tyrer, P., & Johnson, T. (1996). Establishing the severity of personality disorder. *American Journal of Psychiatry, 153*, 1593–1597.

Widiger, T. A., & Clark, L. A. (2000). Toward *DSM–V* and the classification of psychopathology. *Psychological Bulletin, 126*, 946–963.

Widiger, T. A., & Trull, T. J. (2007). Plate tectonics in the classification of personality disorder: Shifting to a dimensional model. *American Psychologist, 62*, 71–83.

Wilberg, T., Hummelen, B., Pedersen, G., & Karterud, S. (2008). A study of patients with personality disorder not otherwise specified. *Comprehensive Psychiatry, 49*, 460–468.

Wong, S., & Hare, R. D. (2005). *Guidelines for a psychopathy treatment program*. Toronto, ON, Canada: Multi-Health Systems.

Zikos, E., Gill, K. J., & Charney, D. A. (2010). Personality disorders among alcoholic outpatients: Prevalence and course in treatment. *Canadian Journal of Psychiatry, 55*, 65–73.

Zimmerman, M., & Coryell, W. (1989). *DSM–III* personality disorders in a nonpatient sample. *Archives of General Psychiatry, 46*, 682–689.

Zimmerman, M., Rothchild, L., & Chelminski, I. (2005). The prevalence of *DSM–IV* personality disorders in psychiatric outpatients. *American Journal of Psychiatry, 162*, 1911–1918.

Qualitative and Quantitative Distinctions in Personality Disorder

AIDAN G. C. WRIGHT

Department of Psychology, The Pennsylvania State University

The categorical–dimensional debate has catalyzed a wealth of empirical advances in the study of personality pathology. However, this debate is merely one articulation of a broader conceptual question regarding whether to define and describe psychopathology as a *quantitatively* extreme expression of normal functioning or as *qualitatively* distinct in its process. In this article I argue that dynamic models of personality (e.g., object relations, cognitive-affective processing system) offer the conceptual scaffolding to reconcile these seemingly incompatible approaches to characterizing the relationship between normal and pathological personality. I propose that advances in personality assessment that sample behavior and experiences intensively provide the empirical techniques, whereas interpersonal theory offers an integrative theoretical framework, for accomplishing this goal.

It is important to understand the structure of psychopathology because this structure clarifies which constructs are meaningful for psychopathologists to study, how to classify and assess individuals with psychiatric difficulties, and how to intervene clinically. The "categorical-dimensional debate" has been historically central to the developing understanding of this structure (Kendell, 1975; Widiger & Trull, 2007). This debate has again taken on heightened significance as the publication of the *Diagnostic and Statistical Manual of Mental Disorders* (5th ed. [*DSM–5*]) is anticipated in 2013. Many have questioned the validity and utility of the categorically defined personality disorders (PDs) in recent editions of the *DSM,* and this has led to suggestions that PD be defined dimensionally using normative personality trait models (Widiger, 1993; Widiger, Livesley, & Clark, 2009; Widiger & Simonsen, 2005). However, significant questions remain about whether personality pathology can be neatly folded into the same dimensions as normal personality functioning (Krueger et al., 2011; Livesley & Jang, 2005). Yet, the debate on whether to define PD as categorically different from or dimensionally continuous with normal personality is but one argument in a broader qualitative–quantitative debate. Qualitative differences are those that are characterized by differences in processes, mechanisms, and structures, whereas quantitative distinctions are characterized by differences in amount or degree. By shifting focus from categorical versus dimensional articulations of personality pathology to qualitative versus quantitative distinctions in functioning, many of the quandaries the field currently faces might be reconciled.

A QUANDARY

The problems with the current categorical classification of PDs have been well documented by many authors (e.g., Clark, 2007; First, 2003; Krueger & Markon, 2006; Widiger & Clark, 2000; Widiger & Samuel, 2005).[1] The consistent finding of high rates of cooccurrence among categorically defined disorders (Krueger & Tackett, 2003; Widiger & Clark, 2000), boundary definitional issues, temporal instability of symptoms (Lenzenweger, Johnson, & Willett, 2004; Skodol, 2008), and the arbitrary nature of symptom cutoffs (Huprich & Bornstein, 2007; Widiger & Clark, 2000) are just some of the problems associated with the categorical approach conceptualized by the *DSM.* Investigators (e.g., Morey et al., 2007; Skodol et al., 2005) have addressed some of these problems by measuring the *DSM* PDs continuously (i.e., as symptom counts) as opposed to categorically (i.e., diagnosed or not). Although this manner of treating the PDs dimensionally increases reliability and predictive power, it sidesteps the fundamental question of whether PD lies on the continuum of normal personality traits and whether there are distinct typologies.

In addition, although the PDs are not explicitly linked to normal personality features in the *Diagnostic and Statistical Manual of Mental Disorders* (4th ed. [*DSM–IV*]; American Psychiatric Association, 1994), the results of numerous programs of research converge on the finding that normative personality traits and PDs are strongly related (Krueger, Markon, Patrick, & Iacono, 2005; Samuel & Widiger, 2008; Saulsman & Page, 2004; Wiggins & Pincus, 1989). When compared to nonclinical control groups, PDs show an elevated profile on certain Five-factor model (FFM) factors (Morey, Gunderson, Quigley, & Lyons, 2000; Morey et al., 2002). Moreover, clinicians can reliably generate FFM profiles for individual PDs and this seems to account for observed patterns of cooccurrence (Lynam & Widiger, 2001). These findings have led some researchers to suggest that PD can be effectively summarized by using the basic dimensions of personality, and, what is more, that PDs are best understood as lying on a continuum with basic personality functioning (Widiger, 1993; Widiger et al., 2009; Widiger & Simonsen, 2005).

---

[1] Due to considerations of space and conceptual clarity, this discussion focuses on personality and PD to the exclusion of the relationship between personality and Axis I disorders. Nevertheless, it is presumed that the arguments presented here similarly apply to these disorders, and there is empirical support for this assumption (e.g., Krueger, 2005).

Nevertheless, despite the appeal of adopting a dimensional approach to describing PD that uses broad, basic personality trait dimensions supplemented by more specific, hierarchically organized subdimensions or facets, considerable problems exist in the ability of this approach to capture the full breadth of phenomenology and phenotypic variation observed in abnormal functioning. Five key problems are associated with adopting a normative trait-based model as the basis for the definition of PD. The first of these problems is *structure*. It is commonly assumed that the structure of personality dimensions in the population adequately captures the personality structure for any given individual. However, individuals might possess widely varying idiographic personality structures (Borkenau & Ostendorf, 1998; Hamaker, Dolan, & Molenaar, 2005; Molenaar & Campbell, 2009; Tracey & Rohlfing, 2010). In other words, popular trait models are based on interindividual differences, and might not be able to fully account for intraindividual structure. Intraindividual structure emerges out of the covariation of functional variables across time, and this has been shown mathematically to be separable from the cross-sectional structure that emerges out of group-based analyses of personality traits (Beckmann, Wood, & Minbashian, 2010; Molenaar, 2004). Thus, although researchers have argued that the structure of normal and abnormal personality is isomorphic on the basis of the emergence of similar factors across normal and clinical samples (O'Connor, 2002), it remains an open question whether individuals with PD differ in intraindividual personality structure in any systematic way from non-PD individuals.

The second problem is *pattern*. Normal trait-based models of PD do not (currently) contain a direct representation of processes and oscillation (or rigid lack of oscillation) between states (Westen, 1995). Extremity (in the statistical sense) on a normal trait does not ipso facto determine whether an individual's behavior will be expressed extremely (e.g., shouting vs. talking), rigidly (i.e., to the exclusion of other behaviors), or maladaptively (i.e., doing a certain behavior when it would be wise to try something else; Wakefield, 2008). Dynamic constructs like affective lability show a complex relationship with traits, which in turn fail to explain the majority of variance in the construct (Kamen, Pryor, Gaughan, & Miller, 2010).

The third problem is *level*. Personality exists at multiple levels of functioning that mutually influence each other (e.g., motivation, cognition, overt behavior; unconscious vs. conscious; John, Robins, & Pervin, 2008). An articulation of the relationships among these levels sharpens the focus on mechanisms that drive personality pathology and augments the description of the purpose of pathological behavior. Overt behavior is given meaning by separating personality into its component processes and understanding functioning at multiple levels. PD is often associated with motivational strivings that manifest in paradoxical behavior. For instance, the overtly hostile aggression sometimes observed in dependent PD would seem anomalous, but it is easily understood if it is recognized as a maladaptive strategy to satisfy the motivation for affiliation (i.e., prevent the other from leaving; Bornstein, 2005).

The fourth problem is *specificity*. Broad dimensions of normative functioning do not explain when and under what circumstances problematic functioning will occur. In other words, it is necessary to know the features of the situation to which an individual is responding (Bornstein, 2003; see also Huprich, 2011/this issue). For example, narcissism predicts aggressive responses to ego threat, but psychopathy predicts aggression in response to physical threat (Jones & Paulhus, 2010). Importantly, normal trait profiles struggle to account for interpretive processes such as an individual's construal of the meaning of situations, events, his or her own behavior, and the behavior of others, all of which are theoretically integral to the concept of PD (Kernberg, 1984; Livesley, 2003; Pincus & Hopwood, in press). These might be more important in predicting behavior than the objectively defined situation (Reis, 2008).

The fifth problem is *coverage* (Trull, 2005). It is not clear whether the majority of variance in pathological personality expression is captured by normal traits (Clark, 2007). Indeed, some of the more aberrant aspects of PD cannot be adequately captured by normal traits alone (e.g., self-mutilation; Benjamin, 1993a). For example, self-injury, an important clinical phenomenon, does not logically follow from extremity on any one or pattern of the commonly assessed trait dimensions, and empirical results confirm that the majority of variance in self-harm is unique and unaccounted for by broader domains of personality (Markon, Krueger, & Watson, 2005). In short, although dimensional trait models of normal personality are systematically related to PD, they cannot fully explain it—when it comes to PD, the whole is more than the sum of its parts.

Therefore, it would seem that the field is faced with a quandary. Normative personality should, by definition, serve as the starting point for understanding and defining PD. This allows for the scientific integration of the study of normal and abnormal processes. And, as expected, normal personality traits show a consistent and replicable relationship with PD. Nevertheless, there remain important aspects in these clinical constructs that are unaccounted for by these models. Given the wealth of empirical results, it is not surprising that the dimensional models that have achieved the most attention propose that PDs exists as an "extreme and maladaptive" manifestation of normal personality traits, and not as separate or distinct categories (Widiger & Simonsen, 2005). And yet, there are actually two parts of this proposal—extremity and maladaptivity. As Wakefield (2008) pointed out, extremity is not necessarily equivalent with maladaptivity (i.e., dysfunction or harm). Moreover, extremity is a purely quantitative distinction, whereas maladaptive (or the notion of a "maladaptive variant") contains an implicit argument for a qualitative difference in process, mechanism, and possibly structure, but certainly functioning, regardless of whether trait extremity is necessary for its manifestation.

A NEW ANALOGY

This distinction between extremity as a quantitative matter of degree and maladaptivity as a qualitative matter of mechanism is critical for the debate about how to best represent PD and for understanding more generally the role of normative personality processes in personality pathology. Analogies can serve as arbiters and guides for whole programs of research (cf. Fernandez-Duque & Johnson, 1999); the analogy that is most often offered to conceptually frame the utility of relating normal to abnormal functioning quantitatively is a medical one—blood pressure (Skodol & Bender, 2009). In this analogy personality dimensions are akin to blood pressure, which is a basic aspect of normal functioning, with everyone falling somewhere along the continuum. Meaningful cutoffs could conceivably be agreed on and established for the definition of extreme or "clinically significant" levels. This analogy is meant to effectively reconcile the need for categorical cutoffs in an area that appears to be dimensionally defined. The blood pressure analogy is a good one in many ways. For one, it is a concept with which most adults are familiar and it is simple and straightforward. More pertinent to PD as potentially represented by extreme normative traits, it includes a full bipolar dimension (see Samuel, 2011/this issue for a discussion of this), as problems are associated both with high and low blood pressure.

However, the blood pressure analogy fails to capture the important qualitative distinctions in process that are not adequately represented by simple quantitative cut scores along linear dimensions. Perhaps this is only a matter of how the analogy is put forth, because what makes extreme blood pressure problematic are qualitatively different processes at the low (i.e., not enough oxygen reaches the brain) and high (i.e., the pressure breaks down the arteries at the bifurcations leading to a buildup of plaques) ends of the continuum. Thus it is not as simple an analogy as it appears on the surface, and further thought reveals interesting new implications—namely, qualitatively distinct processes.

An alternative analogy that offers a distinct perspective on the relationship between normal and abnormal functioning involves the very familiar substance, water (H_2O). Like all physical substances, H_2O is not a static entity, but instead exists in a number of dynamic phases that vary in their internal structure and relationship to the environment. Specifically, although the temperature of H_2O is perfectly continuous and easily measured quantitatively, at two familiar points along this continuum, shifts occur that change H_2O qualitatively as it can take the form of ice, water, or steam. Each of these different phases of H_2O is qualitatively different in its internal relationships between molecules (structure), the manner in which it interacts with other substances (pattern), and its appearance, form, and properties (levels). Additionally, although temperature plays a crucial role, other internal and external variables such as salinity and atmospheric pressure further contribute to determining the phase of the substance (specificity). Regardless of the phase, the internal structure, and the qualitatively distinct properties, all phases are made of the same matter.

The view taken in this article is that the relationship of personality to PD is similar to the relationship among water, ice, and steam. Personality pathology is not merely an arbitrary quantitative cutoff along a continuous distribution, nor is PD a qualitatively distinct "substance" from normal personality. Rather, PD exists as a qualitatively distinct phase along the continuum of basic personality functioning that can be distinguished by an individual's internal psychological structure and the manner in which he or she interacts with the environment. Stated simply, personality and PD are not made of categorically different substances, but they are defined by qualitatively different processes.

EXTENDING THE ANALOGY

Can all that is ice be captured by "extremely cold water?" Can all that is steam be captured by "extremely hot water?" Probably not, because even from a lexical perspective other words (i.e., *ice* and *steam*) have been created to capture this qualitative difference that occurs at each phase shift. Similarly, is pathological narcissism merely "disagreeable extraversion?" Can borderline personality disorder be captured fully by "high neuroticism and low agreeableness and conscientiousness?" The view offered here is that although these trait constellations are

associated with these respective disorders, describing the disorders as constellations of these traits does not fully capture their essence and provides overly simple caricatures of personality pathology, a highly complex clinical phenomenon. A number of empirical studies confirm this by showing that despite significant relationships between normative traits and PD, on average the majority of variance in PD remains unexplained when accounting for traits and even facets (Bagby, Costa, Widiger, Ryder, & Marshall, 2005; Reynolds & Clark, 2001).

Dimensional trait profiles approximate but do not fully articulate the structure of an individual's personality. In part, this is because an individual's trait profile says nothing of the intraindividual relationship between the traits and how the traits interact with each other within an individual across time and situations (Hamaker et al., 2005; Wright, Pincus, & Lenzenweger, 2010). The majority of the research that has linked traits and profiles with psychopathology has done so by correlating traits and disorders or examining the traits and profiles associated with members of different clinical groups. Although this serves to generate meaningful and important results, it does not resolve the issue of specificity of the relationship. Rarely if ever are individuals with a certain trait or profile of traits found, and then subsequently diagnosed. What this leaves us with is the knowledge of what traits might be elevated if a person possesses a diagnosis, but not the reverse. It is not the case that in the population each individual with a given trait profile possesses the same PD diagnosis, or any diagnosis at all for that matter.

Take, for example, the assertion that narcissists are "disagreeable extraverts" (Miller, Gaughan, Pryor, Kamen, & Campbell, 2009). Although it might be the case that certain types of narcissism are associated with this trait profile (but see Samuel & Widiger, 2008, for contrasting results), the reverse is not necessarily true, namely that all disagreeable extraverts (or extraverted antagonists for that matter) are narcissistic. Arguably, what is unique about narcissism is the when, how, and for what purpose extraverted and disagreeable behaviors (and others) are enacted (see, e.g., Morf, Horvath, & Torchetti, 2010; Pincus & Lukowitsky, 2010). Indeed, research shows that narcissism is associated with aggressive behavior, but that aggression among narcissistic individuals tends to be situationally specific (Jones & Paulhus, 2010). What differentiates a narcissist from any given disagreeable extravert is the distinct patterning of behavior (which in turn betrays distinct internal processes and structure), that will be experienced as qualitatively distinct by those with whom they interact, and, importantly, will have implications for intervention and prognosis.

Thus, it is not merely in the what, but also in the how, when, and why that the differences between normal and abnormal personality arise. The maladjustment exists in the process, in other words, the patterning and the purpose for which the individual enacts behaviors. To adequately account for these qualitative differences, dynamic models of personality that include temporal sequences, mental representation of the self and environment, internally experienced drives (e.g., motivations, fears), and regulatory mechanisms are required.[2]

---

[2]The word *dynamic* is used to refer to processes that occur within and between levels of experience. It is not meant to be synonymous with the term *psychodynamic* as has emerged from the psychoanalytic tradition.

Dynamic Models of Personality

If dynamic processes differentiate normal and abnormal personality functioning (i.e., intraindividual structure, behavioral pattern, between-level interactions, and situational specificity), the models used to define and study personality pathology must capture dynamic processes explicitly. However, most research relating normal and abnormal personality is based on static trait conceptualizations of personality. Models that are based on an understanding of personality as an ensemble of structures and processes that include a self-concept, motivations, fears, and self-regulation strategies seem better suited than trait models to capture this distinction.

Two very different theoretical traditions have arrived at strikingly similar systems of personality that are well-suited for these purposes. From the psychodynamic tradition, object-relations models (Fairbairn, 1952; Greenberg & Mitchell, 1983; Kernberg, 1975, 1984) have developed a view of personality as emerging out of interpersonal relationships that are represented mentally and serve as the basis for enduring patterns of relating to others, understanding the world, and responding (see also Luyten & Blatt, 2011). Object relations are units of mental representations of self and other colored by a linking affect state. Key to this viewpoint is the affective link between the way the individuals construe themselves and others in a psychological situation. A strikingly similar description has been offered by social-cognitive theorists under the name Cognitive-Affective Processing System (CAPS; Mischel & Shoda, 1998; Shoda, Mischel, & Wright, 1994). This approach also makes use of elements of personality termed the cognitive-affective processing units, which mediate the encoding of situations and the chosen behavioral responses. These include expectancies, beliefs, goals, and the like, but also emotions. This gives rise to stable *if–then* behavioral signatures that summarize the behavioral contingencies associated with specific interpretations and affective responses to situations. Both object relations and CAPS theories are remarkably similar in their use of mental representation, affective moderation, and behavioral responding that varies as a function of the psychological situation as construed by the individual.

A number of features of dynamic personality models are appealing for defining the distinction between normality and abnormality. For one, they can adequately capture trait-like stability and intraindividual variability. Dynamic models can subsume trait models more readily than trait models can accommodate dynamic models. They accomplish this by allowing for within-situation consistency and across-situation variability. Importantly, the unit of analysis is the psychological situation or the situation as an individual perceives it. An individual's construal of a situation might be a faithful representation of the actual situation or, alternatively, might bear little to no resemblance to what another might describe as occurring, instead representing an idiosyncratic and unique representation (Reis, 2008). Additionally, dynamic models include the interplay between the individual and the environment, allowing for a patterning of these processes. To accomplish this, these models must have a taxonomy that is not limited to an individual's behavior, but also includes the important and salient aspects of situations to which individuals attend and respond. Finally, and perhaps most important, these models tend to be person centered as opposed to variable centered (see Shedler et al., 2010, for a discussion of this issue with respect to PD). Broad variable-based models

have long been plagued by the problem of going from the nomothetic to the idiographic (Molenaar, 2004), an important issue in practical assessment. In contrast, dynamic models are more easily built from the individual up through the use of constructs such as "behavioral signatures" (Mischel & Shoda, 1998), a decidedly person-based nomenclature (e.g., our signature stands in our stead on legal documents).

Object relations and CAPS each bring unique strengths that can be applied to establishing the difference between personality and PD. Object-relations theory has a longer tradition and stems from clinical observation and theory, and therefore possesses a number of established constructs (e.g., splitting, reversals, projective identification) that are familiar to clinicians and that were created specifically for the purpose of capturing the patterns of pathological personality functioning. The CAPS model emerged out of laboratory-based personality science, and therefore offers a language that can be easily translated to experimental research. CAPS has less of a tradition of being applied to psychopathology and PD, although this is changing (Eaton, South, & Krueger, 2009; Pincus, Lukowitsky, Wright, & Eichler, 2009). Cardinal patterns of psychopathology can be anchored to consistent contingent if–then structures of behavioral and emotional responses (thens) in situations the individual experiences as functionally equivalent (ifs). A number of authors have now proposed that the CAPS model would be amenable to characterizing PD pathology (Eaton et al., 2009; Huprich & Bornstein, 2007; Pincus et al., 2009) and empirical findings are beginning to support this view. Rhadigan and Huprich (in press) have found that CAPS if–then signature-based descriptions of the current PDs outperformed trait-based descriptions of the disorders in diagnostic accuracy as rated by clinicians.

Despite the strengths of these dynamic models, they suffer from a lack of an organizing framework for efficiently classifying the psychologically meaningful aspects of situations (Hogan, 2009). Models such as these would benefit greatly from a formal, integrative framework that could serve to classify both the psychologically salient aspects of situations and the behavioral responses an individual enacts. Ideally this would be achieved using a common metric that serves to seamlessly link the internal representation of a situation with other psychological structures such as motivations and goals, and also the enacted behavior in the proximal situation.

The Common Metric: Agency and Communion

What is necessary is a theory of personality that is dynamic, and that can provide the content domains to focus the assessment of the processes and patterns of persons interacting with their environment. Contemporary integrative interpersonal theory (Pincus, 2005; Pincus, Lukowitsky, & Wright, 2010) is well-suited for this task. Rooted in the early theoretical formulations of Sullivan (1953) and Leary (1957), contemporary interpersonal theory has integrated the findings of the neurobiological (Depue & Collins, 1999; Depue & Morrone-Strupinsky, 2005), trait (Wiggins & Trapnell, 1996), social-cognitive (Locke & Sadler, 2007), and motivational (Horowitz et al., 2006; Locke, 2000) literatures to provide a comprehensive scientific model of personality and personality pathology.

A number of recent publications (e.g., Horowitz et al., 2006; Pincus, 2005; Pincus & Hopwood, in press; Pincus et al., 2010; Pincus & Wright, 2010) have detailed the assumptions and propositions of contemporary integrative interpersonal theory (especially as they pertain to psychopathology and personality disturbance) that are only briefly touched on here. Central is the assumption that the most important expressions of personality and its pathology occur in interpersonal situations. The *DSM–IV–TR* (American Psychiatric Association, 2000) lists interpersonal dysfunction as part of the core definitions of each specific PD, and the *DSM–5* proposal affirms this view by defining the general criteria for PD in terms of interpersonal functioning (see also Pincus, 2011). Although the PDs list additional criteria and features beyond those associated with interpersonal dysfunction, much of the symptomatic dysfunction manifests in interpersonal situations (Benjamin, 1993b; Kiesler, 1986). In much the same way that the defining features of steam, ice, and water can be faithfully described by reference to the dynamics of the molecules (e.g., ice is rigid, steam is volatile, and water is stable yet flexible), which has bearing on external relations to the environment (e.g., ice shatters, steam is difficult to contain), so too can personality and its pathology be captured by the dynamics of an individual's interpersonal pattern, both internal via the mental construal of self and other and external in their behavior and approach toward others.

Interpersonal theory uses the broad concepts of agency and communion to provide a structure to define, describe, and classify interpersonal situations. The common metric of agentic and communal dimensions contextualizes both behavior and the salient aspects of situations to which individuals attend and respond (Fournier, Moskowitz, & Zuroff, 2008, 2009; Sadikaj, Russell, Moskowitz, & Paris, 2010).The "interpersonal situation" refers to the in vivo, observable, behavioral exchange between one person and another (or others), and the internal processes and states generated within the mind of those interactants via the capacity for perception, mental representation, memory, fantasy, and expectancy. Normative patterns of interpersonal behavior between interactants (Carson, 1969; Sadler, Woody, & Ethier, 2010) serve as baselines for the field-regulatory pulls of interpersonal behavior (i.e., normative if–then sequences). Chronic deviations from these patterns likely indicate maladaptive functioning and pathology. Patterns of disturbed functioning can be contextualized by linking the perceived agentic and communal characteristics of others in an interpersonal situation (ifs) with the symptomatic or maladaptive behavioral and emotional responses (thens) of the patient. These if–then sequences can be daisy-chained to capture the full complexity of dynamic cycles. Mismatches between the behavior that an individual puts forth and the behavior that is necessary for success in a situation can arise from a failure on the part of the individual to adequately construe the situation or from not being able to call on the appropriate behavioral response (see Eaton et al., 2009, for an elaboration of this issue with the CAPS model).

Building on the content domains of agency and communion, dynamic dimensions are included to specifically articulate the patterned enactment of behaviors (Leary, 1957): moderation versus *intensity* (e.g., talking vs. shouting), flexibility versus *rigidity* (e.g., ability to shift behavior vs. repeating the same behavior over and over), stability versus *oscillation* (e.g., consistency within and across situations vs. unpredictable responses), and accuracy versus *inaccuracy* (i.e., the fit or match of behavior within a situation). Importantly, these dynamic dimensions can be operationalized and quantified with specific reference to interpersonal behavior, and thereby serve as a basis to describe the patterns and processes of disordered personality (e.g., commanding is more dominant than suggesting; variability in dominance across situations; dominant behavior when confronted with dominance; Pincus & Wright, 2010). It is through these dynamic dimensions that we can begin to get an empirical handle on qualitative distinctions in process.

RESEARCHING DYNAMIC PROCESSES: BORDERLINE PERSONALITY DISORDER AS AN EXAMPLE

The key theoretical questions of how personality and PD relate to one another are also inherently questions of methodology. The majority of the research already outlined relating personality to PD uses cross-sectional methods along with self-report personality assessment techniques. These time-honored methods are limited in their ability to assess process (Bornstein, 2003). In the H_2O analogy, this is akin to measuring temperature, but still not knowing whether the phase is ice, water, or steam. However, intensive sampling methods have emerged that, when coupled with advances in statistical modeling, allow for studying the idiographic structure of an individual and the dynamic give-and-take of the individual in his or her environment. Although a variety of approaches certainly exist to assess dynamic processes, some of the more promising approaches seek to capture individuals as they generally behave across a wide variety of situations in naturalistic settings. Referred to variously as Ambulatory Assessment, Intensive Repeated Measurement (IRM), or Ecological Momentary Assessment (EMA), this approach to assessment samples an individual's behavior repeatedly in his or her natural environment (see Ebner-Priemer & Trull, 2009; Moskowitz, Russell, Sadikaj, & Sutton, 2009, for reviews). The power of this approach to capture and statistically model the dynamic interplay of people and their environments is impressive. An additional benefit is that they are robust to the well-known retrospective biases in self-reported functioning (Ebner-Priemer et al., 2006).

A brief review of the manner in which these have been applied to one diagnosis, borderline personality disorder (BPD), demonstrates the power of these approaches to unlock the processes that qualitatively distinguish PD. Russell, Moskowitz, Zuroff, Sookman, and Paris (2007) differentiated individuals with BPD from nonclinical control participants based on intraindividual variability of interpersonal behavior over a 20-day period. Specifically, individuals with BPD and controls reported a similar mean level of agreeable behavior but BPD participants displayed greater variability, vacillating between high and low levels. Results also suggested elevated mean levels of submissive behaviors combined with lower mean levels of dominant behavior that were more variable for individuals with BPD relative to the control participants. In other words, individuals with BPD were consistently more submissive, but also demonstrated acute elevations and declines in dominance. Finally, as predicted, individuals with BPD endorsed higher and more variable levels of quarrelsomeness when compared to controls.

Using a similar assessment approach, Ebner-Priemer et al. (2007) identified group-specific patterns of affective instability when comparing BPD patients to healthy controls, with BPD patients being distinguishable based on rapid and dramatic declines from positive mood states in particular. Moreover, the sequence of experienced emotions (e.g., anxiety followed by anger) differed between these groups (Reisch, Ebner-Priemer, Tschacher, Bohus, & Linehan, 2008). Building on these results,

Trull and colleagues (2008) used EMA to investigate affective instability in BPD with a control group of individuals diagnosed with depressive disorder. Of note is that these two groups did not differ on mean levels of positive or negative affect reported across time. In other words, they exhibited similar trait levels of affect. However, the variability in these scores differentiated the two groups, with BPD patients exhibiting greater variability. Of even more interest is that BPD patients also exhibited more abrupt changes in hostility, fear, and sadness as compared with depressive controls. What these results demonstrate is that it is the temporal patterning and contingency of affective functioning that gives rise to the turbulent experience that clinicians recognize as BPD, even when compared to groups with similarity in overall negative affect. Taken together, the molar results of these studies highlight differences in the underlying processes and beckon further research to find the determinants of those distinctions.

These results have since been extended to include the dynamic interplay between perception in interpersonal situations and affective responding (Sadikaj, Russell, et al., 2010). Results showed that BPD patients, relative to normal controls, exhibited greater negative affect in response to less perceived warmth, and that both positive and negative affect persisted longer across situations. In a recently presented paper, Sadikaj, Moskowitz, Russell, and Zuroff (2010) implemented some of the most articulated models of the processes associated with BPD. Again using EMA techniques, BPD patients were compared with those carrying diagnoses of social phobia (SP). This comparison is particularly interesting because both diagnoses have as core features difficulties with interpersonal perception and responses—in other words, situationally contingent processes. Results showed that for both groups, decreased perceptions of warmth in an interpersonal situation are associated with higher negative affect. However, the association was strongest for anger in BPD and embarrassment for SP. Furthermore, the two groups differed in the behavioral patterns associated with negative affect, with BPD patients becoming more quarrelsome and SP patients becoming more submissive. As Sadikaj, Moskowitz, et al. (2010) noted, the interpersonal dynamics are specific to the clinical groups. It is this type of result that allows for highly articulated and precise description of symptoms, and offers a first look at the internal process that gives rise to these symptoms. This framework points to multiple possible sources of disturbed functioning (e.g., distortions in interpersonal perception and meaning-making processes; maladaptive, underdeveloped, or overvalued interpersonal goals, motives, expectancies, beliefs, and competencies) that allow for the development of specific hypotheses for future research (Pincus et al., 2009).

PROPOSALS FOR FUTURE RESEARCH AND PRACTICE

Dynamic approaches to personality pathology research such as those reviewed and suggested here can offer useful techniques to empirically quantify what makes PD qualitatively different from normal functioning. Methods can now be linked to theory in ways that further the science and practice of assessing personality pathology. Thus, I offer specific directions for empirically defining the relationship between normal personality and PD.

Starting with the least specific, it is predicted that an individual's net amount of variability in interpersonal behavior, affect, cognitions, and motivation will augment average levels of these domains in predicting pathology.[3] Furthermore, the amount of variability will vary by type of pathology. Variability in emotions, self-esteem, and interpersonal behavior is the hallmark of BPD (Schmideberg, 1959), whereas other pathology, say obsessive–compulsive problems, might be better characterized by rigidity in specific domains. Some of the work reviewed in the prior section addresses this directly (Russell et al., 2007; Trull et al., 2008), but these investigations only focused on BPD. More research is necessary on different pathologies.

Net variability can be differentiated from structured variability in describing an individual's pattern of functioning (Ram & Gerstorf, 2009). Structured variability is characterized by a systematic organization or pattern to the variability, whereas net variability refers to gross measures of fluctuation. Thus a more precise prediction is that there are specific patterns of behavior that are associated with maladaptivity (e.g., in a histrionic patient, if there is a perceived lack of attention, then sexually seductive behavior follows). The work outlined earlier by Sadikaj, Moskowitz, and colleagues (2010) and Ebner-Priemer and colleagues (2007; Reisch et al., 2008) has begun to show that structured patterns emerge that are specific to groups. Relatedly, Nock, Prinstein, and Sterba (2009) showed that self-harming behavior is not only variable, but appears to show some situational specificity. But again, this work has primarily been limited to BPD and there is much left to investigate. Structured variability can be investigated in a variety of ways, and a promising avenue is the exploration of intraindividual factor structure and the relationship between intraindividual factors across time. The use of P-technique factor analysis (i.e., applying factor analysis to scores on multiple variables from one individual across multiple time points; Nesselroade & Ford, 1985) holds the potential to elucidate idiographic structure and change through time, especially when it is coupled with techniques such as time-series analysis (e.g., Hamaker et al., 2005). For instance, a feature that is often associated with passive-aggression is the belief that "to cooperate is to subjugate," and it might follow that passive-aggressive individuals view bids from others to collaborate as bids for domination. Across time it would be expected that their perceptions of others' warmth and dominance would covary (i.e., be fused and indistinguishable) such that a factor emerges that blends the two, even when the normative pattern is to perceive interpersonal warmth and dominance in others as separate. This hypothesis can be directly assessed using these techniques. As noted previously, studies that have examined the factor structure of individuals, even when using common trait descriptors, find that there is a great deal of interindividual heterogeneity in factor structure (Borkenau & Ostendorf, 1998; Hamaker et al., 2005; Molenaar & Campbell, 2009). To date, there has been no investigation of this as it pertains to abnormal personality functioning. However, Fournier et al. (2009) demonstrated that intraindividual interpersonal structure across time varies, and this is generally unrelated to broad normative traits, but is related to self-reported depression and self-esteem. Applying these approaches to the investigation of personality pathology and in clinical populations is a highly promising avenue for future research.

---

[3]Note that variability is a continuum, ranging from complete rigidity (i.e., the same behavior across all situations) to wild vacillation that is entirely unpredictable.

The fact that there is evidence of idiographic factor structures and behavioral signatures in turn has bearing on the definition of clinically meaningful groupings of individuals or even taxons (Meehl, 1992), a common (but not isomorphic) adjunct to the categorical-dimensional debate (Waller & Meehl, 1998). Much of the taxometric research is based on scales (e.g., Haslam, 2003), not on a quantification of an individual's dynamic patterning or use of a particular behavioral signature. It could be that by defining a specific if–then process, and then measuring its occurrence over time in individuals, that more clearly defined groups emerge than if dimensional scale scores are used alone. Thus, it is possible that by classifying people based on similarity of individual factor structure or dynamic signatures, more clear groupings or taxa will emerge. More generally, by focusing on specific and testable patterns, a taxonomy of processes might emerge that can be put to good use in the description and differentiation of phenotypic expressions of PD.

Finally, dynamic assessment could eventually play a more direct role in clinical practice. IRM/EMA approaches to personality assessment have not made the jump from use in empirical research to applied assessment. However, as portable yet computationally powerful technology improves (and becomes more affordable), it is easy to imagine the day when an individual patient can be provided a device (or program loaded on his or her own device) that can be used to collect real-time data about targeted assessment issues (e.g., questions about emotion, behavior, specific cognitions) intensively between sessions, thereby providing access to a more detailed analysis of their processes. Using any desktop computer with appropriate software, these data can easily be quantitatively modeled to develop an idiographic personality model of the patient at the outset of treatment, followed by a within-person comparison to the patient's own model at the outset of treatment as the treatment progresses (see, e.g., Hunter, Ram, & Ryback, 2008). This could provide direct tracking of improvement and changes associated with treatment.

QUANTITATIVE AND QUALITATIVE DISTINCTIONS IN THE CONTEXT OF THE *DSM–5*

On the eve of the next edition of the *DSM,* the work groups have now released their proposed revisions, including those for personality and PD. Although not finalized, the proposal appears to have a number of features that are consistent with the observations and arguments offered here. Notably, the work group has suggested a two-step approach that combines discrimination between normal and disordered personality functioning globally, and a separate description of the content areas of dysfunction via traits, facets, and prototypes. The first step in this approach distinguishes the functioning associated with normal and abnormal personality via a general definition of PD. These criteria focus on dysfunction in self-identity and interpersonal relatedness that accords well with contemporary interpersonal theory's ability to serve as the organizational framework (Pilkonis, Hallquist, Morse, & Stepp, 2011; Pincus, 2011). Moreover, much of the language used to define these deficits is inherently process based, which, as is argued here, would seem to be the defining difference between adaptive and maladaptive functioning.

In addition, the work group has proposed a series of maladaptive traits to use to establish the content of the dysfunction. What is important here is that these are maladaptive traits, which bear similarity to the broad domains of normal functioning tapped by basic trait models but are not synonymous (see Krueger & Eaton, 2010; Krueger et al., 2011). Indeed, it is this very distinction between the "normal trait" and the "maladaptive expression" of those traits that this article intends to address. Other maladaptive trait models exist (e.g., Schedule for Nonadaptive and Adaptive Personality [SNAP], Dimensional Assessment of Personality Pathology [DAPP]) that bear significant similarity to the broad domains of normal functioning (Markon et al., 2005; Widiger et al., 2009). However, by employing maladaptive traits the issue of the qualitative distinction between normal and abnormal personality is sidestepped (see also Hopwood, 2011/this issue, for a different perspective on this issue). Facets such as rigid perfectionism or manipulativeness with items that presumably get at the specific processes associated with obsessiveness and taking advantage of others, are, in effect, qualitatively different from normal traits, having the maladaptive processes and functioning embedded within them. The work group's choice to include abnormal traits would seem to be a wise one given the opinions expressed here, but the question remains open as to what connects the normal traits with the abnormal ones.

It bears mentioning that despite the enthusiasm expressed here for dynamic models and associated methodological advances, this article is not a treatise against trait psychology. The intention of this piece is not to undercut or diminish the undeniable advances associated with trait psychology and assessment as they have been applied to the domain of PD. However, it can be difficult for trait models to articulate the "jump" between normal and abnormal functioning, the question at issue here. Traits and traitedness are not incongruous with dynamic models of personality, and the two approaches are best applied in a complementary fashion to the questions addressed here.

CONCLUSION

Sullivan (1954) emphasized that disordered patterns of behavior are deviations and distortions of normal functioning, noting that "We all show everything that any mental patient shows, except for the pattern, the accents, and so on" (p. 183). The use of diagnostic categories ignores the first part of that sentence, whereas the suggestion that pathology exists as mere extreme scores on continuous dimensions of basic personality ignores the second part. The selective attention to quantitative description based purely on the content domains associated with personality traits excludes the highly important process domain that might contain the key to the qualitative distinction between normal and disordered functioning, and between types of disordered functioning. Contemporary interpersonal theory can supply a needed framework for the scientific study of personality and its disorder, and, when coupled with dynamic assessment methodology, the elusive aspects of what differentiates the two can hopefully be understood and inform *DSM–5.1* and beyond.

ACKNOWLEDGMENTS

Preparation of this article was supported by Grant F31MH087053 from the National Institute of Mental Health. I thank Rachel L. Bachrach, Nicholas R. Eaton, Christopher J. Hopwood, Mark R. Lukowitsky, Aaron L. Pincus, Michael J. Roche, and Gentiana Sadikaj for helpful comments on earlier drafts of this article. I am grateful for conversations with Peter C. M. Molenaar which influenced the thinking behind this piece.

REFERENCES

American Psychiatric Association. (1994). *Diagnostic and statistical manual of mental disorders* (4th ed.). Washington, DC: Author.

American Psychiatric Association. (2000). *Diagnostic and statistical manual of mental disorders* (4th ed., text revision). Washington, DC: Author.

Bagby, R. M., Costa, P. T., Jr., Widiger, T. A., Ryder, A. G., & Marshall, M. (2005). *DSM–IV* personality disorders and the five-factor model of personality: A multi-method examination of domain- and facet-level predictions. *European Journal of Personality, 19,* 307–324.

Beckmann, N., Wood, R. E., & Minbashian, A. (2010). It depends how you look at it: On the relationship between neuroticism and conscientiousness at the within- and the between-person levels of analysis. *Journal of Research in Personality, 44,* 593–601.

Benjamin, L. S. (1993a). Dimensional, categorical, or hybrid analyses of personality: A response to Widiger's proposal. *Psychological Inquiry, 4,* 91–95.

Benjamin, L. S. (1993b). *Interpersonal diagnosis and treatment of personality disorders.* New York, NY: Guilford.

Borkenau, P., & Ostendorf, F. (1998). The big five as states: How useful is the five-factor model to describe intraindividual variations over time? *Journal of Research in Personality, 32,* 202–221.

Bornstein, R. F. (2003). Behaviorally referenced experimentation and symptom validation: A paradigm for 21st-century personality disorder research. *Journal of Personality Disorders, 17,* 1–18.

Bornstein, R. F. (2005). *The dependent patient: A practitioner's guide.* Washington, DC: American Psychological Association.

Carson, R. C. (1969). *Interaction concepts of personality.* Chicago, IL: Aldine.

Clark, L. A. (2007). Assessment and diagnosis of personality disorder: Perennial issues and an emerging reconceptualization. *Annual Review of Psychology, 58,* 227–257.

Depue, R. A., & Collins, P. F. (1999). Neurobiology of the structure of personality: Dopamine, facilitation of incentive motivation, and extraversion. *Behavioral and Brain Sciences, 22,* 491–569.

Depue, R. A., & Morrone-Strupinsky, J. V. (2005). A neurobehavioral model of affiliative bonding: Implications for conceptualizing a human trait of affiliation. *Behavioral and Brain Sciences, 28,* 313–395.

Eaton, N. R., South, S. C., & Krueger, R. F. (2009). The cognitive-affective processing system (CAPS) approach to personality and the concept of personality disorder: Integrating clinical and social-cognitive research. *Journal of Research in Personality, 43,* 208–217.

Ebner-Priemer, U. W., Kuo, J., Kleindienst, N., Welch, S. S., Reisch, T., Reinhard, I., ... Bohus, M. (2007). State affective instability in borderline personality disorder assessed by ambulatory monitoring. *Psychological Medicine: A Journal of Research in Psychiatry and the Allied Sciences, 37,* 961–970.

Ebner-Priemer, U. W., Kuo, J., Welch, S. S., Thielgen, T., Witte, S., Bohus, M., & Linehan, M. M. (2006). A valence-dependent group-specific recall bias of retrospective self-reports: A study of borderline personality disorder in everyday life. *Journal of Nervous and Mental Disease, 194,* 774–779.

Ebner-Priemer, U. W., & Trull, T. J. (2009). Ecological momentary assessment of mood disorders and mood dysregulation. *Psychological Assessment, 21,* 463–475.

Fairbairn, W. R. (1952). *Psychoanalytic studies of the personality.* Oxford, UK: Routledge & Kegan Paul.

Fernandez-Duque, D., & Johnson, M. L. (1999). Attention metaphors: How metaphors guide the cognitive psychology of attention. *Cognitive Science, 23,* 83–116.

First, M. B. (2003). Psychiatric classification. In A. Tasman, J. Kay, & J. Lieberman (Eds.), *Psychiatry* (2nd ed., Vol. 1, pp. 659–676). New York, NY: Wiley.

Fournier, M. A., Moskowitz, D. S., & Zuroff, C. (2008). Integrating dispositions, signatures, and the interpersonal domain. *Journal of Personality and Social Psychology, 94,* 531–545.

Fournier, M., Moskowitz, D. S., & Zuroff, D. (2009). The interpersonal signature. *Journal of Research in Personality, 43,* 155–162.

Greenberg, J. R., & Mitchell, S. M. (1983). *Object relations in psychoanalytic theory.* Cambridge, MA: Harvard University Press.

Hamaker, E. L., Dolan, C. V., & Molenaar, P. C. M. (2005). Statistical modeling of the individual: Rationale and application of multivariate stationary time series analysis. *Multivariate Behavioral Research, 40,* 207–233.

Haslam, N. (2003). The dimensional view of personality disorders: A review of the taxometric evidence. *Clinical Psychology Review, 23,* 75–93.

Hogan, R. (2009). Much ado about nothing: The person–situation debate. *Journal of Research in Personality, 43,* 249.

Hopwood, C. J. (2011/this issue). Personality traits in the *DSM–5. Journal of Personality Assessment, 93,* 398–405.

Horowitz, L. M., Wilson, K. R., Turan, B., Zolotsev, P., Constantino, M. J., & Henderson, L. (2006). How interpersonal motives clarify the meaning of interpersonal behavior: A revised circumplex model. *Personality and Social Psychology Review, 10,* 67–86.

Hunter, J. A., Ram, N., & Ryback, R. (2008). Use of satiation therapy in the treatment of adolescent-manifest sexual interest in male children: A single-case, repeated measures design. *Clinical Case Studies, 7,* 54–74.

Huprich, S. K. (2011/this issue). Contributions from personality- and psychodynamically oriented assessment to the development of the *DSM-5* personality disorders. *Journal of Personality Assessment, 93,* 354–361.

Huprich, S. K., & Bornstein, R. F. (2007). An overview of issues related to categorical and dimensional models of personality disorder assessment. *Journal of Personality Assessment, 89,* 3–15.

John, O. P., Robins, R. W., & Pervin, L. A. (2008). *Handbook of personality* (3rd ed.). New York, NY: Guilford.

Jones, D. N., & Paulhus, D. L. (2010). Different provocations trigger aggression in narcissists and psychopaths. *Social and Personality Psychology Science, 1,* 12–18.

Kamen, C., Pryor, L. R., Gaughan, E. T., & Miller, J. D. (2010). Affective lability: Separable from neuroticism and the other big four? *Psychiatric Research, 176,* 202–207.

Kendell, R. C. (1975). *The role of diagnosis in psychiatry.* Oxford, UK: Blackwell Scientific.

Kernberg, O. F. (1975). *Borderline conditions and pathological narcissism.* New York, NY: Jason Aronson.

Kernberg, O. F. (1984). *Severe personality disorders: Psychotherapeutic strategies.* New Haven, CT: Yale University Press.

Kiesler, D. J. (1986). The 1982 interpersonal circle: An analysis of *DSM–III* personality disorders. In T. Millon & G. L. Klerman (Eds.), *Contemporary directions in psychopathology: Toward the* DSM–IV (pp. 571–597). New York, NY: Guilford.

Krueger, R. F. (2005). Continuity of axes I and II: Toward a unified model of personality, personality disorders, and clinical disorders. *Journal of Personality Disorders, 19,* 233–261.

Krueger, R. F., & Eaton, N. R. (2010). Personality traits and the classification of mental disorders: Toward a more complete integration in *DSM–5* and an empirical model of psychopathology. *Personality Disorders: Theory, Research, and Treatment, 1,* 97–118.

Krueger, R. F., Eaton, N. R., Clark, L. A., Watson, D., Markon, K. E., Derringer, J., ... Livesley, W. J. (in press). Deriving an empirical structure of personality pathology for *DSM–5. Journal of Personality Disorders, 25,* 170–191.

Krueger, R. F., & Markon, K. E. (2006). Reinterpreting comorbidity: A model-based approach to understanding and classifying psychopathology. *Annual Review of Clinical Psychology, 2,* 111–133.

Krueger, R. F., Markon, K. E., Patrick, C. J., & Iacono, W. G. (2005). Externalizing psychopathology in adulthood: A dimensional-spectrum conceptualization and its implications for *DSM–V. Journal of Abnormal Psychology, 114,* 537–550.

Krueger, R. F., & Tackett, J. L. (2003). Personality and psychopathology: Working toward the bigger picture. *Journal of Personality Disorders, 17,* 109–128.

Leary, T. (1957). *Interpersonal diagnosis of personality.* New York, NY: Ronald.

Lenzenweger, M. F., Johnson, M. D., & Willet, J. B. (2004). Individual growth curve analysis illuminates stability and change in personality disorder features: The Longitudinal Study of Personality Disorders. *Archives of General Psychiatry, 61,* 1015–1024.

Livesley, W. J. (2003). *Practical management of personality disorder.* New York, NY: Guilford.

Livesley, W. J., & Jang, K. L. (2005). Differentiating normal, abnormal, and disordered personality. *European Journal of Personality, 19,* 257–268.

Locke, K. D. (2000). Circumplex scales of interpersonal values: Reliability, validity, and applicability to interpersonal problems and personality disorders. *Journal of Personality Assessment, 75*, 249–267.

Locke, K. D., & Sadler, P. (2007). Self-efficacy, values, and complementarity in dyadic interactions: Integrating interpersonal and social-cognitive theory. *Personality and Social Psychology Bulletin, 33*, 94–109.

Luyten, P., & Blatt, S. J. (2011). Integrating theory-driven and empirically-derived models of personality development and psychopathology: A proposal for *DSM–V*. *Clinical Psychology Review, 31*, 52–68.

Lynam, D. R., & Widiger, T. A. (2001). Using the five-factor model to represent the *DSM–IV* personality disorders: An expert consensus approach. *Journal of Abnormal Psychology, 110*, 401–412.

Markon, K. E., Krueger, R. F., & Watson, D. (2005). Delineating the structure of normal and abnormal personality: An integrative hierarchical approach. *Journal of Personality and Social Psychology, 88*, 139–157.

Meehl, P. E. (1992). Factors and taxa, traits and types, differences of degree and differences of kind. *Journal of Personality, 60*, 117–174.

Miller, J. D., Gaughan, E. T., Prior, L. R., Kamen, C., & Campbell, W. K. (2009). Is research using the NPI relevant for understanding Narcissistic Personality Disorder? *Journal of Research in Personality, 43*, 482–488.

Mischel, W., & Shoda, Y. (1998). Reconciling processing dynamics and personality dispositions. *Annual Review of Psychology, 49*, 229–258.

Molenaar, P. C. M. (2004). A manifesto on psychology as idiographic science: Bringing the person back into scientific psychology, this time forever. *Measurement, 2*, 201–218.

Molenaar, P. C. M., & Campbell, C. G. (2009). The new person-specific paradigm in psychology. *Current Directions in Psychological Science, 18*, 112–117.

Morey, L. C., Gunderson, J., Quigley, B. D., & Lyons, M. (2000). Dimensions and categories: The "big five" factors and the *DSM* personality disorders. *Assessment, 7*, 203–216.

Morey, L. C., Gunderson, J., Quigley, B. D., Shea, M. T., Skodol, A. E., McGlashan, T. H., . . . Zanarini, M. C. (2002). The representation of borderline, avoidant, obsessive-compulsive, and schizotypal personality disorders by the five-factor model. *Journal of Personality Disorders, 16*, 215–234.

Morey, L. C., Hopwood, C. J., Gunderson, J. G., Skodol, A. E., Shea, M. T., Yen, S., . . . McGlashan, T. H. (2007). Comparison of alternative models for personality disorders. *Psychological Medicine, 37*, 983–994.

Morf, C. C., Horvath, S., & Torchetti, L. (2010). Narcissistic self-enhancement: Tales of (successful?) self-portrayal. In M. D. Alicke & C. Sedikides (Eds.), *Handbook of self-enhancement and self-protection* (pp. 399–424). New York, NY: Guilford.

Moskowitz, D. S., Russell, J. J., Sadikaj, G., & Sutton, R. (2009). Measuring people intensively. *Canadian Psychology, 50*, 131–140.

Nesselroade, J. R., & Ford, D. H. (1985). P-technique comes of age: Multivariate, replicated, single-subject designs for research on older adults. *Research on Aging, 7*, 46–80.

Nock, M. K., Prinstein, M. J., & Sterba, S. (2009). Revealing the form and function of self-injurious thoughts and behaviors: A real-time ecological assessment study among adolescents and young adults. *Journal of Abnormal Psychology, 118*, 816–827.

O'Connor, B. P. (2002). The search for dimensional structure differences between normality and abnormality: A statistical review of published data on personality and psychopathology. *Journal of Personality and Social Psychology, 83*, 962–982.

Pilkonis, P. A., Hallquist, M. N., Morse, J. Q., & Stepp, S. D. (2011). Striking the (im)proper balance between scientific advances and clinical utility: Commentary on the *DSM–5* proposal for personality disorders. *Personality Disorders: Theory, Research, and Treatment, 2*, 68–82.

Pincus, A. L. (2005). A contemporary integrative interpersonal theory of personality disorders. In J. Clarkin & M. Lenzenweger (Eds.), *Major theories of personality disorder* (2nd ed., pp. 282–331). New York, NY: Guilford.

Pincus, A. L. (2011). Some comments on nomology, diagnostic process, and narcissistic personality disorder in the *DSM–5* proposal for personality and personality disorders. *Personality Disorders: Theory, Research, and Treatment, 2*, 41–53.

Pincus, A. L., & Hopwood, C. J. (in press). A contemporary interpersonal model of personality pathology and personality disorder. In T. A. Widiger (Ed.), *The Oxford handbook of personality disorders*. New York, NY: Oxford University Press.

Pincus, A. L., & Lukowitsky, M. R. (2010). Pathological narcissism and narcissistic personality disorder. *Annual Review of Clinical Psychology, 6*, 421–446.

Pincus, A. L., Lukowitsky, M. R., & Wright, A. G. C. (2010). The interpersonal nexus of personality and psychopathology. In T. Millon, R. Kreuger, & E. Simonsen (Eds.), *Contemporary directions in psychopathology: Scientific foundations for DSM–V and ICD–11* (pp. 523–552). New York, NY: Guilford.

Pincus, A. L., Lukowitsky, M. R., Wright, A. G. C., & Eichler, W. C. (2009). The interpersonal nexus of persons, situations, and psychopathology. *Journal of Research in Personality, 43*, 264–265.

Pincus, A. L., & Wright, A. G. C. (2010). Interpersonal diagnosis of psychopathology. In L. M. Horowitz & S. Strack (Eds.), *Handbook of interpersonal psychology: Theory, research, and therapeutic interventions* (pp. 359–381). Hoboken, NJ: Wiley.

Ram, N., & Gerstorf, D. (2009). Time-structured and net intraindividual variability: Tools for examining the development of dynamic characteristics and processes. *Psychology and Aging, 24*, 778–791.

Reis, H. T. (2008). Reinvigorating the concept of situation in social psychology. *Personality and Social Psychology Review, 12*, 311–329.

Reisch, T., Ebner-Priemer, U. W., Tschacher, W., Bohus, M., & Linehan, M. M. (2008). Sequences of emotions in patients with borderline personality disorder. *Acta Psychiatrica Scandinavica, 118*, 42–48.

Reynolds, S. K., & Clark, L. A. (2001). Predicting dimensions of personality disorder from domains and facets of the five-factor model. *Journal of Personality, 69*, 199–222.

Rhadigan, C., & Huprich, S. K. (in press). The utility of the Cognitive Affective Processing System in the diagnosis of personality disorders: Some preliminary evidence. *Journal of Personality Disorders*.

Russell, J. J., Moskowitz, D. S., Zuroff, D. C., Sookman, D., & Paris, J. (2007). Stability and variability of affective experience and interpersonal behavior in borderline personality disorder. *Journal of Abnormal Psychology, 116*, 578–588.

Sadikaj, G., Moskowitz, D. S., Russell, J. J., & Zuroff, D. C. (2010, June). *On the dynamic association between interpersonal perception, interpersonal behavior, and affect: Effects of social anxiety and borderline personality disorder*. Paper presented at the 13th annual meeting of the Society for Interpersonal Theory and Research, Philadelphia, PA.

Sadikaj, G., Russell, J. J., Moskowitz, D. S., & Paris, J. (2010). Affect dysregulation in individuals with borderline personality disorder: Persistence and interpersonal triggers. *Journal of Personality Assessment, 92*, 490–500.

Sadler, P., Woody, E., & Ethier, N. (2010). Complementarity in interpersonal relationships. In L. M. Horowitz & S. Strack (Eds.), *Handbook of interpersonal psychology: Theory, research, and therapeutic interventions* (pp. 123–141). Hoboken, NJ: Wiley.

Samuel, D. B. (2011/this issue). Assessing personality in the *DSM–5*: The utility of bipolar constructs. *Journal of Personality Assessment, 93*, 390–397.

Samuel, D. B., & Widiger, T. A. (2008). A meta-analytic review of the relationships between the five-factor model and *DSM–IV–TR* personality disorders: A facet level analysis. *Clinical Psychology Review, 28*, 1326–1342.

Saulsman, L. M., & Page, A. C. (2004). The five-factor model and personality disorder empirical literature: A meta-analytic review. *Clinical Psychology Review, 23*, 1055–1085.

Schmideberg, M. (1959). The borderline patient. In S. Arieti (Ed.), *American handbook of psychiatry* (Vol. 1, pp. 398–416). New York, NY: Basic Books.

Shedler, J., Beck, A., Fonagy, P., Gabbard, G. O., Gunderson, J., Kernberg, O., . . . Westen, D. (2010). Personality disorders in *DSM–5*. *The American Journal of Psychiatry, 167*, 1026–1028.

Shoda, Y., Mischel, W., & Wright, J. C. (1994). Intraindividual stability in the organization and patterning of behavior: Incorporating psychological situations into the idiographic analysis of personality. *Journal of Personality and Social Psychology, 67*, 674–687.

Skodol, A. E. (2008). Longitudinal course and outcome of personality disorders. *Psychiatric Clinics of North America, 31*, 495–503.

Skodol, A. E., & Bender, D. S. (2009). The future of personality disorders in the *DSM–V? American Journal of Psychiatry, 166*, 388–391.

Sullivan, H. S. (1953). *The interpersonal theory of psychiatry.* New York, NY: Norton.

Sullivan, H. S. (1954). *The psychiatric interview.* New York, NY: Norton.

Tracey, T. J. G., & Rohlfing, J. E. (2010). Variations in the understanding of interpersonal behavior: Adherence to the interpersonal circle as a moderator of the rigidity psychological well-being relation. *Journal of Personality, 78*, 711–746.

Trull, T. J. (2005). Dimensional models of personality disorder: Coverage and cutoffs. *Journal of Personality Disorders, 19*, 262–283.

Trull, T. J., Solhan, M. B., Tragesser, S. L., Jahng, S., Wood, P. K., Piaskecki, T. M., & Watson, D. (2008). Affective instability: Measuring a core feature of borderline personality disorder with ecological momentary assessment. *Journal of Abnormal Psychology, 117*, 647–661.

Wakefield, J. (2008). The perils of dimensionalization: Challenge in distinguishing negative traits from personality disorders. *Psychiatric Clinics of North America, 31*, 379–393.

Waller, N. G., & Meehl, P. E. (1998). *Multivariate taxometric procedures: Distinguishing types from continua.* Thousand Oaks, CA: Sage.

Westen, D. (1995). A clinical-empirical model of personality: Life after the Mischelian ice age and the NEO-lithic era. *Journal of Personality, 63*, 495–524.

Widiger, T. A. (1993). The *DSM–III–R* categorical personality disorder diagnoses: A critique and an alternative. *Psychological Inquiry, 4*, 75–90.

Widiger, T. A., & Clark, L. A. (2000). Toward *DSM–V* and the classification of psychopathology. *Psychological Bulletin, 126*, 946–963.

Widiger, T. A., Livesley, W. J., & Clark, L. A. (2009). An integrative dimensional classification of personality disorder. *Psychological Assessment, 21*, 243–255.

Widiger, T. A., & Samuel, D. B. (2005). Diagnostic categories or dimensions? A question for the *Diagnostic and statistical manual of mental disorders–Fifth edition. Journal of Abnormal Psychology, 114*, 494–504.

Widiger, T. A., & Simonsen, E. (2005). Alternative dimensional models of personality disorder: Finding a common ground. *Journal of Personality Disorders, 19*, 110–130.

Widiger, T. A., & Trull, T. J. (2007). Plate tectonics in the classification of personality disorder: Shifting to a dimensional model. *American Psychologist, 62*, 71–83.

Wiggins, J. S., & Pincus, H. A. (1989). Conceptions of personality disorder and dimensions of personality. *Psychological Assessment: A Journal of Consulting and Clinical Psychology, 1*, 305–316.

Wiggins, J. S., & Trapnell, P. D. (1996). A dyadic-interactional perspective on the five-factor model. In J. S. Wiggins (Ed.), *The five-factor model of personality: Theoretical perspectives* (pp. 88–162). New York, NY: Guilford.

Wright, A. G. C., Pincus, A. L., & Lenzenweger, M. F. (2010). Modeling stability and change in Borderline Personality Disorder symptoms using the Revised Interpersonal Adjective Scales–Big Five (IASR–B5). *Journal of Personality Assessment, 92*, 501–513.

A Comparison of Passive–Aggressive and Negativistic Personality Disorders

Christopher J. Hopwood[1] and Aidan G. C. Wright[2,3]

[1]Department of Psychology, Michigan State University
[2]Department of Psychology, The Pennsylvania State University
[3]Western Psychiatric Institute and Clinic, Pittsburgh, Pennsylvania

Passive–aggressive personality disorder (PAPD) has historically played an important role in clinical theorizing and was diagnosable prior to the *Diagnostic and Statistical Manual of Mental Disorders* (4th ed. [*DSM–IV*]; American Psychiatric Association, 1994), in which the construct was relabeled negativistic (NEGPD), expanded to include negative affective symptoms, and appendicized. In this study we tested the hypothesis that the expansion of PAPD to include content related to negative moods and nonspecific personality pathology compromised its discriminant validity. In an undergraduate sample ($N = 1,215$), a self-report measure of PAPD was only moderately related to NEGPD and showed less diagnostic overlap with other personality disorders than NEGPD. Furthermore, a conjoint factor analysis yielded a strong first factor (moodiness) that appeared less specific to passive–aggressive behavior than 3 other factors (irresponsibility, inadequacy, and contempt). We conclude that future research on this potentially important clinical construct should focus on core passive–aggressive features and abandon the negativistic content that has been added to it in successive editions of the *DSM*.

The term *passive–aggressive* was first used clinically during World War II to describe soldiers who refused to comply with officers' demands (Millon, 1981). However, the concept has been central to clinical theorizing, for instance in the form of anal or masochistic character types (Abraham, 1925; Fenichel, 1945; Reich, 1949), for nearly a century and has been featured in personality disorder (PD) models from a variety of contemporary theoretical orientations (Beck, Freeman, Davis, & Associates, 2003; Benjamin, 1993; Fine, Overholser, & Berkoff, 1992; Lazarus, 1971; McCrae, 1994; Millon, 1981; Stone, 1993). Clinicians and clinical theorists seem to continue to value the concept. For instance, Benjamin (1993) recommends routine assessment of passive–aggressive features because of the potential for passive–aggressive behavior to undermine the successful treatment of other primary (e.g., Axis I) conditions.

In the first edition of the *Diagnostic and Statistical Manual of Mental Disorders* (*DSM*; American Psychiatric Association, 1952), passive–aggressive personality disorder (PAPD) was conceptualized as having three types. Passive–dependent patients were helpless, indecisive, and clingy. This type eventually became dependent PD. The passive–aggressive type was pouty, stubborn, inefficient, and prone to procrastination and obstruction. The aggressive type was irritable, destructive, and resentful, with an underlying dependency thought to differentiate these behaviors from antisocial personality. Features of the latter two types were merged in the *DSM–II* (American Psychiatric Association, 1968), in which PAPD symptoms included obstructionism, pouting, procrastination, intentional inefficiency, and stubbornness, each of which were thought to reflect hostility that the individual was unable to express openly.

The retention of PAPD in the *DSM–III* (American Psychiatric Association, 1980) was controversial because some work group members believed that passive–aggressive symptoms reflected a specific behavioral response to particular situations rather than a broad personality syndrome (Millon, 1981; Wetzler & Morey, 1999). It was retained, but unlike other *DSM–III* PDs, clinicians could only diagnose PAPD if the patient did not meet criteria for any other PD. Symptoms included resistance to demands for adequate social or occupational performance in the form of procrastination, dawdling, stubbornness, intentional inefficiency, and apparent forgetfulness. In the *DSM–III–R* (American Psychiatric Association, 1987), PAPD criteria were expanded to include more negative emotional features such as sulking, irritability, and argumentativeness in addition to passive–aggressive behaviors, and the exclusion criterion was dropped.

In *DSM–IV* (American Psychiatric Association, 1994), the diagnostic criteria were expanded further, the disorder was renamed *negativistic* (NEGPD), and it was appendicized. Symptoms included passive resistance to routine social or occupational tasks, complaints of being misunderstood, sullen argumentativeness, criticism and scorn of authority, envy and resentment of the relatively fortunate, exaggerated complaints of personal misfortune, and alternation between hostility and contrition. Millon (1993), who championed the decision to expand and rename PAPD as a member of the *DSM–IV* PD work group, offered several rationales, including that (a) the disorder had not received sufficient acceptance in the clinical literature, (b) its content was too narrow and behavioral, (c) passive–aggressive behavior was too situational to reflect a syndrome, (d) the term implies a particular motivation in a time when PD criteria were descriptive, thus diagnosis would require clinical inference, and (e) PAPD overlapped too much with other disorders.

The proposed solution was to focus on "negativistic attitudes" thought to underlie passive–aggressive behavior. The general argument of this article is that the increasing focus on negativism that characterized the PAPD, and eventually NEGPD, diagnosis over time significantly altered and decreased the specificity and clinical utility of the construct. It is ironic that this move, which might have spared PAPD from the diagnostic graveyard in the *DSM–III–R* and *DSM–IV,* might have led to its ultimate demise, as represented by indifference to the construct in most contemporary research and the *DSM–5.* Currently the prevailing mood is to cut PD diagnoses, and constructs that are not commonly researched and do not offer demonstrably unique clinical value are the first on the chopping block (Skodol et al., 2011).

Indeed, NEGPD might have contributed to the problems described by Millon (1993) at least as much as it has helped to solve them. Regarding acceptance in the clinical literature, Wetzler and Morey (1999) noted that passive–aggressive behavior was as acceptable among researchers and clinicians as most other PDs during the time of *DSM–III* and *DSM–III–R,* but it has been studied much less often than most other PDs since that time. Although passive–aggressive behavior is narrow and behavioral, it is understood in clinical theory to be driven by certain relatively stable personality dynamics (e.g., Beck et al., 2003; Benjamin, 1993; Kernberg, 1985; Stone, 1993). Thus, the critique that *DSM–III–R* symptoms were too narrow and behavioral might say more about the atheoretical approach of the *DSM–III* than passive–aggressive personality per se. The notion that pre–*DSM–IV* passive–aggressive personality is too situational to reflect a syndrome conflicts with the relatively high prevalence rates of *DSM–III–R* PAPD (Morey, 1988), given that symptoms must be persistent to achieve the diagnosis. Furthermore, recent evidence that PD symptoms are generally less stable than was previously thought (Lenzenweger, Johnson, & Willett, 2004; Morey et al., 2007) make stability a questionable criterion for the validity of PD constructs. That the level of inference required to diagnose PAPD was seen as problematic says more about the descriptive focus of the *DSM–III* and *DSM–IV* than the construct itself, and we would suggest that this issue is more effectively framed as a measurement question: Can PAPD be reliably measured? Seen this way, mixing in content that is not directly related to the theoretical construct would likely make reliable measurement more challenging, not less (see Bradley, Shedler, & Westen, 2006, for an alternative approach to measuring PAPD).

In this article, we focus primarily on Millon's fifth reason for expanding PAPD: its overlap with other disorders. Diagnostic overlap, a serious problem with all *DSM–III* and *DSM–IV* PDs, is driven primarily by the tendency for many PDs to share certain features, and in particular a tendency to experience negative emotions and to be interpersonally antagonistic (Samuel & Widiger, 2008). Thus adding criteria involving moodiness, antagonism, and feeling misunderstood to any disorder would tend to decrease its discriminant validity. We therefore suspect that adding negativistic content to PAPD lessened discriminant validity and decreased its unique potential to describe patients.

Folding content related to nonspecific personality pathology into the PAPD diagnosis also might have decreased the likelihood of identifying its core features by creating "noise" in the PAPD "signal." Research on the structure of NEGPD is ambiguous, with some covariance analyses suggesting multidimensionality (Rotenstein et al., 2007) and others suggesting a single dimension (Hopwood et al., 2009). However, no study yet has conducted a conjoint analysis of PAPD and NEGPD features. Given that criteria were both expanded in content and trimmed in number in the transition from PAPD to NEGPD, a conjoint analysis of PAPD and NEGPD criteria will permit the identification of more dimensions than an analysis of the criteria of only one operationalization, and will facilitate distinctions between dimensions that appear to be closer or more distal to the theoretical core of passive aggression.

Identifying underlying dimensions will also permit an examination of the correlates of the various features of PAPD and NEGPD. Recent research suggests that the disorder is influenced by both genes (Czajkowski et al., 2008) and an abusive environment (Grover et al., 2007; Hopwood et al., 2009), predictive of clinical outcomes such as presence of anxiety disorder (Johnson, Cohen, Kasen, & Brook, 2006; Rotenstein et al., 2007), suicidal behavior (Joiner & Rudd, 2002), and dysfunction (Hopwood et al., 2009), and linked to poor response to treatment of other disorders (Fricke et al., 2006). In terms of personality features, research suggests that PAPD is related to concerns about autonomy (Morse, Robins, & Gittes-Fox, 2002), and is associated with higher levels of neuroticism, manipulativeness, and aggression and lower levels of agreeableness and conscientiousness (Hopwood et al., 2009). However these correlations do not speak to the potential for different underlying components of the construct to have varying relations with criterion variables. Furthermore, this research is unable to evaluate the degree to which criterion relations are a function of nonspecific features that PAPD and NEGPD share with many other PDs as opposed to their being explained by specific aspects of passive–aggressive personality.

In summary, despite the historical relevance of passive aggression to a number of influential clinical theories, empirical research on the construct is limited (Blashfield & Intoccia, 2000; Boschen & Warner, 2009) and the diagnosis has been abandoned by the *DSM.* We hypothesize that the saturation of the PAPD diagnosis with nonspecific distress and interpersonal dysfunction that is common across PDs but not particular to passive–aggressive behavior contributed to this trajectory. We also suspect that passive aggression is a unique and clinically important construct despite historical problems in operationalizing it, and believe that PAPD is worthy of further investigation. Thus we aim to begin the process of building an empirical basis for future decisions about the nosological status of passive–aggressive personality by articulating what is and what is not uniquely PAPD. Specifically, our goal is to evaluate the impact of the negativistic content that has been added to it in the last two editions of the *DSM,* and to begin the process of separating this negativistic content from PAPD.

We first correlated *DSM–III–R* PAPD and *DSM–IV* NEGPD with one another and with other *DSM–IV* PDs. We hypothesized that the emphasis of NEGPD on symptoms involving a general propensity to experience negative emotions reduced the syndrome's discriminant validity, such that correlations with other PDs would be uniformly higher for NEGPD than for PAPD. We next evaluated the structure of passive–aggressive personality pathology via conjoint factor analysis of PAPD and NEGPD symptoms. We then related the dimensions revealed by this analysis to a number of clinically relevant outcomes, including PDs, mood, attachment style, and interpersonal problems, to evaluate the differential relations among passive–aggressive features. This conjoint structure and criterion associations were exploratory given the absence of comparable analyses in previous research. Nevertheless, we generally expected some dimensions to be more closely linked to theoretical conceptions of passive–aggressive behavior, whereas others we expected to reflect nonspecific distress and dysfunction (i.e., "negativism").

METHOD

Participants

We sampled 1,453 undergraduates who were compensated with course credit for participating in this study approved by the institutional review board. Of these, 1,215 responded to at least 95% of all study items and had scores that were less than 2.5 SDs higher than a community mean on a scale measuring random responding (Morey's [1991] Personality Assessment Inventory Infrequency scale), and were thus retained for further analyses. The average age was 19.02 ($SD = 1.68$); 644 (53.0%) were female, and 1,042 (85.8%) were non-Hispanic Caucasian.

Measures

We administered the Personality Diagnostic Questionnaire–4+ (PDQ–4+; Hyler, 1994), a self-report questionnaire with a true–false item response format and items that correspond directly to DSM content, to measure NEGPD ($\alpha = .58$, average corrected interitem $r = .30$) and the PDQ–R (Hyler, Skodol, Kellman, Oldham, & Rosnick, 1990) to measure $DSM–III–R$ PAPD ($\alpha = .60$, interitem $r = .27$). On average respondents reported having 1.80 ($SD = 1.59$) of 7 possible NEGPD symptoms and 2.26 ($SD = 1.85$) of 9 possible PAPD symptoms. The PDQ–4+ was also used to assess other $DSM–IV$ PDs, which were treated as criterion variables (Mdn $\alpha = .57$, Mdn of average corrected interitem correlations $= .29$). These somewhat low values might be due to factors such as the multidimensionality of some PDs, binary response format, and limitations of the DSM criteria in terms of content coverage. Importantly for the current study, low internal consistencies did not appear to be due to the potential for range restriction in student samples, as on average students had around four PAPD or NEGPD symptoms, variabilities were substantial, and skew tended to be modest ($Mdn = .73$). This is consistent with previous research that shows relatively higher rates of PD endorsement on questionnaire relative to interview assessments (Hyler et al., 1990) as well as heightened rates of PD psychopathology among young adults (Grant et al., 2004). It is also reassuring that internal consistency appears to have limited impacts on criterion-validity estimates (McCrae, Kurtz, Yamagata, & Terraciano, 2010; Schmitt, 1996).

We also administered three non-PD criterion measures. The Revised Experiences in Close Relationships scale (Fraley, Waller, & Brennan, 2000) is a 36-item measure of the anxiety ($\alpha = .75$, interitem $r = .49$) and avoidance ($\alpha = .76$, interitem $r = .50$) dimensions of attachment. The Inventory of Interpersonal Problems–Short Circumplex (Soldz, Budman, Demby, & Merry, 1995) is a 32-item measure of interpersonal problems with a total score reflecting overall interpersonal distress ($\alpha = .88$, interitem $r = .60$) and indicators of difficulties related to agency and communion based on linear combinations of eight circumplex octant scores (Mdn $\alpha = .79$). The trait version of the 20-item Positive Affect Negative Affect Scales (Watson, Clark, & Tellegen, 1988) was used to measure dimensions reflecting propensities for negative (e.g., anger, sadness, shame; $\alpha = .88$, interitem $r = .60$) and positive (e.g., happiness, excitement, joy; $\alpha = .88$, interitem $r = .62$) emotions.

TABLE 1.—Correlations of $DSM–III–R$ passive–aggressive, $DSM–IV$ negativistic, and other $DSM–IV$ personality disorders.

$DSM–IV$ Criterion Disorder	$DSM–III–R$ Passive–Aggressive	$DSM–IV$ Negativistic	Steiger's Z
Negativistic	.52**	—	
Paranoid	.38**	.52**	5.77**
Schizoid	.30**	.30**	0.00
Schizotypal	.38**	.45**	2.81*
Histrionic	.33**	.45**	4.75**
Narcissistic	.37**	.52**	6.16**
Borderline	.44**	.61**	7.51**
Antisocial	.37**	.41**	1.58
Avoidant	.36**	.43**	2.77*
Dependent	.40**	.46**	2.43*
Obsessive–Compulsive	.28**	.40**	4.62**

Note. $DSM–III–R$ = Diagnostic and Statistical Manual of Mental Disorders (3rd ed., revised; American Psychiatric Association, 1987); $DSM–IV$ = Diagnostic and Statistical Manual of Mental Disorders (4th ed.; American Psychiatric Association, 1994).
*$p < .01$. **$p < .001$.

Analyses

We first correlated PAPD and NEGPD to one another and to other $DSM–IV$ PDs to test their overlap and discriminant validity. We tested differences between dependent correlations using Steiger's (1980) z test at Type I error probabilities of .01 and .001. We next conducted a conjoint factor analysis on the tetrachoric correlation matrix of PAPD and NEGPD items in M$plus$. Weighted least squares (mean and variance adjusted) estimation was applied to account for the nonnormality of dichotomous items. We requested an oblique geomin rotation to achieve a desirable balance between factor complexity and interpretability (Sass & Schmitt, 2010). Scales were constructed based on the results of this analysis. These scales were then related to outcome criteria via bivariate correlations and multiple regression models to investigate the nomological net of passive–aggressive features. Given the large number of analyses and relatively large sample size, we used Type I error rates of .001 and focused interpretively on effect sizes in this family of analyses.

RESULTS

Correlations between PDs are listed in Table 1. The correlation between PAPD and NEGPD was somewhat modest (.52), suggesting that the change from PAPD to NEGPD was substantial. In fact, this value is significantly lower than the correlation between NEGPD and borderline PD ($z = 3.86$, $p < .001$), and is equal to correlations between NEGPD and paranoid and narcissistic PDs.

Our first hypothesis was that PAPD would demonstrate superior discriminant validity to NEGPD. Overall, 9 out of 10 correlations were larger for NEGPD than PAPD (binomial probability $< .01$), with eight of these differences being statistically significant at $p < .01$. On average, the NEGPD correlations were greater than the PAPD correlations by .09. To provide context for interpreting these correlations, we note that the average of the intercorrelations between all of the personality disorders was .41, and the standard deviation of these intercorrelations was .09. A majority of the correlates for PAPD were within 1 SD of this mean, whereas we found that three correlations for NEGPD (with paranoid, narcissistic, and borderline PDs) were more than 1 *SD* higher than the mean. Each of these coefficients is also more than .10 larger than the corresponding correlation for PAPD, a difference that is in each case statistically significant at $p < .001$.

We next conducted a conjoint factor analysis of PAPD and NEGPD symptoms. A four-factor solution was selected as the first four factors appeared to be interpretable and had eigenvalues >1. The fit of this model was excellent (root mean square error of approximation = .03, 90% confidence interval [.025, .039]; comparative fit index = .98). Although the fifth factor also had an eigenvalue >1 (1.04), one of its factors was almost completely influenced by a single item (NEGPD: "Others consider me moody or 'hot-tempered'") that also showed a sizable loading (.40) on another factor. We consequently retained a four-factor solution.

Eigenvalues, geomin-rotated factor pattern coefficients, and factor correlations for this model are given in Table 2. The first factor had pattern coefficients greater than .40 on four NEGPD and three PAPD criteria involving negative emotions, resentment, and moodiness. Three PAPD and one NEGPD criteria that reflect irresponsibility, such as forgetting or procrastinating undesirable responsibilities and working slowly or poorly, comprised the second factor. The third factor had sizable loadings on three PAPD criteria that, when reverse scored, appear to reflect work-related insecurity, credit-seeking, and inadequacy. The fourth factor included two NEGPD and three PAPD criteria referring to feeling underappreciated, authority conflicts or need for approval at work, and contempt.

Scores were computed for each of these factors by summing corresponding items (i.e., those in bold in Table 2). Alphas for the factors were as follows: moodiness = .67 (corrected average interitem $r = .38$), irresponsibility = .61 (interitem $r = .39$), inadequacy = .57 (interitem $r = .39$), and contempt = .47 (interitem $r = .26$). Some of these values are lower than might be desirable, likely because of problems related to the *DSM* and PDQ as discussed earlier as well as the limited saturation of these apparent subdimensions of passive–aggressive personality pathology in this measure and corresponding low number of items for each factor. Again, it is noteworthy that internal consistency values in this range have a limited effect on criterion validity (Schmitt, 1996). Table 3 shows bivariate correlations between these factors and criterion variables, as well as R^2 values and β weights from multiple regression models in which the four conjoint PAPD and NEGPD scale scores predicted each criterion variable.

Of particular relevance to study hypotheses, moodiness demonstrates the strongest overlap with other PDs. Moodiness also showed the strongest correlations with negative affectivity, anxious attachment, and generalized interpersonal problems. This pattern is consistent with the hypothesis that the broadening of the passive–aggressive construct to include negativistic symptoms worsened discriminant validity by saturating PAPD with criteria involving a general tendency to experience distress and dysfunction. As such, the best clues as to what is unique about passive–aggressive personality might lie in the composition and correlates of the other three dimensions.

Contempt and irresponsibility also showed consistent overlap with other PDs, although this overlap was of a lesser magnitude than that of moodiness, particularly for irresponsibility. Contempt was most strongly related to paranoid, schizotypal, and narcissistic PDs. It was also associated with negative affectivity, coldness, avoidant attachment, and interpersonal distress. This pattern suggests that it shares with moodiness a propensity for negative affectivity, but it is differentiated based on interpersonal characteristics. Whereas moodiness connotes more generalized interpersonal problems, contempt is more specific to interpersonal coldness, insecurity, and mistrust. This pattern suggests that mistrustful, idiosyncratic, and self-focused rumination about others' unjust or abusive behavior and consequent contempt might be a core aspect of passive–aggressive personality.

Irresponsibility showed the strongest correlations with antisocial PD, and also had unique associations with low positive affect and attachment avoidance. This factor seems to involve an immature aspect of personality in which negative emotions or interpersonal disruptions characteristically lead to irresponsible behavior. The management of distress through ineffective interpersonal behavior and neglect of responsibilities is a central aspect of most theories of passive aggression.

Inadequacy had the weakest correlations with PDs, and in fact regression coefficients were mostly negative, suggesting perhaps a suppression effect in the regression models that indicates a very weak relation between inadequacy and generalized personality pathology. It also correlated negatively with positive

TABLE 2.—Results from conjoint factor analysis of passive–aggressive and negativistic personality disorder symptoms.

	1	2	3	4
Eigenvalues	4.88	2.16	1.44	1.11
Pattern coefficients				
Others have complained that I do not fulfill my obligations. (N)	.01	**.62**	.11	.05
I am not understood or appreciated. (N)	.27	.17	−.05	**.36**
People think I am moody and have a temper. (N)	**.56**	−.04	.21	.11
I do not like supervisors telling me how I should do my job. (N)	.14	.14	.03	**.56**
I resent people who are luckier than me. (N)	**.50**	.03	−.07	.25
I complain about my difficulties. (N)	**.68**	−.07	.08	.00
I am sometimes so nasty to others that I have to apologize later. (N)	**.60**	−.02	−.06	−.11
I procrastinate too much. (P)	−.03	**.79**	.05	.05
I get irritable with people rather than openly refusing to do something they want. (P)	**.58**	.21	.05	−.02
I screw things up for people whom I resent. (P)	**.43**	**.44**	−.05	−.01
I don't like it when people want me to do things that are not my job. (P)	**.54**	.14	.03	.09
I am forgetful about things I do not like doing. (P)	.28	**.54**	−.03	−.06
People appreciate my hard work. (P) (R)	−.04	.03	**.45**	**.40**
I am grateful for suggestions about how I could improve my work performance. (P) (R)	.00	−.05	**.56**	**.52**
People see me as a worker who does my fair share. (P) (R)	.02	.05	**1.15**	−.04
I could do a better job than my supervisors. (P)	.00	−.07	−.05	**.53**
Factor correlations				
2	.41			
3	−.01	.18		
4	.32	.22	.12	—

Note. All items are paraphrased from the Personality Diagnostic Questionnaire, which is copyrighted by Steven Hyler, and do not reflect actual item content. (N) indicates *Diagnostic and Statistical Manual of Mental Disorders* (4th ed.; American Psychiatric Association, 1994) negativistic criteria; (P) indicates *Diagnostic and Statistical Manual of Mental Disorders* (3rd ed., rev.; American Psychiatric Association, 1987) passive–aggressive criteria; (R) indicates item was reverse-scored prior to analysis. The fifth eigenvalue = .99. The correlation matrix on which this analysis was conducted is available on request. Note that it is possible with certain rotations, including Geomin, to observe pattern coefficients >1, as is the case here for one coefficient on the third factor. Values > .39 in bold.

TABLE 3.—Bivariate and partial associations of passive–aggressive/negativistic features with personality disorders, mood, attachment styles, and interpersonal problems.

	R^2	Moodiness		Irresponsibility		Inadequacy		Contempt	
		r	β	r	β	r	β	r	β
Personality disorders									
Paranoid	.31*	.49*	.42*	.27*	−.03	.11*	−.15*	.37*	.34*
Schizoid	.13*	.23*	.07	.24*	.15*	.16*	−.05	.31*	.28*
Schizotypal	.27*	.37*	.16*	.34*	.18*	.12*	−.20*	.40*	.43*
Antisocial	.19*	.34*	.16*	.38*	.26*	.12*	−.03	.26*	.16*
Borderline	.37*	.58*	.48*	.38*	.07	.13*	−.07	.34*	.22*
Histrionic	.21*	.45*	.39*	.29*	.06	.07	−.04	.20*	.10
Narcissistic	.26*	.45*	.35*	.29*	.04	.09	−.16*	.34*	.32*
Avoidant	.22*	.44*	.35*	.30*	.08	.12*	−.04	.27*	.17*
Dependent	.25*	.48*	.38*	.37*	.15*	.14*	.05	.23*	.05
Obsessive–Compulsive	.22*	.42*	.37*	.23*	−.01	−.04	−.24*	.21*	.25*
Mood									
Negative affect	.22*	.43*	.36*	.29*	.07	.19*	.08	.28*	.11
Positive affect	.16*	−.24*	−.07	−.33*	−.28*	−.24*	−.20*	−.21*	.00
Attachment styles									
Avoidance	.07*	.10*	−.07	.23*	.23*	.16*	.06	.18*	.11
Anxiety	.14*	.37*	.36*	.18*	−.03	.10*	.01	.20*	.09
Interpersonal problems									
Interpersonal Distress	.23*	.45*	.36*	.32*	.08	.13*	−.02	.28*	.16*
Agentic problems	.03*	.15*	.20*	.01	−.11	.05	.02	.08	.03
Communal problems	.05*	−.01	.06	−.09	−.07	−.19*	−.10	−.19*	−.13*

Note. R^2 and β values are from regression models in which the four passive–aggressive/negativistic scales predicted the criterion scale in the left-most column.
*$p < .001$.

affectivity. Overall, this pattern suggests that inadequacy connotes a depressive and self-defeating tendency to be somewhat disorganized and affectively dull. One might question the centrality of this factor to passive–aggressive personality. Indeed, there are psychometric reasons to be skeptical. First, this pattern of weak correlations in general and negative correlations with PDs might simply reflect that the existence of the inadequacy factor is mostly due to the reverse-scored items on the PDQ. Second, this factor is heavily influenced by a single item involving the degree to which others view the respondent as being a good worker. Thus it is possible that it relates to actual work performance or concern with impressions, independent of the potentially passive–aggressive influences on that performance or concern.

DISCUSSION

This study was designed to evaluate the overlap of *DSM–III–R* PAPD and *DSM–IV* NEGPD to determine the effects of broadening diagnostic criteria and toward identifying core dimensions of passive–aggressive personality. Overall, our results suggest (a) modest correspondence between PAPD and NEGPD, (b) that the broadening of the construct to include more criteria involving generalized negative affectivity and dysfunction might have been detrimental in terms of discriminant validity, and (c) that core dimensions of passive–aggressive personality, at least in terms of *DSM* criteria, involve immature, irresponsible behavior, inner feelings of inadequacy and need for acknowledgment, and ruminative resentment about and contempt for authority figures.

Even though the *DSM–III–R* PAPD criteria included some "negativistic" features, the modest correspondence between

NEGPD and PAPD suggests substantial construct redefinition from *DSM–III–R* to *DSM–IV*. Of course this was intentional, and might have even served in the short term to save the diagnosis. However, it is also possible that this redefinition and the decision to place NEGPD in the *DSM–IV* appendix might have affected the lack of research on PAPD since the publication of *DSM–IV* despite the importance of passive–aggressive behavior in several clinical theories. Indeed, although there has been some research on the construct as previously described, most PAPD research has been the result of broader studies that assessed all PDs and in which PAPD was not the central construct of interest. There has been very little, if any, programmatic research on the construct. To the extent that passive–aggressive personality features are clinically important and risk being lost altogether in future editions of the diagnostic manual, it might be important for researchers to focus more on historical conceptions of passive–aggressive behavior than negativism.

This is particularly true because the oversampling of symptoms related to negative affectivity and generalized interpersonal dysfunction in the criteria appears to have compromised the discriminant validity of the disorder. NEGPD had stronger correlations with PDs than PAPD across the board. The first factor from our conjoint analysis, moodiness, was made up of NEGPD and PAPD items with negativistic content, and showed strong and consistent correlations with other PDs. This factor also had the strongest average correlation with other conjoint factors and correlated with generalized distress in the form of attachment anxiety, interpersonal problems, and negative affectivity. As such, it appears that the inclusion of these items significantly compromises the discriminant validity of passive–aggressive personality, as the items do not clearly reflect passive aggression, but instead indicate nonspecific personality dysfunction.

The fact that this was the first factor extracted and that more criteria showed strong pattern coefficients with it than any other factor demonstrate the extent to which PAPD was saturated with negativistic content, beginning in the *DSM–III–R* and continuing to a greater extent in *DSM–IV*. It is striking that 57% of NEGPD symptoms primarily involve moodiness. Future researchers interested in potentially unique aspects of passive–aggressive personality should conceptualize the construct independent of this nonspecific factor, and in general should focus on feelings, thoughts, and behaviors that are theoretically specific to passive aggression.

Based on this study, three such features might be worthy of further consideration. First, passive–aggressive individuals might tend to engage in irresponsible or unproductive behavior as a way of expressing negative emotions or interpersonal grievances. Second, this behavior could relate to an inner insecurity regarding one's value or worth, particularly with respect to authority figures. Third, passive–aggressive people might ruminate about how others treat them unfairly or disrespect them, and develop a deep but perhaps unexpressed sense of resentment and contempt.

We caution that the degree to which the nature of passive–aggressive personality can be understood based on the results of this study is constrained by the use of *DSM* criteria to operationalize the construct. We used *DSM* criteria because our primary purpose was to evaluate the impact of the change in conceptualization over the course of successive issues of the *DSM*, not to derive a canonical structure of PAPD moving forward. The *DSM* criteria are limited in a number of ways in terms of identifying the core features of passive–aggressive personality. For instance, the lack of motivational content in the atheoretical *DSM* renders pathological behaviors context-free. Simply having contempt or feeling inadequate or being irresponsible might or might not be sufficient to be labeled passive–aggressive. Irresponsibility is only passive–aggressive if it is meant to communicate a negative interpersonal message or expresses latent anger; irresponsibility can also be a function of attention problems, motivation, or disorganization associated with other forms of pathology. Similarly, many forms of personality pathology involve feelings of contempt (e.g., paranoid, antisocial) and inadequacy (e.g., dependent, avoidant). However, the cognitive context of these feelings likely depends on the underlying personality. For instance, whereas the dependent person might feel inadequate due to the belief that he or she might lose the affection of close others if he or she does not do something to appease them, the passive aggressive person might feel inadequate due to his or her history and expectations of being humiliated. Thus the motivations to either maintain attachment (in the case of dependency) or retain autonomy and respect (in the case of passive aggression) contextualize the symptom, and without this context the meaning of the symptom is obfuscated. Future research should use measures of passive–aggressive personality that incorporate motivational dynamics and the contents of cognitive attributions as a way of distinguishing the meaning of behaviors that are descriptive of but not uniquely passive aggressive. Notably, the *DSM–III* criteria were both behaviorally specific and implied a specific dynamic: PAPD was diagnosed if the person showed resistance to occupational and social performance through procrastination, dawdling, stubbornness, intentional inefficiency, or "forgetfulness" (American Psychiatric

Association, 1980, p. 329). Perhaps the *DSM–III* would be a good place to restart.

Another issue with item content involves the importance of work. The term passive–aggressive was conceived in an occupational (military) context, and many behavioral examples of and *DSM* criteria for passive aggression involve the failure to comply with job-related expectations. Two of the factors from this study, inadequacy and contempt, appear to be mostly specific to occupational situations. However, Millon (1993) and others have argued that, to be a PD, associated behaviors should generalize beyond a particular setting. For example, obsessive–compulsive personality is strongly associated with workaholism, perfectionism, and other occupation-relevant behaviors, but it is also associated with a particular interpersonal style that is observable across settings. Future research should explore the degree to which passive–aggressive behavior depends on the context, and in particular the extent to which it generalizes from work to other situations.

This study was limited by our use of questionnaires among undergraduates. This convenient method permitted the collection of data on a number of variables in a fairly large sample. Although there was sufficient variability in PD symptoms for covariance analyses and the large sample contributed to small confidence intervals, results might not generalize to other assessment methods or other kinds of samples. Replication in clinical samples would be informative. Although the PDQ corresponds to the *DSM* in terms of criterion content and number, it is possible that meanings shift slightly from the *DSM* to PDQ and thus a different structure and pattern of correlates would emerge from diagnostic interviews based precisely on the *DSM*. Additionally, self-reports and interviews of PD often show somewhat modest agreement. Future research should employ multiple methods across diverse samples to replicate and extend these results.

There were additional issues with our measurement strategy. For instance, there might have been limited content coverage for some of the dimensions that underlie personality pathology, such as those identified here in the conjoint structure of PAPD and NEGPD. This likely contributed to, among other things, low scale internal consistencies. Future research should employ methods that go beyond *DSM* criteria to more adequately examine such dimensions. Another issue was the presence of a factor (3) with exclusively reverse-scored items. It is not clear how this factor might differ substantively from the others given this method artifact, particularly because some of its items have fairly direct positively worded analogs that load on other factors. Finally, although the use of a number of external validating variables was a strength of this study, it would be beneficial for future research on the underlying structure of PAPD to include a wider array of criterion variables, particularly including other psychopathology constructs and measures of general personality functioning.

In conclusion, in this study we evaluated the impact of expanding *DSM* PAPD criteria to include more negativistic content. Overall, this expansion appears to have compromised discriminant validity, perhaps contributing to the loss of potentially unique and clinically important aspects of passive–aggressive behavior in the *DSM–5*. We acknowledge that studying a construct such as PAPD is against the current stream of diagnostic cutting in the *DSM*. We also recognize that the *DSM–5* trait-specified proposal might permit an articulation of PAPD for interested clinicians and researchers, although we do not expect the dynamics of passive–aggressive behavior to ever fully be captured by traits (see Wright, 2011). More specifically, we view the two traits suggested for depicting PAPD—depressivity and hostility (www.dsm5.org), to primarily indicate negativism as opposed to passive–aggressive behavior. Evaluating the ability of proposed *DSM–5* traits to account for passive–aggressive and other forms of pathological behavior is an important area of ongoing research (Hopwood, Thomas, Markon, Wright, & Krueger, in press).

Although there is insufficient research to recommend PAPD for inclusion in the diagnostic manual at this time, we believe that there is sufficient theoretical work and research to suggest that the construct is worthy of further investigation. A first step in this research involves identifying and focusing on content that is unique to the diagnosis, a process we have initiated in this study. The capriciousness of the diagnostic manual does not bear on the validity of any particular diagnostic construct. Thus PAPD's absence from the *DSM–5* should not impede research; however, given the history of the *DSM*'s impact on PD research, it probably will. This is all the more reason to continue studying passive–aggressive behavior, and perhaps the vacuum left by its abandonment in the *DSM* could spur novel conceptualizations.

ACKNOWLEDGMENTS

Portions of this study were presented at the annual meeting of the Society for Personality Assessment, Boston, MA, March 2011, and the annual convention for the Association for Behavioral and Cognitive Therapies, San Francisco, CA, November 2010. We thank Jessica Sims and Katherine Thomas for their help on earlier drafts of this article, and Aaron Pincus for his assistance with data collection. This research was supported in part by a grant (F31MH087053, to Aidan G. C. Wright) from the National Institute of Mental Health, Washington, DC. The views expressed herein are solely those of the authors.

REFERENCES

Abraham, K. (1925). The influence of oral erotism on character-formation. *International Journal of Psychoanalysis, 6*, 247–258.

American Psychiatric Association. (1952). *Diagnostic and statistical manual of mental disorders*. Washington, DC: Author.

American Psychiatric Association. (1968). *Diagnostic and statistical manual of mental disorders* (2nd ed.). Washington, DC: Author.

American Psychiatric Association. (1980). *Diagnostic and statistical manual of mental disorders* (3rd ed.). Washington, DC: Author.

American Psychiatric Association. (1987). *Diagnostic and statistical manual of mental disorders* (3rd ed., rev.). Washington, DC: Author.

American Psychiatric Association. (1994). *Diagnostic and statistical manual of mental disorders* (4th ed.). Washington, DC: Author.

Beck, A. T., Freeman, A., Davis, D. D., & Associates. (2003). *Cognitive therapy of personality disorders* (2nd ed.). New York, NY: Guilford.

Benjamin, L. S. (1993). *Interpersonal diagnosis of personality disorders*. New York, NY: Guilford.

Blashfield, R. K., & Intoccia, V. (2000). Growth of the literature on the topic of personality disorders. *American Journal of Psychiatry, 157*, 472–473.

Boschen, M. J., & Warner, J. C. (2009). Publication trends in individual DSM personality disorders: 1971–2015. *Australian Psychologist, 44*, 136–142.

Bradley, R., Shedler, J., & Westen, D. (2006). Is the appendix a useful appendage? An empirical examination of depressive, passive–aggressive (negativistic), sadistic, and self-defeating personality disorders. *Journal of Personality Disorders, 20*, 524–540.

Czajkowski, N., Kendler, K. S., Jacobson, K. C., Tambs, K., Rosyamb, E., & Reichborn-Kjennerud, T. (2008). Passive–aggressive (negativistic) personality disorder: A population-based twin-study. *Journal of Personality Disorders, 22*, 109–122.

Fenichel, O. (1945). *The psychoanalytic theory of neurosis*. New York, NY: Norton.

Fine, M. A., Overholser, J. C., & Berkoff, K. (1992). Diagnostic validity of the passive aggressive personality disorder: Suggestions for reform. *American Journal of Psychotherapy, 46*, 470–784.

Fraley, R. C., Waller, N. G., & Brennan, K. A. (2000). An item-response theory analysis of self-report measures of adult attachment. *Journal of Personality and Social Psychology, 78*, 350–365.

Fricke, S., Moritz, S., Andresen, B., Jacobsen, D., Kloss, M., Rufer, M., & Hand, I. (2006). Do personality disorders predict negative treatment outcome in obsessive–compulsive disorders? A prospective 6-month follow-up study. *European Psychiatry, 21*, 319–324.

Grant, B. F., Hasin, D. S., Stinson, F. S., Dawson, D. A., Chou, S. P., Ruan, W. J., & Pickering, R. P. (2004). Prevalence, correlates, and disability of personality disorders in the United States: Results from the National Epidemiologic Survey on Alcohol and Related Conditions. *Journal of Clinical Psychiatry, 65*, 948–958.

Grover, K. E., Carpenter, L. L., Price, L. H., Gagne, G. G., Mello, A. F., Mello, M. F., & Tyrka, A. R. (2007). The relationship between childhood abuse and adult personality disorder symptoms. *Journal of Personality Disorders, 21*, 442–447.

Hopwood, C. J., Morey, L. C., Markowitz, J. C., Pinto, A., Skodol, A. E., Gunderson, J. G., . . . Sanislow, C. A. (2009). The construct validity of passive–aggressive personality disorder. *Psychiatry: Interpersonal and Biological Processes, 72*, 256–268.

Hopwood, C. J., Thomas, K. M., Markon, K. E., Wright, A. G. C., & Krueger, R. F. (in press). DSM–5 personality traits and DSM–5 personality disorders. *Journal of Abnormal Psychology*.

Hyler, S. E. (1994). *The Personality Diagnostic Questionnaire 4+*. New York, NY: New York State Psychiatric Institute.

Hyler, S. E., Skodol, A. E., Kellman, H. D., Oldham, J., & Rosnick, L. (1990). The validity of the Personality Diagnostic Questionnaire: A comparison with two structured interviews. *American Journal of Psychiatry, 147*, 1043–1048.

Johnson, J. G., Cohen, P., Kasen, S., & Brook, J. S. (2006). Personality disorders evident by early adulthood and risk for anxiety disorders during middle adulthood. *Anxiety Disorders, 20*, 408–426.

Joiner, T. E., Jr., & Rudd, M. D. (2002). The incremental validity of passive–aggressive personality symptoms rivals or exceeds that of other personality symptoms in suicidal outpatients. *Journal of Personality Assessment, 79*, 161–170.

Kernberg, O. F. (1985). *Severe personality disorders*. New Haven, CT: Yale University Press.

Lazarus, A. (1971). *Behavior therapy and beyond*. New York, NY: McGraw-Hill.

Lenzenweger, M. F., Johnson, M. D., & Willett, J. B. (2004). Individual growth curve analysis illuminates stability and change in personality disorder features: The longitudinal study of personality disorders. *Archives of General Psychiatry, 61*, 1015–1024.

McCrae, R. R. (1994). A reformulation of Axis II: Personality and personality-related problems. In P. T. Costa, Jr. & T. A. Widiger (Eds.), *Personality disorders and the Five-factor model of personality* (pp. 303–310). Washington, DC: American Psychological Association.

McCrae, R. R., Kurtz, J. E., Yamagata, S., & Terraciano, A. (2010). Internal consistency, retest reliability, and their implications for personality scale validity. *Personality and Social Psychology Review, 15*, 28–50.

Millon, T. (1981). *Disorders of personality: DSM–III Axis II*. New York, NY: Wiley.

Millon, T. (1993). Negativistic (passive–aggressive) personality disorder. *Journal of Personality Disorders, 7*, 78–85.

Morey, L. C. (1988). Personality disorders in *DSM–III* and *DSM–III–R*: Convergence, coverage, and internal consistency. *American Journal of Psychiatry, 145*, 573–577.

Morey, L. C. (1991). *Personality Assessment Inventory professional manual*. Odessa, FL: Psychological Assessment Resources.

Morey, L. C., Hopwood, C. J., Gunderson, J. G., Skodol, A. E., Shea, M. T., Yen, S., . . . McGlashan, T. H. (2007). Comparison of alternative models for personality disorders. *Psychological Medicine*, *37*, 983–994.

Morse, J. Q., Robins, C. J., & Gittes-Fox, M. (2002). Sociotropy, autonomy, and personality disorder criteria in psychiatric patients. *Journal of Personality Disorders*, *16*, 549–560.

Reich, W. R. (1949). *Character analysis* (3rd ed.). New York, NY: Farrar, Straus, & Giroux.

Rotenstein, O. H., McDermut, W., Bergman, A., Young, D., Zimmerman, M., & Chelminski, I. (2007). The validity of *DSM–IV* passive–aggressive (negativistic) personality disorder. *Journal of Personality Disorders*, *21*, 28–41.

Samuel, D. B., & Widiger, T. A. (2008). A meta-analytic review of the relationships between the five-factor model and *DSM–IV–TR* personality disorders: A facet level analysis. *Clinical Psychology Review*, *28*, 1326–1342.

Sass, D. A., & Schmitt, T. A. (2010). A comparative investigation of rotation criteria within exploratory factor analysis. *Multivariate Behavioral Research*, *45*, 73–103.

Schmitt, N. (1996). Uses and abuses of coefficient alpha. *Psychological Assessment*, *8*, 350–353.

Skodol, A. E., Clark, L. A., Bender, D. S., Krueger, R. F., Livesley, W. J., Morey, L. C., . . . Oldham, J. M. (2011). Proposed changes in personality and personality disorder assessment and diagnosis for *DSM–5* Part I: Description and rationale. *Personality Disorders: Theory, Research, and Treatment*, *2*, 4–22.

Soldz, S., Budman, S., Demby, A., & Merry, J. (1995). A short form of the Inventory of Interpersonal Problems Circumplex scales. *Assessment*, *2*, 53–63.

Steiger, J. H. (1980). Tests for comparing elements of a correlation matrix. *Psychological Bulletin*, *87*, 245–251.

Stone, M. H. (1993). *Abnormalities of personality: Within and beyond the realm of treatment*. New York, NY: Norton.

Watson, D., Clark, L. A., & Tellegen, A. (1988). Development and validation of brief measures of positive and negative affect: The PANAS scales. *Journal of Personality and Social Psychology*, *47*, 1063–1070.

Wetzler, S., & Morey, L. C. (1999). Passive–aggressive personality disorder: The demise of a syndrome. *Psychiatry*, *62*, 49–59.

Wright, A. G. C. (2011). Qualitative and quantitative distinctions in personality disorder. *Journal of Personality Assessment*, *93*, 370–379.

Index

T - #0074 - 160425 - C0 - 276/216/8 [10] - CB - 9780415634533 - Gloss Lamination